An Introduction to General Pathology

This book is dedicated to the late Professor W.G. Spector of St Bartholomew's Hospital, who devised and wrote the first two editions and who was one of the first teachers to believe that understanding rather than memorising the key disease processes is the best way to learn pathology.

For Churchill Livingstone:

Commissioning editor: Timothy Horne
Project editor: Barbara Simmons
Project controller: Frances Affleck
Design direction: Erik Bigland
Artist: David Gardner

An Introduction to General Pathology

Tim D. Spector MB BS MSc MD FRCP
Consultant Rheumatologist and Director of the Twin and Genetic
Epidemiology Unit, St Thomas' Hospital, Guy's and St Thomas'
Hospital Trust, London

John S. Axford BSc MD FRCP
Reader and Consultant Physician in Rheumatology and Clinical
Immunology, Department of Cellular and Molecular Sciences,
St George's Hospital Medical School, London

FOURTH EDITION

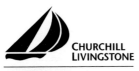
CHURCHILL
LIVINGSTONE

EDINBURGH LONDON NEW YORK PHILADELPHIA
ST LOUIS SYDNEY TORONTO 1999

CHURCHILL LIVINGSTONE
An imprint of Harcourt Brace and Company Limited

Churchill Livingstone, 1–3 Baxter's Place, Leith Walk,
Edinburgh EH1 3AF

© Longman Group Limited 1977, 1980
© Longman Group UK Limited 1989
© Harcourt Brace and Company Limited 1999

First edition 1977
Second edition 1980
Third edition 1989
Fourth edition 1999

ISBN 0443 048843

British Library of Cataloguing in Publication Data
A catalogue record for this book is available from the British
Library.

Library of Congress Cataloging in Publication Data
A catalog record for this book is available from the Library
of Congress.

Medical knowledge is constantly changing. As information
becomes available, changes in treatment, procedures,
equipment and the use of drugs become necessary. The
authors and publisher have, as far as it is possible, taken care
to ensure that the information given in the text is accurate
and up-to-date. However, readers are strongly advised to
confirm that the information, especially with regard to drug
usage, complies with current legislation and standard of
practice.

The
publisher's
policy is to use
**paper manufactured
from sustainable forests**

Printed in China

Preface

This book is intended primarily for students of Medicine, Dentistry and Veterinary science; it should prove useful to a wide range of scientists wishing to understand or keep up with the essential disease processes. Although concise, the book contains enough information for readers to achieve a satisfactory standard in exams where general pathology forms a part; this includes the MB or MD course as well as a variety of postgraduate exams.

Over twenty years have passed since the first edition was written – a time which has seen pathology pass from gross descriptions of disease to detailed cell biology and more recently to the explosion of knowledge generated by molecular biology. All of these processes are integral processes of the body's defence system and the book has been extensively rewritten with figures added and redrawn and includes new chapters on genetics to keep up with these changes. The book also now has key points for each chapter and a glossary of terms. However, the aim of this book remains the same – to enable students to learn general pathology by understanding it, and to do so as painlessly as possible.

The moral of the book, which is also the key to the understanding of disease, is that pathology is a by-product of evolution, a footnote to the history of natural selection.

London   T.S.
1999   J.A.

Acknowledgement

We should like to thank Susan Henderson and Christel Barnetson for help in the preparation of the manuscript and colleagues who have helped with previous editions, particularly Professor Peter Hall.

T.S.
J.A.

Contents

1 Understanding pathology

What is pathology?

Defining pathology is simple. It is the study of disease—but what is disease? It is often defined as disability, or in terms of visible changes in bodily organs, but this avoids the issue. In the normal, non-pathological state our existence depends upon thousands of adjustments which the homeostatic mechanisms of our bodies make every second, as our outside medium oscillates between overheated rooms and cold windy streets and as our internal milieu changes from a need to conserve water due to thirst to a need to excrete water due to swallowing several pints of beer. This continuous process of monitoring and adjustment, which lasts from our first to our last hours, is the substance of the science of *physiology*, the study of adaptation to the body's ever-changing internal and external needs.

By contrast, *pathology is the study of disordered functions*, i.e. inadequate adaptation to changes in the external and internal environment. In simple terms pathology is the scientific study of the way things go wrong.

Pathology as failure of adaptation

Failure of adaptation as seen in pathology may take one of two forms. It may be a simple inability to respond adequately, i.e. in the face of a truly overwhelming infection for which the body has no answer. Or, usually, disease is partly the result of an adaptive mechanism being turned against the host instead of working to his benefit. For example, antibodies appeared in vertebrates as an aid to the destruction of harmful parasites such as bacteria; they are, however, also a significant cause of disease, because if the host's tissues become in any way

1

altered they may themselves be mistaken as alien and invoke a destructive antibody response, as in various allergic disorders.

Survival mechanisms and disease

The major killing disease of western man is *ischaemic heart disease,* due mainly to atheroma by which the inner part of the wall of arteries becomes infiltrated by fat from the blood. This is an inevitable consequence of the fact that this part of the arterial wall normally receives its nourishment by diffusion of nutrients from the blood. If the wall incorporated tiny blood vessels the diffusion process would be unnecessary but the artery would be too weak to withstand the force of the blood pressure.

As Figure 1.1 clearly shows, cancer comes close behind cardiovascular disease as a major cause of death in developed countries. If the organs of the body contained no stem cells capable of mitotic division, cancer would be rare. But if there were no stem cells, cell renewal would be impossible and our life span would be enormously shortened.

Thrombosis allies itself with atheroma as a major cause of death both in cardiovascular disease and in cerebrovascular disease (strokes); its essence is the formation of clumps of blood platelets. One might then ask why natural selection has not eliminated platelet clumping. The answer is that the aggregation of these little blood cells is one of the most important bodily devices for the arrest of bleeding.

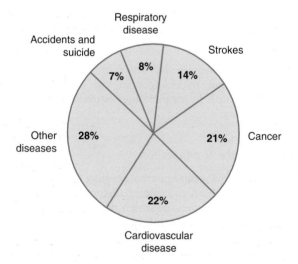

Fig. 1.1 Major causes of death in developed countries (World Health Organization 1996).

Any mutant not able to produce platelets or to clump them effectively would quickly die. In this instance, as in many others, fatal pathology is an unfortunate but inevitable consequence of a process essential for life. This emphasis on disease as the other side of the coin of survival is deliberate. The main conceptual problem which medical students encounter in pathology is the attempt to reconcile opposites such as the dual role of antibodies in defending and attacking the body. If it is accepted in advance that this duality is the hallmark of most disease processes the subject becomes much easier to understand. The reason for the double-edged nature of many survival mechanisms is that natural selection can act only on individuals young enough to reproduce. What happens to such individuals in later life cannot be influenced by natural selection. So the young have antibodies against bacteria while in middle age antibodies can cause thyroid disease and rheumatoid arthritis. The young are saved from haemorrhage by having sticky platelets which in middle age may kill them by causing coronary thrombosis.

In middle age most disease consists of the unwanted side effects of homeostatic mechanisms. What ill effects nature fails to achieve, man introduces by way of environmental hazards such as cigarettes, industrial pollutants and medicines. In the young, disease is more likely to result from a straightforward aberration of nature such as failure to produce some vital enzyme.

Themes in pathology

Pathology cannot be said to have laws, in the same way that thermodynamics has laws, but it does have recurrent themes:

1. As already discussed, disease often originates from a perversion of a survival mechanism.

2. Failures of adaptation tend to be self-reinforcing and progressive. In other words, once a pathological process has started 'one damn thing leads to another'. This is best seen in long-lasting (or chronic) illness and is often due to the inappropriate triggering of homeostatic mechanisms, e.g. unwanted retention of sodium in kidney disease.

3. When the body responds quickly to unfavourable environmental events the response is often overdone. In normal circumstances if more leukocytes are needed the bone marrow produces the appropriate amount; in pathological circumstances a great excess is released from the marrow.

4. Pathological duels, e.g. those between bacteria and man, tend to be fought to a draw rather than outright victory. The reason for this paradox is that natural selection favours such a conclusion for parasite and host.

Classification of disease

Reflection on the themes outlined above provides the beginning of a conceptual basis for pathology but still leaves the student confronted with a bewildering variety of diseases. It may be convenient to consider these as belonging to one of four broad categories. This simple classification is based primarily on the bodily defect or response rather than on the causation of disease. The classification consists of *inflammation, degeneration* and *neoplasia*, and a fourth group which cuts across the other three, namely *congenital* or *inherited disease*. These terms will be defined in the appropriate place.

KEY POINTS

- Pathology is the study of disordered function.
- Pathology may result from:
  — failure to respond adequately
  — perversion of a survival mechanism.
- Alteration of a survival mechanism tends to be self-reinforcing and over-compensatory, resulting in a chronic disease state.
- Disease may be classified by bodily defect or response as:
  — congenital
  — inflammatory
  — degenerative
  — neoplastic.

2 | Infection: man and his symbiotes

Symbiosis

Human disease is commonly caused by infection with microorganisms but the relationship between man and microbe is widely misunderstood. It is not one of defender (man) and invader (microbe) but rather one of *symbiosis*, a term meaning living together. The bodily contact between man and microorganism is one part of the broad interdependence between species that we call *ecology*, defined in 1959 by Odium as the study of the function and structure of nature.

It is no longer consistent with the evidence to think of man defending himself against bacterial invasion. This error grows from the scientific attitude developed in the 17th century and reinforced over the next 200 years, in which man was placed at the centre of natural science while the observer stood back and recorded his relationship with his environment. We are now wary of imagining the body's reaction to microbes as a gift for the preservation of man. A look at the evidence shows us that nature is impartial and its concern is as much for bacteria and viruses as for ourselves. Germs differ from man only in the level of organisation which they exhibit. Like man, some of their reactions are protective whilst others appear self destructive depending, as we shall see, on circumstances. It follows that the majority of terms such as parasitism no longer serve a useful function, merely describing a symbiotic situation in which no advantage to the host is apparent.

Pathogenicity and virulence

It is customary to speak of *pathogenic* and *non-pathogenic* organisms, the words implying a capacity to produce disease. Although bacteria do vary in this respect, the term is meaningless in the general sense since almost any organism can produce severe disease if the conditions are right, and almost any pathogen can live in peaceful symbiosis in a disease-free host. A word often used synonymously with pathogenicity is *virulence*, which means the disease-producing capability of an organism at different doses.

Infection

Infection itself is a word used in many different ways revealing confusion in our concepts of the relationship between man and germs. Sometimes it means that microbes produce overt signs of damage. Sometimes it signifies the mere presence of microorganisms whether they are normally present or not, for example:

- The urine is normally sterile, but if bacteria are present urinary infection is diagnosed even if evidence of damage or disease is absent.
- If signs of disease are present one would speak of a bacterial infection of the skin, even though it was known that this part of the skin in that individual normally harboured bacteria of the same strain.
- A surgeon would think of the normal large bowel as being infected simply because of the massive bacterial flora it invariably contains.

All infection is better thought of as a variation on the theme of symbiosis. Of the alterations taking place the most important is the change in population of the resident microbial flora and the second most important is the deficiency in those bodily mechanisms which normally limit the type and extent of microbial cohabitation with man.

Koch's postulates

When infection occurs, in the sense of microbial organisms causing demonstrable disease, it is important for obvious reasons to establish which particular organism is responsible. To do this with complete certainty Koch's postulates should in theory be fulfilled. These postulates are:

1. that the microorganism be obtained from the pathological lesions it is thought to have caused
2. that it be isolated in pure culture uncontaminated by other forms of life which might complicate the experiment
3. that the pure culture be injected into animals and the predicted disease develop
4. that the microorganisms be isolated again from these experimentally induced lesions and be shown to be identical with those originally isolated from the human patient.

However it is often not possible to satisfy all Koch's postulates even in infections where no doubt exists as to the causative organisms; classic examples are syphilis and hepatitis C.

Classification of microorganisms which may cause disease

It is now appropriate to list the microorganisms which are symbiotes of man and which may produce disease. These are listed in ascending order of complexity and degree of organisation:

Prions

These are a group of proteins that can be infectious in certain rare circumstances. They are often found in brain and nervous tissue. Examples of prion diseases include kuru, scrapie and Jakob–Creutzfeldt disease, a variant of which is commonly known as 'mad cow disease'.

Viruses

These are very small organisms, seen only with the electron microscope. Their size ranges from 28 nm (a nanometre is 1 millionth of a mm) to 450 nm. They are composed of a core of either RNA or DNA (but never both) and a protein coat called the capsid. They are obligatory intracellular symbiotes, i.e. they can only multiply within the susceptible cells of a host. They can, however, survive outside cells in a resting form for long periods even under unfavourable conditions. They are the main cause of many diseases of man, ranging from smallpox to the common cold, and have a role in causing cancer. They can infect animal, plant or bacterial cells and may be subdivided on this basis.

Rickettsiae

These are often classified as a form of bacteria. They are larger than viruses although a subspecies, the *Coxiella*, are small enough, like viruses, to pass through fine filters, also like viruses being resistant to heat and disinfectants. Rickettsiae contain RNA and DNA plus proteins, and resemble viruses in being obligatory intracellular symbiotes but, like bacteria, are visible under the light microscope and can reproduce by binary fission, i.e. by simply dividing into two. Rickettsiae can survive for months outside the body and cause many severe diseases, notably typhus. Like viruses they may spread disease with the aid of insect carriers, e.g. mosquitoes. Chlamydiae are similar to rickettsiae but deserve special mention because they cause the important diseases trachoma, non-specific urethritis and reactive arthritis.

Bacteria

These are larger (0.5–0.8 μm) and more highly organised than viruses, containing DNA, RNA, a cell wall and a complete biosynthetic, respiratory and energy yielding apparatus. With their complex chemical structure they have the capacity to proliferate outside cells by binary fission, that is they are not obligatory intracellular symbiotes. However, some species, such as *Mycobacterium tuberculosis*, are facultative intracellular symbiotes, i.e. they proliferate better inside cells than outside. Many bacteria survive in a resting form in unfavourable environmental conditions such as dust.

In pathology it is traditional to divide bacteria into two broad categories on the arbitrary basis of whether or not they retain a Gram stain. *Gram-positive bacteria* are those which retain a Gram stain (gentian or methyl violet) after alcohol treatment. *Gram-negative bacteria* are those that lose the stain and take up a carbol fuchsin counterstain. They also subdivide by virtue of shape, e.g. round cocci, elongated bacilli or spiral shaped spirochaetes, and in other ways such as whether they function in aerobic or anaerobic conditions.

Mycoplasma

These are closely allied to bacteria but less highly organised, being facultative intracellular symbiotes without a cell wall. Like bacteria they can be grown on artificial cell-free culture media and they are a cause of atypical pneumonias, e.g. *Mycoplasma pneumoniae*.

Protozoa

These are highly organised but unicellular organisms of which the amoeba is the prototype. Disease-producing protozoa include plasmodia (malaria), *Trichomonas*, *Toxoplasma*, *Leishmania* (kala-azar), trypanosomes (sleeping sickness) and *Entamoeba histolytica* (amoebic dysentery). Protozoa are the most important cause of tropical diseases.

Fungi

These are plants devoid of roots, stem or leaf. Unlike the algae they have no chlorophyll so they are obligatory symbiotes. They reproduce by spores which germinate and send out branching hyphae. Fungi rarely produce more than superficial disease in man unless there is a major breakdown in host mechanisms, such as occurs in diseases leading to reduced immunity.

Helminths

These are worms. They may cause disease at a variety of stages in their life cycle. The main categories are:

- nematodes
- cestodes
- trematodes.

The most important diseases that they cause occur in hot, non-industrialised countries, e.g. schistosomiasis caused by a trematode.

KEY POINTS

- Man and microorganisms have a general symbiotic relationship which can break down and result in infection.
- The likelihood of infection depends on a number of host factors and the virulence of the organisms.
- The major classes of symbiotic organisms include:
  — viruses
  — bacteria
  — protozoa
  — fungi
  — helminths.

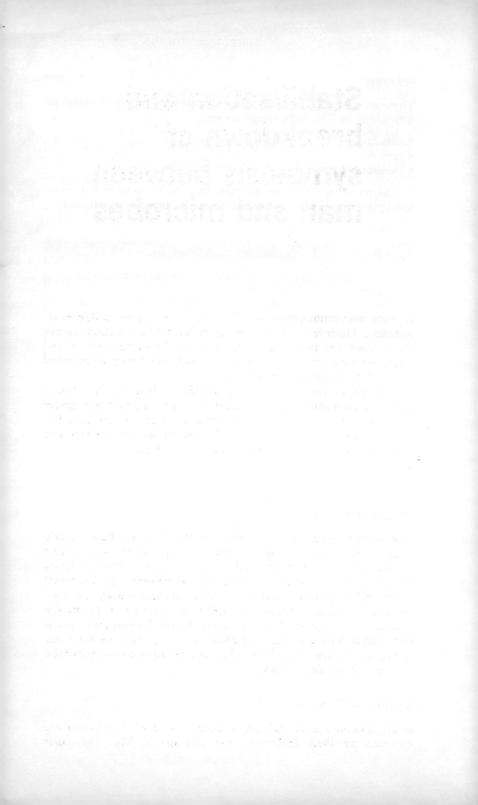

3 Stabilisation and breakdown of symbiosis between man and microbes

A more conventional title for this chapter would be resistance to infection. However, although in everyday terms infection means disease caused by microorganisms, the phrase 'resistance to infection' gives, as we shall see, a misleading picture of the relationship between man and his microbial companions.

One of the many false images surrounding infection is that of man moving permanently through a cloud of dangerous germs as if the air we breathe were an aerosol of pathogenic bacteria. In fact, the microbes are present not in the air but on the surface of floors and furniture and, especially, on the surface of our bodies.

Bacteria and the skin

Integrity of the skin

The primary defence against invasion of the tissues by these bacteria is our intact, cornified skin. This is easily shown by a simple experiment commonly performed by nature in which children's knees are temporarily denuded of their cornified epithelium by a physical injury such as a graze. Such a wound may become heavily colonised by bacteria which give rise to a local tissue reaction, including the formation of pus (p. 103). Two bacterial species, *Staphylococcus aureus* and *Streptococcus pyogenes*, are especially likely to participate but neither could have invaded the tissues and damaged the tissue had the skin surface remained intact.

Chemical defences

Apart from the mechanical barrier afforded by tightly interlocked and cornified stratified epithelium, the skin has at least two other mechanisms for controlling bacterial populations. There is normally a coating of long-chain saturated fatty acids which by virtue of their chemical composition discourage the growth of all but a few species of organisms. In particular *Strep. pyogenes* is killed by exposure to them. These substances are most important at weak points where the skin is moist and poorly keratinised and contains many hair follicles, e.g. the armpits. In these parts there is normally an abundant flora of bacteria of low pathogenicity, e.g. *Staphylococcus albus* or diphtheroids. It is very likely that here, as elsewhere, the sitting tenants, by pre-empting local supplies of nutriment, discourage colonisation by bacteria which, although more dangerous to the host, are less well adapted to live in the local conditions. This inhibition of the growth of new invaders may be due to metabolic products of the resident flora. Thus poorly pathogenic streptococci may produce hydrogen peroxide which kills diphtheria bacilli. Similarly, *Lactobacillus acidophilus* in the vagina ferments glycogen and raises the local acidity to such a degree as to prevent the growth of all organisms except those specially adapted to survive in such unusual conditions. A similar mechanism operates in the bowel of the newborn infant in which the growth of potential harmful bacteria is inhibited by acidic products of the fermentation of lactose achieved by *Lactobacillus bifidus,* the local resident.

Competition between bacteria

It is apparent that one of the most powerful mechanisms for preventing invasions of tissues by disease-producing organisms is competition between the various bacterial species inhabiting the area. This interesting aspect of ecology is well illustrated by the unfortunate consequences which can occur after treatment of patients with antibiotics. Thus dosage with penicillin may kill off the streptococci resident in the throat but allow a massive growth of fungi to occur, having previously only been present in very small numbers. It would seem therefore that successful symbiotes, i.e. bacteria that normally live in tissues, do not usually produce disease (to do so would destroy the host which shelters them), and by virtue of their numbers, monopoly of territory and food supply and better adaptation to the local environment are important in preventing colonisation by other strains, some of which could be highly pathogenic. This happy situation has evolved primarily for their benefit and not for that of the host although it remains a good example of symbiosis.

Certain bacteria can cause infection only in the presence of another organism, so-called *infective synergy.* This often leads to severe diseases such as gangrene and often occurs when the normal environment is altered.

The population dynamics of bacteria can be governed by quite highly developed competitive mechanisms such as the colicins formed by the bacteria *Escherichia coli*. They are unusual in that they are specified by extra chromosomal genes and they kill susceptible *E. coli* but never the strain which produces the colicin. Colicins are bactericidal by splitting off fragments of RNA in the ribosomes. The host cell is protected because of simultaneous production of colicin inhibitor.

Shedding of squames

It has been suggested that continual shedding of squames by the epithelium of the skin is a defensive device for keeping down its bacterial population since resident bacteria, e.g. staphylococci, are shed with squames. However it seems more in accord with the evidence, e.g. the spread of skin bacteria in operating theatres, to regard such shedding as a means of disseminating germs and allowing the organisms access to fresh pastures. Paradoxically then, while the regulation of bacterial populations by bacteria themselves always protects the host, the characteristics of host skin epithelium may either protect the patient or help to propagate bacteria.

The role of mucus

An even more equivocal role is that played by the sticky mucus secreted by the cells of pulmonary bronchi. This substance kills bacteria or inhibits their growth and also acts as a mechanical trap, a kind of fly paper, preventing access of germs to the underlying bronchial cells. When mucus secretion ceases due to changes in the cells producing it, a lung infection may occur. There is no doubt, therefore, that mucus secretion is a defensive mechanism against bacteria. On the other hand, small droplets of mucus coughed up into the atmosphere are one of the most effective vehicles for spread of microorganisms to other individuals. In this instance the mucus provides the virus or bacteria with sufficient mass to transport them to neighbouring hosts or to horizontal surfaces where they form droplet nuclei with dust. These nuclei of dust and mucus stirred up by air currents or movement are one of the most important ways in which organisms spread from person to person.

An excess of mucus secretion may promote rather than hamper bacterial growth. This is well seen in chronic bronchitis (defined as having a productive cough for more than 3 months a year; p. 118). Patients suffering from this condition frequently develop pulmonary infection due to a variety of bacteria and it is possible that stagnation of excess mucus may assist in this. Abnormally sticky mucus, such as occurs in the inherited disease of cystic fibrosis, is also associated with frequent severe bacterial lung infections. These diseases show how survival mechanisms can be turned against the host, in the first case by cigarette smoking and possibly air pollution and in the second by unfavourable genetic mutation.

Saliva

Like mucus, saliva is bactericidal and part of the host's strategy for controlling bacterial flora. Like mucus too, saliva helps the spread of infection, especially respiratory viruses, by acting as a vehicle propelled by coughing, sneezing and spitting.

Factors predisposing to infection

It is obvious (see Table 3.1) that all these mechanisms—skin, saliva and mucus respectively—not only protect the host but also facilitate the infection of other hosts and therefore protect the microorganisms from possible extinction. It is only when we get to the integrity of the surface cells themselves that we can speak of a protective mechanism operating solely in favour of the host. The importance of an intact cell surface is shown by the effects of viral invasion of the respiratory tract causing destruction of the cells which line the trachea and bronchi. With removal of this lining barrier, bacteria are free to invade and multiply in the lung itself. This process of bacterial infection secondary to viral destruction of the bronchial lining cells has cost the lives of countless people from pneumonia.

Table 3.1   The double-edged nature of defence mechanisms against microbial infection

Host mechanism	Survival value for host	Survival value for microorganism
Mucus secretion	Traps and kills some bacteria	Spreads bacteria and viruses in droplets
Saliva secretion	Kills some bacteria	Spreads bacteria and viruses in droplets
Cough and sneeze reflexes	Expel bacteria from respiratory tract	Spreads bacteria and viruses
Shedding of squamous epithelium	Discards bacteria from skin	Spreads bacteria on shed squames
Acidic secretion	Prevents growth of most bacteria	Protects normal bacterial inhabitants
Intact integument of surface cells	Prevents entry of bacteria	Portal of entry for viruses via receptor sites on cells

These defensive breaches apart, the entry of pathogenic bacteria into the tissues and their subsequent multiplication depend on factors that are often unpredictable. Viruses are more fortunate in that cells have on their surface a variety of receptor molecules as part of the normal chemical constituents of the cell wall, some of which bind specifically to receptors on the viral surface.

In the case of bacteria, a breakdown in the self-regulating population control may be a key factor in initiating infective disease. Thus, a rapidly growing virulent strain may colonise part of the body at the expense of the existing and more indolent bacterial population. This could follow a change in local conditions favouring growth of the virulent strain or their arrival in massive numbers. Natural selection would ensure that the virulent organisms conquered. This means that the virulent organisms may already be at the site or be transported from another site. For example *Staphylococcus aureus* may move from the nose to a surgical wound or *Pseudomonas aeruginosa* from the gut to the urinary tract.

Alternatively the germ may enter the body from the environment. The environment may be the soil, as in the case of tetanus, or, as in the case of gonorrhoea, another human being. Transmission by way of humans is by infected patients or carriers. The carrier is a very important vehicle and demonstrates how dangerous organisms may live in symbiosis in a disease-free host. In some symbiotic systems a plausible explanation can be found. For example the larvae of nemoritis are not taken up by the phagocytes (p. 27) of the moth Ephestia and thus survive in the host. If the larvae are washed in solvents to remove their fatty coat they are phagocytosed and destroyed. Here the carrier status is presumably due to the chemical properties of the larvae. The problem in human–bacterial relationships is why some individuals should exhibit the carrier state, i.e. harbour enough organisms to infect others without themselves suffering disease, while others do not.

The carrier state is an example of stable symbiosis, at least as far as the individual carrier is concerned. Some viruses however may be carried in this harmless fashion in apparently stable symbiosis then emerge to produce disease in an individual in which they live. The classic example is the virus of herpes zoster which lives in symbiosis for many years and may then proliferate, destroy cells and cause the unpleasant condition shingles with which it is associated.

KEY POINTS

- An intact cell surface, e.g. the skin or the lining of the respiratory tract, is an important defence against infection. Damage to these defences, e.g. by viral infection, predisposes to bacterial infection.
- The skin is also protected by acidic secretions and competition between bacteria.
- Mucus and saliva afford natural protection against infection but also allow further transmission of microorganisms.
- The carrier state is one whereby dangerous organisms can live in symbiosis with the disease-free host.

4 Microbial factors in man and disease

Bacterial toxins

Once established by whatever means, a variety of methods are available for disease-producing bacteria to express virulence, i.e. to break down symbiosis and damage the host (Table 4.1). Toxins play an important role in virulence. Most bacteria must multiply in the tissues to cause damage, but others need only gain a foothold and produce toxins to cause harmful effect. Toxins are potent cell-damaging agents. They are classified as *exotoxins* or *endotoxins*, depending on whether the substance is secreted externally or remains part of the organism.

Table 4.1   Methods by which bacteria express their virulence

Toxins	
Exotoxins	Increase cell wall permeability (e.g. *Staphylococcus aureus*)
	Bipartite toxins activated after entry into host (e.g. diphtheria)
Endotoxins	Lipid A portion of cell wall (in Gram-negative bacteria) activates cytokine release (p. 66), coagulation and complement cascade
Fimbriae/pili	Enable attachment to the host mucosa (e.g. *Neisseria gonorrhoeae*)
Aggressins	Alter the local environment of a the host to reduce defence, e.g. coagulase, streptokinase and collagenase (e.g. *Streptococcus pyogenes*)
Shedding of body	Inactive portions are used to mop up antibody (p. 38) (e.g. pneumococci)
Slippery surface	To avoid phagocytosis (e.g. pneumococci)

Exotoxins

The true classical exotoxins include some of the most powerful poisons known, such as those of tetanus, botulism and diphtheria. In other potentially lethal infections, such as those due to streptococci and staphylococci, toxins play a secondary role.

Host factors

The virulence of diphtheria is governed largely by the degree of toxin production and this in turn depends on many subtle factors. The gravis strain is more harmful than the mitis variety; this is partly because the relatively high iron content of human tissues inhibits toxin production by mitis organisms but not by gravis bacteria. The gravis strain grows more quickly in a high iron environment and so forms a thick layer, the outermost organisms being protected from the high iron concentration of host tissues, the iron being removed by the innermost layers. From the viewpoint of the diphtheria bacillus, the gravis strain is successfully adapted to survive in human hosts.

Toxin production, however, is not really part of the survival mechanism, and death of the host is an accidental by-product. The diphtheria organism uses iron to make cytochrome B from porphyrin and protein that it synthesises. It is only in iron-deficient environments that this pathway is diverted to toxin production. Thus too much iron prevents bacterial growth and hinders toxin production whereas iron depletion diverts the organisms to toxin production.

In the case of *Shigella dysenteriae*, which may cause food poisoning and paralysis, an excess of iron hampers production of the nerve toxin because an amount of iron above that required for cytochrome synthesis inhibits the formation of toxin. Here we have an example of a single host factor (iron concentration) affecting a single bacterial factor by two different mechanisms.

Bacteriophages

Toxin production by diphtheria organisms is governed by another mechanism, namely bacteriophages. A bacteriophage is a virus which is a symbiote of bacteria; what bacteria are to man, bacteriophages are to bacteria. Most bacteriophages destroy bacteria (lysis) when the appropriate strains meet, but sometimes the two coexist, this being attributed to a *temperate bacteriophage* and to production by the host cell of a repressor substance which prevents lysis.

Bacteria may be changed by a temperate phage inserting its DNA into host bacterial DNA, the phage then being known as a *prophage*. When a non-toxin-producing variety of diphtheria bacterium is infected by an appropriate temperate bacteriophage, the host organisms may be changed to a toxin-producing strain, the process of lysogenic conversion being attributable to a DNA transplant from the phage. If the bacterial cells suffer some form of injury the repressor substance is weakened and the phage is 'induced' and becomes lysogenic. The host cell is then destroyed and a mixture of phage and host DNA liberated. This mixture may be incorporated into a mature phage particle which may then infect a new host bacterium. The new host then receives not only phage genes but also bacterial genes from another and possibly somewhat different bacterium, thereby undergoing a non-sexual genetic exchange and possibly acquiring new and important characteristics, e.g. resistance to antibiotics. Lysogenic conversion to toxin production may occur also in staphylococci and streptococci.

Action of exotoxins

Bacterial exotoxins appear to work in two main ways:

1. in the form of *cytolytic toxins* which alter cell permeability
2. as *bipartite toxins* that bind to a receptor with one portion, allowing the release of the other portion into the host cytoplasm.

Bipartite exotoxins are actually activated by enzyme cleavage within the host target cell, e.g. diphtheria, cholera, pertussis. This conversion of an innocuous precursor to a harmful form by the host is hard to reconcile with a teleological view of the relationship between men and microbes. The lethal effect of diphtheria toxin appears to be related to its ability to inhibit protein synthesis in host cells. Cholera toxin induces uncontrollable diarrhoea by stimulating the enzyme adenyl cyclase in the wall of the bowel.

It is often difficult to separate the cause and effect relationship of toxins as local changes could represent the primary action of the toxin or could be the result of other effects occurring even earlier and hitherto undetected. Another problem that arises in the study of antitoxins (p. 43) is the fact that different results are obtained in the whole animal, in isolated tissue cells and in broken up cells. Antitoxin prevents diphtheria toxin from interfering with protein synthesis in isolated cells but has no effect when cell-free systems are used. In other words the antitoxin appears to stop the toxin from penetrating the cell and the whole animal; however, the main action of the antitoxin appears to be to facilitate ingestion of toxin by leukocytes, therefore preventing the toxin from reaching vital parts such as the heart muscle.

Undoubtedly, one of the main dangers of bacterial toxin to the host is the small amount needed to kill. Even if you survive an attack of tetanus you are not immune to a second attack because the amount needed to kill is less than that needed to produce immunity (p. 37).

Endotoxins

Endotoxins produce their effect through the lipid A portion of their liposaccharide cell wall (in Gram-negative bacteria). Lipid A is an extremely potent activator of a number of inflammatory mechanisms including the complement system (p. 38).

Aggressins

As well as toxins, certain bacteria contain *aggressins*—bacterial enzymes which alter the local environment to the benefit of the organism. Examples of this mechanism include streptokinase (from *Strep. pyogenes*) which dissolves fibrin, and coagulase (from *Staph. aureus*) which forms a barrier against the local defence mechanisms.

Fimbriae

Some strains of bacteria, e.g. *E. coli* and neisseriae, have been found to have hair-like filaments or fimbriae which assist them to attach themselves to body surfaces, with obvious survival benefits to these particular strains.

Other bacterial factors

1. Pneumococci (a cause of pneumonia) shed part of their substance to mop up antibody which might otherwise destroy them (p. 37).
2. Other bacteria have slippery surfaces which prevent their uptake by host phagocytes (p. 27), the situation akin to the larvae and moth mentioned earlier.
3. Bacteria can also damage the host directly by stimulating an *immune reaction* which may over-respond (p. 37).

Viruses

The mode of attack of viruses is probably better understood than that of bacteria. Although viruses can adhere non-specifically to host cells, the specific infectivity of a particular virus for a particular cell type, which is a characteristic feature of viral infections (e.g. polio virus and nerve cells, smallpox virus and skin cells), is due to the presence on host cells of specific receptors which fit neatly into the viral attachment proteins on the surface of the virus. Only cells that carry these particular receptors are susceptible to viral infections. The process whereby viruses attach themselves to susceptible cells is known classically as *adsorption*.

Entry into cells

Following adsorption the virus enters the cells through two main mechanisms (Fig. 4.1). The first is known as *receptor-mediated endocytosis* by which, following the triggering of receptors on the cell surface, the virus is taken into the cell by formation of a vesicle (endosome) where replication can occur.

The other known method involves glycoproteins on the viral surface called haemagglutinins; these attach the virus to the surface. If certain host cell proteases are present the viral membrane is fused to the surface and penetrated, allowing viral entry and subsequent replication. This host protease accounts for whether or not the virus will be pathogenic.

Viral synthesis

The naked nucleic acid core, now safely within the cell, is ready to begin the rapid synthesis of more virus. The viral nucleic acid begins its takeover very quickly and within one to two hours it is being synthesised in the cell as a result of new transcription from the

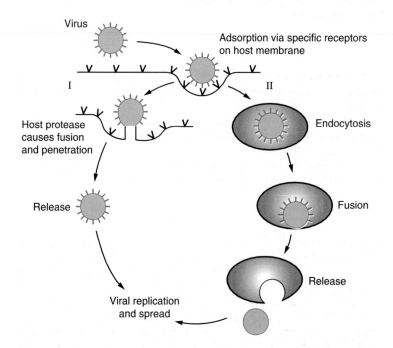

Fig. 4.1 Method of entry of viruses, via either (I) host proteases or (II) receptor-mediated endocytosis.

invading viral DNA (or RNA polymerase in the case of RNA viruses). This process too may be accelerated by host cell polymerase. The outcome of this activity is the synthesis of new RNA templates which direct the formation of new enzymes, including DNA polymerase in the case of DNA viruses. Thus viral DNA, RNA, coat proteins, enzymes or lipids are synthesised within the host cell (the stage of *synthesis*). From these components are assembled within the host cell a new virus particle (*maturation*). Because of the total disruption of its own metabolic process the cell ruptures and releases newly assembled virus (the *release* phase). In the whole of nature it would be hard to find a more economical and efficient mechanism.

Cell death

Efficiency and economy in this case relate to the virus rather than the host, since the infected cell is generally destroyed during the process outlined above. In tissue culture infected cells round up and float off the surface to which they were attached. In the body, before the cells show signs of disintegration, they often exhibit what are known as *inclusion bodies*; these have been shown to be the site of viral synthesis in the cell, appearing as areas in the cytoplasm or nucleus with abnormal staining properties.

The precise way in which viral invasion kills cells varies somewhat. In general, rather more is involved than a takeover of cell metabolism with consequent 'running-down' of the latter. Polio virus for example shuts down RNA synthesis in the cell within minutes of infection, probably by coding the production of a viral protein that inhibits the enzyme responsible for the synthesis. Polio virus also initiates the synthesis of viral capsid proteins which are lethal for the cell even before inhibition of RNA synthesis could be effective. Many other viruses, e.g. adenovirus and herpes, produce cytotoxic proteins during the early stages of viral synthesis which lead to the cessation of various vital cell activities such as the maintenance of normal membrane permeability, known as a *cytopathic* effect.

Viruses can also induce new antigens to appear on the surface of cells. Normally this leads to their destruction as 'foreign cells' by the immune system. However, if the immune system does not respond appropriately a carrier state can develop to the advantage of the virus and the host.

A particular virus may therefore kill a particular cell by a variety of uncomfortably efficient methods. Fortunately, at least one of the proteins the cell is induced to synthesise, namely interferon, is a potent non-specific antiviral agent, and plays a major role in terminating viral infection (p. 46). So on this occasion the duality of response so typical of pathology favours the host rather than the infecting symbiote.

Other effects of viruses

Viruses also have effects on cells other than simple killing. They cause them to fuse, thereby facilitating passage of virus from cell to cell. They can also lead to cell transformation, an ambiguous sounding term with special relevance to cancer, which will be dealt with in later sections (p. 277).

KEY POINTS

- Bacteria have a variety of methods for expressing their virulence which include:
  — the production of endo- and exotoxins
  — aggressins
  — specialised methods for adhering to cell surfaces via fimbrial adhesins
  — serum resistance
  — antiphagocytic properties.
- Viruses enter cells either by triggering specific receptors or by adhering to the surface and encountering specific host proteases which break down the viral protein coat.
- Both methods are highly specific and lead to the synthesis of new RNA and DNA, maturation of new virus particles and their subsequent release on the death of the infected cell.
- Viruses kill cells by a variety of means; most common is the alteration of cell permeability.

5 Phagocytosis

In Chapter 3 we discussed some of those bodily properties which, without being directed against any specific microbe, helped to prevent an unfavourable trend in symbiotic relationships. These stratagems are known collectively as *non-specific immunity*.

Specific immunity

Due to the process of evolution there has also developed a more refined system for achieving the same end. This system is called *specific immunity* because some degree of special recognition is always involved and sometimes the immunity may not extend beyond the particular bacterium or virus which elicited it. Its existence has given rise to the massive scientific enterprise, or perhaps one should say industry, of immunology.

The study of specific immunity began with the observation that people who survived certain diseases, such as smallpox, never suffered a second attack, i.e. they were immune to that particular disease while remaining susceptible to others. The observation that certain illnesses produce some kind of antidote to the malady in question long antedated the discovery of bacteria and their association with disease.

Specific immunity involves both body cells and body fluids. The cellular element consists of lymphocytes, whose role is described later (p. 37), and phagocytes.

Phagocytosis

Phagocytosis is the ingestion of particulate matter, especially bacteria, into the cytoplasm of cells. As can be learned from the study of the humble amoeba, phagocytosis is a fairly general property of cells. In practice only two kinds of cell in the human body are truly and avidly phagocytic. These professional phagocytes are the *polymorphonuclear leukocyte* and the *macrophage*. These cells will ingest alien particles in the total absence of any previous contact with them, although their ability to undertake phagocytosis is greatly improved by the presence of chemical substances—*antibodies*—which the body has produced as a result of such contact. The augmentation of cellular uptake by antibody specific for the particular particle is the main justification for describing phagocytosis as part of specific, as opposed to non-specific, immunity.

Opsonisation

The process whereby substances improve phagocytosis is called opsonisation. Opsonisation is vital in host defence and is probably the most important function of antibody. The process consists of the opsonin molecule attaching itself both to the phagocyte surface and to the bacterium, thereby acting as a kind of glue. This is important because a firm attachment of the bacterium to the cell surface must precede its ingestion; such attachment is always the initial stage of phagocytosis. The surface of professional phagocytes has two special binding sites or receptors for opsonins. One is the Fc receptor which binds the antibodies (principally IgG, see p. 42) and the other is the C3 receptor which attaches to part of the C3 fragment of complement (p. 39) which, like IgG, acts as an opsonin.

Both of these receptors are important in the adherence and phagocytosis of the microorganisms; if both are present phagocytosis is further enhanced.

There is no known disease in which phagocytosis itself is defective. Whenever there is a fault in the host leading to failure to ingest bacteria, the fault invariably lies in the opsonisation system.

The polymorphonuclear leukocytes (granulocytes)

These cells are formed in the bone marrow and depending on the staining properties of the granules (*lysosomes*) in the cytoplasm are classified as neutrophil, eosinophil or basophil. The neutrophil is the only variety of major importance as a phagocyte. It has lost the capacity for mitotic division and is the end product of a sequence of division and maturation in precursor cells, of which the earliest recognisable form is the myeloblast, itself derived from a bone marrow stem cell.

The mature polymorphonuclear leukocyte (polymorph) has a characteristic multi-lobed nucleus from which its name is derived. These cells spend less than 48 hours in the circulation before they migrate into the tissues under the influence of chemotactic factors. In the tissues they may phagocytose unwanted or foreign material and

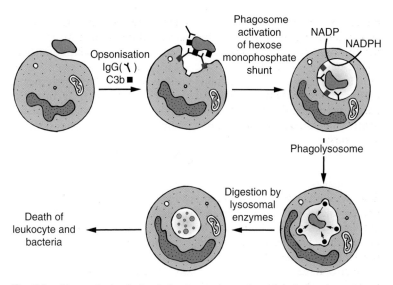

Fig. 5.1 Phagocytosis of a bacterium by a polymorphonuclear leukocyte.

eventually die. They exhibit the characteristics of professional phagocytes:

- an adhesive cell membrane, so that the cell sticks firmly to surfaces such as glass
- mobility with the aid of amoeboid pseudopodia
- a generous supply of lysosomes, which are cytoplasmic vesicles full of digestive enzymes.

For phagocytosis to take place the bacterium or other particle must come into contact with the leukocyte surface. The cell membrane then invaginates and two arms of cytoplasm (pseudopods) engulf the particles so that they become included in the cell cytoplasm, lying in a membrane-lined vacuole called a *phagosome*. Adjacent lysosomes then fuse with the phagosome and discharge their enzymes into it forming a *phagolysosome*. This may result in death and dissolution of the bacteria and the leukocyte itself. The process is depicted in Figure 5.1.

The macrophage

Polymorphs are short-lived, disposable cells, most of them dying soon after phagocytosing bacteria, even if the latter are killed and digested. The other major phagocyte, the macrophage, is a very different proposition with a capacity for longer life and mitotic division. This cell, too, is derived from a bone marrow precursor and circulates in the blood as a monocyte. It is discussed further in a later section (p. 107). Regarding its phagocytic powers, however, there are no very striking differences from those described for the polymorphonuclear leukocyte.

Where the two cell populations are mixed the polymorphs ingest most types of particles quickly. Larger particles, such as tubercle bacilli, are phagocytosed by the macrophages, the polymorphs being relatively helpless. With the partial exception of macrophages derived from the lung, phagocytosis by macrophages is independent of oxygen but inhibited by blockage of glycolysis.

The most striking difference between granulocytes and macrophages is that macrophages may survive for months or even years with phagocytosed material inside them, as opposed to the 'kill and be killed' technique of the polymorph. Otherwise the formation of phagolysosomes is similar in the two cell types except that in the macrophage vesicles from the Golgi apparatus, as well as lysosomes, contribute enzymes to the destructive process.

Macrophages will take up many different sorts of particles including carbon or plastic spherules. It is justifiable therefore to ask whether phagocytosis by these cells should not be considered as non-specific immunity. Two points must be made:

1. Macrophages come into contact with a wide range of tempting particles within their own host, e.g. healthy red blood corpuscles, but somehow recognise them and resist the urge to ingest them.

2. There is a wide difference in the avidity with which particles are swallowed. This is true even of the macrophages of invertebrates where antibodies as we know them (p. 38) are not present. As an example, macrophages (haematocytes) from moth larvae were found to phagocytose sheep erythrocytes treated with a variety of chemical agents, e.g. tannic acid, whereas the same cells treated with other chemicals, e.g. sucrose, were taken up hardly at all. Sheep red cells treated with mouse antibody, or aged sheep red cells were ingested by mouse macrophages but not by moth macrophages. Thus invertebrate macrophages not only exhibit specific recognition of particles, but also recognise different receptors from those recognised by mouse macrophages. In addition to this form of discrimination it is likely that fluid recognition factors, a rudimentary form of antibody (p. 38), are present in the haemolymph of insects. It is probable therefore that specific immunity in man is evolved from a more primitive form now seen in contemporary invertebrates.

The phagocytosis by macrophages of dead host cells is one of the major routes for disposal of insoluble bodily debris. In spite of its importance this latter process is not well understood, the problem being how macrophages recognise an effete red cell from a healthy one. It is appropriate to use the red cell as an example because it is macrophages which digest dead red corpuscles and make their constituents available for reutilisation. Ageing may alter the surface composition or diminish the negative charge on the corpuscular surface, or make the cell more rigid, all of which may lead to phagocytosis. Alternatively, the circulation may contain specific binding antibodies which attach to the effete but not to the healthy cells and then link the corpuscle to the macrophage for phagocytosis. The macrophage surface has three types of receptor:

1. Fc
2. C3 fragment (p. 39)
3. a non-specific receptor available for objects such as denatured red cells.

It can be seen, therefore, to be very fully equipped for its phagocytic role and its contribution to inflammation, repair and immunity.

The mononuclear phagocyte system

If bacteria are injected into the vein of an animal they circulate briefly but then disappear from the blood. If injected subcutaneously they are removed somewhat more slowly from the affected area. If instilled into the respiratory tract, they remain for a while in the lungs and are then cleared. The same is true of the peritoneal cavity. All these statements depend of course on the bacteria not being sufficiently virulent or numerous to kill the host rapidly. Clearance of bacteria from body spaces and fluids is true also of other types of particle, colloidal carbon often being used to demonstrate this phenomenon.

The process is due to the presence in key sites of large numbers of macrophages. It is still customary to talk of the dispersed collections of macrophages as the *reticuloendothelial system*—a name which was given for historical reasons and is no longer applicable. Contemporary workers in the field prefer the term *mononuclear phagocyte system* since neither reticulin (collagen fibrils found in connective tissue) nor endothelium (cells lining blood vessels or lymphatics) is relevant to phagocytosis.

The origin and maturation of macrophages

Mononuclear phagocytes are formed in the bone marrow from a precursor cell called the promonocyte, derived in turn from the haemopoietic stem cell. The promonocyte matures into a monocyte which circulates in the blood. The monocyte enters a variety of tissue compartments becoming as it does so a macrophage (Table 5.1). The transition from monocyte to macrophage is accompanied by a large increase in the phagocytic, digestive and synthetic apparatus in the

Table 5.1   The mononuclear phagocytic system

Bone marrow	Precursor stem cell
	Promonocyte
Blood	Monocyte
Tissues	
Connective tissue (histiocyte)	
Lymph nodes	
Spleen sinus	
Bone marrow (resident macrophages)	
Liver (Kupffer cells)	Macrophage
Peritoneum (serosal macrophages)	
Pleura	
Lung (alveolar macrophages)	
Bone (osteoclasts)	
Brain (microglia)	
Gastrointestinal tract	Langerhans cells
Genitourinary tract	Dendritic cells
Synovia	

cell. In particular the cytoplasm enlarges, phagosomes appear, the membrane becomes more elaborate, lysosomes become more numerous, the Golgi apparatus enlarges and rough endoplasmic reticulum develops.

This process of development is due to the stimulation of the monocytes and young macrophages by factors in their new environment. The mature cell which finally emerges is known as a *stimulated macrophage*.

Macrophages appear as free cells throughout the body as more specialised cells which are all related but which demonstrate considerable heterogeneity. They are seen in the spleen and bone marrow, the liver (Kupffer cells), the sinusoidal lining cells of the spleen, and lymph nodes. Other members are the osteoclast of bone and the microglia of the central nervous system. Their exact relationship with Langerhans cells and dendritic antigen presenting cells is still somewhat unclear.

Monocytes spend 20–30 hours in the blood stream. In the tissues, once transformed to macrophages, their turnover time in the normal uninjured condition is rather slow and they are probably replaced at intervals of several months. There is likely to be considerable variation in this depending on the local conditions and site.

The mononuclear phagocyte system, as we have seen, can be traced back to invertebrates. It is vital for the host because it sequesters microbes within its cells and therefore prevents them getting access to important tissues such as the brain or heart, or achieving release into the circulation. In addition, the cells of the system, like polymorphonuclear phagocytes, have developed special characteristics which enable them to kill and digest potentially harmful microorganisms.

The killing of microbes within phagocytes

Prevention of infectious disease due to bacteria is essentially the stabilisation of the relationship between man and microorganisms. The most important part of the stabilisation process is undoubtedly the phagocytosis and intracellular killing of the organisms. That this statement can be made so dogmatically is due to the experiments performed by nature on man. In the disease of hypogammaglobu-linaemia, antibodies (p. 39) may be almost non-existent and infections frequent. However in the disease of agranulocytosis, where polymorphs are virtually absent but antibodies normal, infections are even more frequent, more severe and more often fatal. It seems that inside the body microorganisms are seldom killed in any way other than bactericidal action inside the cytoplasm of polymorphs and macrophages.

Phagocytosis is accompanied by the so-called *respiratory burst*, which includes a three-fold increase in oxygen consumption and a ten-fold increase in the activity of the hexose monophosphate shunt pathway as well as increased glycolysis, RNA turnover and lipid synthesis. Studies with metabolic inhibitors show that glycolysis and not oxidative respiration provides the energy for phagocytosis, an obvious advantage since leukocytes often work in areas of low oxygen tension. Polymorphs are well supplied with glycogen as an energy source. The process of phagocytosis can however be hampered by factors such as a local environment of excessive ionic strength and deficiency of certain cations such as magnesium, as well as a variety of serum factors.

Formation of free radicals

Following the respiratory burst, molecular oxygen is converted to the superoxide anion within the phagolysosome. This occurs in the presence of NADPH oxidase. The *superoxide anion* is an oxygen atom with an extra electron. This unstable or free radical is called reactive because it can either donate or receive an electron. When two superoxides combine in the presence of the catalyst superoxide dismutase (SOD), hydrogen peroxide and oxygen are produced. With the granular enzyme myeloperoxidase and halide anions the highly reactive and toxic hypohalide anions are produced. Although most of these products are cytotoxic to some extent the resultant HOCl is believed to be the final oxidant that does most damage. These pathways are outlined in Figure 5.2.

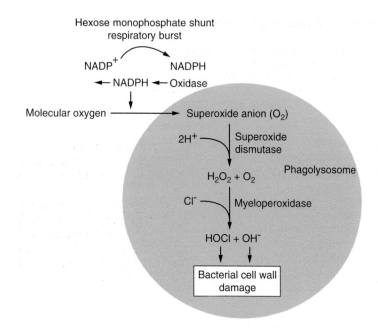

Fig. 5.2   Mechanism of oxygen-dependent bacterial killing in a phagocyte.

The importance of these mechanisms is illustrated by the fact that phagocytosis is much less efficient in the presence of a respiratory poison such as cyanide and in the absence of myeloperoxidase. Nature has produced two diseases, both genetically determined, which are associated with frequent bacterial infection. In the first (*chronic granulomatous disease*) there is a deficiency in the enzyme system (probably cytochrome B245 in phagocytes) which produces the respiratory burst; in the second it is myeloperoxidase itself which is lacking and this produces a milder condition.

The most important free radicals, which are part of a family of reactive molecules known collectively as *reactive oxygen intermediates*, are those generated by the reduction of molecular oxygen to water. These include the superoxide anion (O_2^-'), the perhydroxide radical (HO_2'), the peroxide anion (as in H_2O_2), the hydroxide radical (OH') and the hydroxide anion (OH^-). They have a number of mechanisms by which they can cause cell injury; these are listed in Table 5.2. Because of this wide range of abilities they are now being recognised as having a key role in such diverse conditions as radiation injury (p. 299), reperfusion ischaemia, drug-induced haemolytic anaemias, paracetamol and carbon tetrachloride poisoning, neonatal respiratory distress syndrome due to high concentration of oxygen, and ageing

Table 5.2   Properties of free radicals

1. Can produce cell injury by generating other free radicals.
2. Can peroxidise lipids in cell membranes (i.e. mitochondria).
3. Can cause strand breaks in DNA.
4. Can alter redox potential of cells and release calcium.

(p. 355). They also play a key role in a number of inflammatory diseases, such as gout and rheumatoid arthritis. As well as causing cell injury, free radicals may also play a part in the regulation of the inflammatory response in chronic granulomas (p. 113).

As free radicals appear to be produced continuously by a number of cells, protective mechanisms are necessary to prevent damage to the host. The activation involves antioxidants such as alpha tocopherol (a part of vitamin E), glutathione and the enzymes superoxide dismutase and catalase. Obviously the activation of free radical formation could be a powerful therapeutic tool in a number of diseases.

Other bactericidal mechanisms

A number of other bactericidal mechanisms are present in granulocytes:

1. The acidity in the phagolysosomes is very high due to accumulation of lactic acid as a result of enhanced glycolysis. The resulting low pH (3.5–4) is lethal for some bacteria.
2. The cells also contain an enzyme—lysozyme—capable of attacking the cell walls of living bacteria and killing them, especially if complement (p. 38) or H_2O_2 or ascorbic acid (vitamin C) is also present.
3. The lysosomes contain cationic proteins such as *lactoferrin,* which is lethal for some bacteria.
4. Hydrogen peroxide by itself may kill bacteria without the help of catalase.

Macrophages too produce superoxide when stimulated, although less efficiently than granulocytes. Macrophages lack myeloperoxidase but contain catalase and GSH (reduced glutathione) peroxidase, both of which could catalyse the bactericidal effects of H_2O_2. As in granulocytes, H_2O_2 and peroxidase may kill bacteria directly or by formation of free halide radicals or aldehydes. The aldehydes would be derived from spontaneous breakdown of unstable products of lipid peroxidation, the lipid being present in cell constituents such as membranes.

These mechanisms are set out in Table 5.3.

Table 5.3   Mechanisms of intracellular killing of microorganisms

High acidity in phagosomes	Lactic acid accumulation due to increased glycolysis
Lysozyme	Secreted by cell
Lactoferrin	Present in lysosomes
Superoxide anion	Generated after phagocytosis
H_2O_2	Generated after phagocytosis
Catalase	Present in cell
H_2O_2 + catalase	
Aldehydes	Formed after peroxidation of cell lipids by H_2O_2
Free halide radicals	Formed from iodine or chloride in cell by H_2O_2 and myeloperoxidase or GSH peroxidase

Activated macrophages

One aspect of bacterial killing by macrophages that has been looked at in detail is the more rapid dispatch of large bacteria such as tubercle bacilli after a previous contact of the host with the microorganism in question. Thus macrophages from animals previously infected with tubercle bacilli show a greatly enhanced capacity to kill phagocytosed tubercle bacilli and are known as activated (or cytolytic macrophages). The phenomenon is relatively non-specific in that, once it has developed, the accelerated lethality extends to other comparable organisms such as *Listeria monocytogenes*. The basis of this augmented macrophage activity is largely dependent on the efforts of another cell population, the T lymphocytes (p. 44). This can be shown by transferring such lymphocytes from an animal immunised against tuberculosis to a non-immunised recipient. These macrophages thereupon kill tubercle bacilli more proficiently than they did previously.

The phagocytosis and killing of microorganisms by macrophages in response to activation by specifically immunised T lymphocytes is one of the most important manifestations of *cell-mediated immunity*. This term means that the circulating antibody plays no apparent role in the reaction concerned. By contrast, the polymorphonuclear leukocytes do not participate in cell-mediated immunity but are instead aided in their phagocytic role by opsonising antibodies and complement, i.e. by antibody-mediated immunity. Resistance to tuberculosis is almost certainly due to cell-mediated immunity.

Effects of phagocytosis detrimental to the host

In spite of being the most important defence mechanism against microbes, phagocytosis is no exception to the rule that all such mechanisms may work to the detriment of the host.

Abscess

Granulocytes which phagocytose destructive bacteria such as streptococci or staphylococci may be destroyed by them in vast numbers. Their liquefied bodies accumulate at the site of the bacterial invasion forming an abscess. This collection of pus involves much destruction of the tissue and toxic effects on the patient. In addition it may also act as a fluid carrier spreading living bacteria to parts of the body not previously infected. An abscess is also very often painful and the patient may well feel that not only medical science, but also nature herself, sometimes provides a cure that is worse than the disease.

Liberation of lysosomal enzymes

Another consequence of phagocytosis which is harmful to the host is the secretion and liberation from the phagocyte of lysosomal enzymes. Escape of these catalysts causes cellular destruction and inflammation. The excruciating pain of gout is due to phagocytosis of urate crystals and subsequent rupture of lysosomes and discharge of their contents into the joint, resulting in damage to the joint.

Facultative intracellular organisms

Particularly ambiguous is the relationship between macrophages and those bacteria which thrive better inside them than outside them. These are called facultative intracellular organisms; they include the important bacilli which cause tuberculosis, leprosy and syphilis. They are largely ignored by granulocytes and must be dealt with by macrophages. Although many are killed and digested within these cells, others survive and multiply in the cell cytoplasm; they are then carried by the mobile macrophages to all parts of the body, where satellite infections may be set up. In tuberculosis, this form of dissemination is a frequent cause of death if antibiotics are not available.

KEY POINTS

- Phagocytosis is one of the most important methods of defence against microorganisms.
- The two major types of phagocytic cells in the body are polymorphonuclear leukocytes and macrophages.
- Phagocytosis is enhanced by opsonisation whereby antibodies to the IgG and complement fragments attach themselves to the microorganism and facilitate adherence of the phagocyte.
- Intracellular killing occurs in phagolysosomes and involves the production of free radicals and a number of cytolytic enzymes.
- Free radicals are molecular species containing electrons unpaired in spin. They are believed to cause cell death by several means and are increasingly thought to play an important role in a number of disease states.

6 Immunity, antibodies and complement

The control of symbiotic relationships between mammals and microorganisms depends largely on specific immunity which, as we have seen, has cellular and fluid (humoral) components. The word 'humoral' is an historical relic and means fluid substance circulating in the blood stream. '*Humoral immunity*' refers to the presence of antibodies—proteins produced as a result of the introduction of substances which the body recognises as foreign (antigen).

The most striking thing about antigens and antibodies is their mutual specificity. The antibody which a particular antigen causes to be formed may react only with the particular overall configuration which the antigen exhibits and with no other. The overall configuration of the antibody-combining part of the antigen appears to be even more important than its chemical nature. If, however, other substances contain the same molecular groupings as the antigen, these may react with the antibody. Bacteria are composed of many different chemical groupings, so contain more than one antigen and will usually give rise to a number of antibodies of different specificity. All, however, will combine with the bacterial body so that the heterogeneity of their chemical specificity will not be obvious.

Most antigens are proteins but not all chemical substances are antigenic. Even a small molecule may become antigenic if combined with a protein, the antigen then being called a *hapten*. In addition some carbohydrates and lipids are antigenic, both in the pure state and when part of a protein molecule. It is rare for a substance of molecular weight less than 5000 daltons to be an effective antigen other than as a hapten. A hapten may be defined as a small molecule which on its own cannot induce antibody synthesis, but will combine with antibody once formed.

Immunoglobulins

Immunoglobulins are a group of related glycoproteins called antibodies. There are five subgroups of immunoglobulins—IgG, IgM, IgA, IgE and IgD—which are discussed in more detail later. The molecule consists of an Fc (fragment crystallisable) portion which binds to the cell surface and activates complement, and the Fab (fragment antigen binding) portion which contains 'light and heavy' polypeptide chains and combines specifically with the antigen which elicited the immunoglobulin (Fig. 6.1).

Complement

Complement is the historically hallowed name for a family of proteins in plasma which cooperates with ('complement') antibodies. The complement system consists of many components and is easily distinguished from antibody since, unlike the latter, it is quickly destroyed by moderate heating. This susceptibility to raised temperature is a characteristic of enzyme reactions culminating in the activation of an esterase which can attack and dissolve the phospholipid wall of bacteria and tissue cells.

There are three other comparable cascades important in pathology which are responsible respectively for blood coagulation (p. 225), kinin formation (p. 96) and fibrinolysis (p. 221).

When antibody combines with a bacterium or other antigen the resultant complex triggers off the cascade of reactions which constitutes activation of the complement pathway. Activated complement is also known as *'fixed' complement* because, when it is all

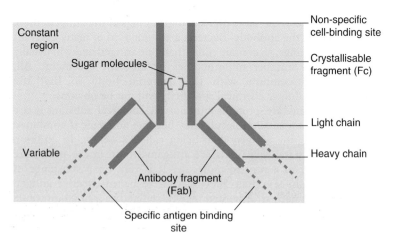

Fig. 6.1   The immunoglobulin molecule.

used up, its activity in that particular sample of serum is no longer demonstrable, none being available for further antigen–antibody reactions. Combination of antigen and antibody activates complement by the *'classical' pathway* in which all the complement components are involved. Complement can also be activated, however, by the phylogenetically older *'alternate' pathway*, triggered by the presence of certain foreign particles or molecules not of an antibody nature and in which certain steps of the cascade are bypassed (Fig. 6.2).

The surfaces of polymorphs and macrophages contain receptors for at least some components of complement. As a result complement is bound not only to the antibody molecule but also to the cell wall of the phagocyte and possibly also to bacteria themselves. The various components of the complement cascade have different functions but involve three main types of reaction:

1. interaction with cell surface receptors leading to phagocytosis
2. production of biologically active components
3. membrane damage via the membrane attack complex.

The third complement (written C3) is the only one involved in phagocytosis. Some components, notably C3 and C5, split into a small portion (C3a and C5a) and a larger fragment (C3b and C5b)

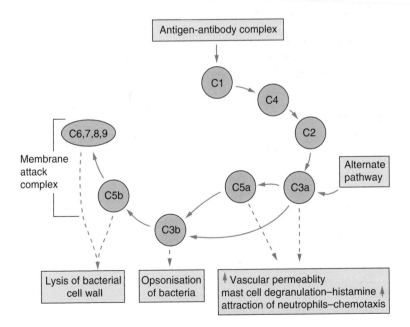

Fig. 6.2 Activation and major functions of the complement pathway.

which have different actions. C3a and C5a are vasoactive peptides which cause vasodilatation and increased vascular permeability, activating mast cells and basophils and releasing histamine (anaphylotoxin), kinins and leukotrienes, leading to further inflammation. C3b is the most important contribution of the complement system to opsonisation. C3b facilitates adherence of bacteria, viruses and neutrophils to monocytes and macrophages. It also facilitates phagocytosis of certain bacteria by neutrophils, monocytes and activated macrophages. C5a is the major chemotactic factor for neutrophils and it also activates neutrophils by triggering the respiratory burst, increases vascular permeability directly via mast cell degranulation, and causes smooth muscle contraction. The final products of the cascade, C5–9 (membrane attack complex), when activated, lyse cell or bacterial membranes (Fig. 6.2).

The destructive potential of complement is kept in check by the elaborate nature of the cascade, by the very short life span of the individual activated components and by a system of natural inhibitors in the plasma.

Opsonisation

The word opsonisation is derived from the Greek 'to prepare for the table'. The most important role of the antibody/complement system is to facilitate the phagocytosis of bacteria. Coating of the surface of foreign particles by complement promotes phagocytosis. Patients who have all the antibodies they need but who have only a few phagocytic leukocytes quickly die of infection. The surface of undamaged bacteria often has characteristics which make phagocytosis difficult, these no doubt having evolved through natural selection. However, the immunoglobulin IgG attaches itself to the chemical groupings of the bacterial surface by virtue of closely matching, reciprocal molecular configuration, and the bacterial/antibody complex will bind easily to the leukocyte surface because of the presence on that surface of matching receptors for the free portions of the immunoglobulin molecule, the so-called Fc portions seen in Figure 6.3. IgM is also an opsonin but seems more likely to adhere to the phagocyte surface by non-specific binding.

With antibody and complement bound to each other and independently to the bacteria and leukocyte surfaces, the complement system provides a 'belt and braces' mechanism for securing bacteria to the membrane of the phagocyte, as shown in Figure 6.3.

Opsonisation is a form of specific immune adherence and it is important because once a bacterium is attached to the outer membrane of a phagocyte it is drawn into the interior of the cell (Fig. 6.4), where it can be killed and ingested as described in Chapter 5. Killing and digestion depend upon the respiratory burst and on the discharge of the contents of the lysosomes into the vacuole where the bacterium lies, as shown in Figure 6.5. Complement plays a role here too since it will be taken in with the bacterium and may then lyse it

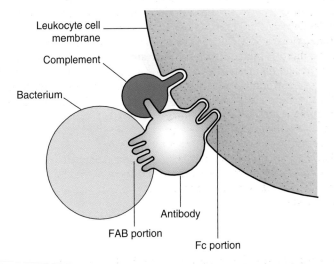

Fig. 6.3   Trapping of bacteria on leukocyte surface by antibody and complement (opsonisation).

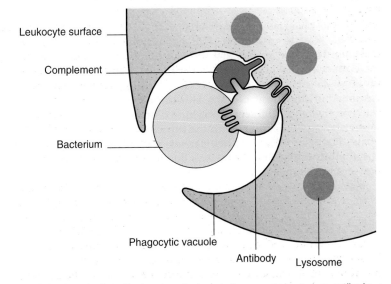

Fig. 6.4   Invagination of leukocyte cytoplasm to incorporate bacterium, antibody and complement.

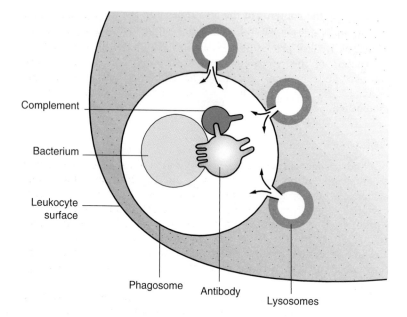

Complement

Bacterium

Leukocyte
surface

Phagosome   Antibody   Lysosomes

Fig. 6.5 Discharge of lysosomal contents into phagocytic vacuole.

directly or activate another enzyme, lysozyme, which has a similar effect.

If the host has had previous contact with the type of bacterium to be phagocytosed, opsonins should be plentiful or at least rapidly provided. However, even if there has been no such contact there are sufficient opsonins in the plasma to ensure phagocytosis. This is due to the so-called *natural antibody*. Natural antibody may result from previous but unnoticed contact with the antigen, or chance cross-reactivity with a different antigen, or may be a non-antibody substance, e.g. 'properdin', with the capacity to activate complement by the alternate pathway. When patients are found to have defective phagocytosis of bacteria it is always due to a fault in one or more of the serum factors described above rather than in the leukocytes themselves.

Specific properties and functions of antibodies

IgG

IgG is the major component in most antibody responses, contributing 70–75% of the total immunoglobulin pool with a molecular weight of 150 000. It deals with bacteria in a number of ways: by acting as an opsonin and by causing them to clump together (aggregate) and making them more easily phagocytosed. It also activates complement which, as well as promoting phagocytosis, can lead to extracellular destruction of the microorganisms by the C5–9 membrane attack complex. IgG crosses the placenta and is responsible for the protection of the fetus until its own immune system becomes established.

Antitoxins

Antibodies such as IgG which detoxify bacterial exotoxins are known as *antitoxins*. Antibodies combine with the soluble toxins which some bacteria produce, thus acting as antibodies to the toxin. Most bacterial toxins are enzymes, and the combination of toxin and antibody leads to masking of the active sites of the enzyme and resultant inactivation. The combination may result also in an insoluble reaction product with the precipitation of the antigen. Antibodies can also be raised against plant or animal enzymes, e.g. uricase.

In diseases where much of the damage to the host is caused by bacterial toxins it may be life saving to administer antitoxic antibody to the patient as part of the treatment (*passive immunisation*). These antibodies are produced in large quantities by administering the antigen to horses and then collecting blood from the animals. To prevent the toxin from killing the horses, it is modified by chemical treatment to form a toxoid. It is now customary to give these toxoids directly to children so that they form their own antibodies, an example of the use of *active immunisation* to prevent disease, in this case diphtheria or tetanus.

IgM

IgM is of very high molecular weight (900 000 daltons) and is too big to cross the placental barrier. It is often the first antibody to appear after entry of bacterial or viral antigens, contributing approximately 10% of the total pool. Its large size and multiple binding sites make it a powerful agglutinator and opsonin, an activator of complement.

IgA

IgA makes up 15–20% of the pool; it has a weight of 32 000 daltons and is found mostly at the surface of the mucous membranes. It has a special structure ('the secretory piece') which allows it to be secreted at particular sites such as the salivary glands and the gastrointestinal tract. It plays a major role in preventing infection via the external seromucous body surfaces. It is a poor opsonin and probably works by coating bacteria and preventing their attachment to the epithelial lining. It can activate the alternate complement pathway.

IgE

IgE has a molecular weight of 188 000 daltons and has two major roles. The first is in certain allergic diseases such as hayfever and asthma (p. 61) where in the presence of antigen it can activate mast cells and lead to inflammation (p. 95). It also plays a vital role in host defence against parasitic infections, particularly helminths (worms), by the attraction of circulating eosinophils.

IgD

IgD is a lymphocyte membrane protein, present in only trace amounts and weighing 185 000 daltons. Its exact function is unclear but it appears to play a role in B-cell differentiation.

The protective role of the various immunoglobulins is summarised in Table 6.1.

Cell-mediated immunity

This was discussed briefly at the end of Chapter 5. By definition, it is specific immunity which does not depend upon antibody or complement but is instead due to a subtle interplay between macrophages and T lymphocytes, and largely confined to these two cell types. It is therefore easily distinguished conceptually from

Table 6.1   Role of the immunoglobulin subclasses in host defence

Immunoglobulin	Major roles
IgG	1. Antitoxin 2. Opsonin 3. Neutralisation of virus in blood 4. Protection of fetus and neonate
IgM	1. Agglutinator (of bacteria) 2. Opsonin
IgA	1. Prevents bacterial adhesion to mucous membranes 2. Antitoxin 3. Antiviral agent on mucous membranes
IgE	1. Antiparasitic by degranulating mast cells and attracting eosinophils 2. Involved in hypersensitivity reactions

antibody-mediated immunity which depends upon antibody and complement and on phagocytes.

Although antibody-mediated immunity may be passively transferred between individuals by serum alone, cell-mediated immunity can only be transferred by sensitised T lymphocytes, and not by serum.

Cell-mediated immunity essentially involves the combination of antigen, phagocyte and T cell. The T cell cannot respond directly to the antigen but requires a cell to present the antigen. The cell that serves this function is a phagocyte (usually a macrophage), and is known not surprisingly as an *antigen presenting cell*. Recognition by the T cell is by means of a receptor on its surface which interacts with the antigen of the antigen presenting cell (see Fig. 6.6). In addition T cells also recognise other antigens on its surface; these are surface glycoproteins coded for by a gene sequence within the major histocompatibility complex (MHC), known as *histocompatibility antigens* (p. 75).

As a host defence mechanism, cell-mediated immunity is of vital importance in the killing of fungi and large bacteria such as *Mycobacterium tuberculosis*, *Listeria monocytogenes*, *Brucella abortus* and *Mycobacterium leprae* which grow well inside cells and are resistant to destruction. The killing of these bacteria is performed within the cytoplasm of macrophages after these large phagocytes have been

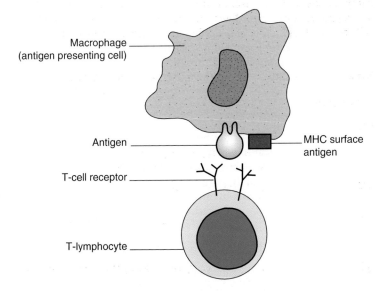

Fig. 6.6   The T cell and antigen recognition.

Table 6.2   Effector mechanisms of specific host immunity against bacteria and parasites

Type of immunity Target	Mechanism
Cell-mediated	
Large bacteria, e.g. tubercle bacillus	Intracellular killing after phagocytosis by T-cell activated macrophages
Fungi	Extracellular killing by secretory products of T-cell activated macrophages
Helminths and protozoa	Control of eosinophils and mast cells by sensitised T cells
Antibody-mediated	
Most bacteria	Opsonisation of IgG or IgM leading to phagocytosis by polymorphs and macrophages
Extracelluar bacteria	Extracellular destruction by IgM or IgG-activated complement
	Destruction on mucous membranes by complement, after binding by IgA
Helminths and protozoa	Extracellular destruction by contents of mast cells degranulated by IgE

non-specifically activated by specifically sensitised T cells. It is also likely that activated macrophages secrete bactericidal substances (e.g. H_2O_2 or lysozyme) into their micro-environment so that targets may be killed extracellularly. This certainly seems to be the case when T-cell activated macrophages kill neoplastic cells as described in Chapter 28. The most important features of antibody-mediated and cell-mediated immunity are set out in Table 6.2.

Immunity to viral infection

The defensive response of the host to viral invasion is complex. This is not surprising because when the viruses reach harbour inside host cells it becomes impossible to attack the virus without also damaging host tissues. Fortunately viruses can sometimes be eliminated extracellularly on mucous membranes or in the blood before major cellular colonisation has occurred.

Interferon

The first line of defence against viruses is interferon. Interferons are a family of glycoproteins secreted by various cell types and are important in limiting the spread of viral infection. There are three types, *IFN* α + β and *IFN* γ, produced by activated T lymphocytes. Interferon released from virally infected cells binds to receptors on neighbouring cells inducing these cells to make antiviral proteins. IFN is also a powerful inhibitor of cell growth, can modulate immune responses and enhances natural killer cell activity (NK cells).

NK cells are large granular lymphocytes which are capable of killing a number of virally-infected and transformed cells to which they have not been previously sensitised. IFN α also has the capacity to activate macrophages, thereby modifying the response to injury.

IgA secreted by epithelial cells will react to viral antigens, if immunisation or previous infection has occurred, and eliminate viruses with the aid of activated complement. In the blood stream IgG performs a similar function, again with the aid of complement. Viruses can also activate complement by the alternate pathway without the aid of antibody and thus precipitate their own destruction.

Once inside host cells, the virus may still be killed by IgG antibody reacting to a combination of viral and host cell surface antigen. The reaction activates complement which destroys both cell and virus. This process is called ADCC (*antibody-dependent cell-mediated cytotoxicity*). Obviously, antibody-mediated immunity is most likely to be effective against viruses after a previous infection or immunisation has made specific immunoglobulin quickly available. In first infections, cell-mediated immunity is usually more important. There is also evidence that cytotoxic T lymphocytes are important in the body defence against some virus infections by killing the cell in which the virus is replicating.

In cell-mediated immunity to virus infection, the target is not a phagocytosed bacillus but the combination of viral and host antigens presented by the intracellular virus, especially at the cell surface. Another important difference is that in cell-mediated immunity provoked by bacteria, macrophages do the killing at the bidding of T cells. In viral infections, a special breed of 'killer' T cells themselves destroy the virus-infected cells although they may be aided by macrophages. In both cases, chemical substances (*lymphokines*) released by T cells probably mediate the respective effects, i.e. there are cytotoxic lymphokines and macrophage-activating lymphokines (p. 66). The methods of antiviral protection are summarised in Table 6.3.

Effects of immune processes harmful to the host

An important example of cell-mediated immunity to virus infection is provided by serum hepatitis, i.e. destruction and inflammation of the liver caused by the hepatitis B virus. This virus is by itself not destructive to the liver cells it invades and in which it proliferates; it is said therefore to be non-cytotoxic. However the cell-mediated

Table 6.3   Methods of host protection against viruses

Site	Antiviral agent	Mechanism
Extracellular	Interferon	Produces antiviral proteins in environment
		Produces killer (NK) cells
	IgA (on mucous membranes)	Reacts with complement to produce phagocytosis
	IgG (in blood), complement	Direct activation
Intracellular		
In sensitised host	IgG reacting to host + viral antigens (humoral immunity)	Antibody-dependent cell-mediated cytotoxicity (ADCC)
No previous exposure	T-cell recognition of host + viral antigen (cell-mediated immunity)	Cytotoxic (killer) T cells
		Activated macrophages

reaction it provokes kills numerous liver cells together with their cohabiting virus. Thus the immune response not only eliminates the invader but also produces almost all the detectable manifestations of the disease, including the possibility of death from liver failure. There are many other examples of virus disease, e.g. measles or smallpox, in which the unpleasant or lethal manifestations are due to the cell-mediated immune response to the viral infection.

In addition the antibody-mediated viral immunity discussed above often contributes its quota of tissue damage. This is usually due to the circulating complexes of viral antigen and IgG (p. 62), and the blood vessels or renal glomeruli are likely to be damaged by them. This happens in hepatitis B infections.

The one antiviral defence mechanism which does not appear to be harmful to the host is the production by the infected cells of interferon.

KEY POINTS

- Humoral immunity involves production of antibodies against proteins or haptens whose main role is to bind to protein, activate complement and facilitate phagocytosis via opsonisation.
- The role of complement is to aid phagocytosis, activate inflammatory pathways and destroy cell walls via the membrane attack complex.
- IgG and IgA also have a role as antibodies against bacterial exotoxins as antitoxins.
- Cell-mediated immunity is useful against intracellular bacteria. It involves the presentation of antigen on the cell surface of a macrophage which is recognised by a T cell which then activates a series of cytotoxic reactions.
- Viruses are dealt with by a variety of methods including interferon, IgA, IgG, antibody-dependent cell-mediated cytotoxicity and cell-mediated immunity.

7 The function of lymphocytes

The role of lymphoid tissue

Although it is conventional to divide specific immunity into cellular and humoral components, antibodies which contribute to the humoral element themselves owe their existence to the development of a particular cell system, the lymphoid tissue, which manufactures the immunoglobulins.

The lowest vertebrate to possess a recognisable lymphoid system is the lamprey. The complement system appeared later in evolution than the lymphoid tissue and is first recognisable in the paddle fish.

In mammals, including man, the lymphoid tissue is located in the lymph nodes (also known as lymph glands) all over the body, e.g. in the neck, axilla and mesentery. Lymphoid tissue is present also in the spleen, bone marrow and intestinal wall and in small amounts in other organs such as the lungs. The thymus gland too is part of the lymphoid system. In most instances the lymph nodes are the most important sites of antibody production. These bean-shaped organs are fed by protein-containing extravascular fluid known as *lymph* which arrives at the periphery of the node and is drained off at the hilum. In the substance of the lymph node the lymph filters through a network of sinusoids lined by cells of the mononuclear phagocyte system (p. 29). These cells trap bacteria very efficiently and as a result lymph glands readily become inflamed during bacterial infection of the tissue draining into them. This mopping up effect, though painful, often prevents generalised dissemination of large numbers of bacteria in the blood stream, a potentially lethal situation known as *septicaemia*.

It is obvious that the lymph nodes are well placed to catch antigens and therefore ideal sites for the production of antibodies. The spleen plays a similar role for antigens arriving by the blood stream as opposed to the lymph. On arrival at the node antigen is taken up by the mononuclear phagocytes, and in fact most antigens need to be digested by macrophages for antibody formation to proceed.

B cells

The essential process in the manufacture of antibodies is the mitotic proliferation of a particular family (clone) of lymphocytes known as B cells with the inherited capability to respond to a particular antigen by proliferating and expressing antibody of a single specificity. During the process of immunoglobulin synthesis they tend to proliferate and produce other B cells or they may change their appearance from that of a small lymphocyte to that of a plasma cell which is not capable of further replication.

The specific proliferative response of B cells to individual antigens is known as *clonal selection*. The particular antigen is recognised only by those B cells capable of responding to it. Other clones ignore its presence. Recognition is achieved by the simple means of the lymphocyte having on its surface a sample of the immunoglobulin it will manufacture when the appropriate antigen arrives. Antigen and antibody sample recognise each other and this is the signal for the activated clone to proliferate and produce antibodies (Fig. 7.1).

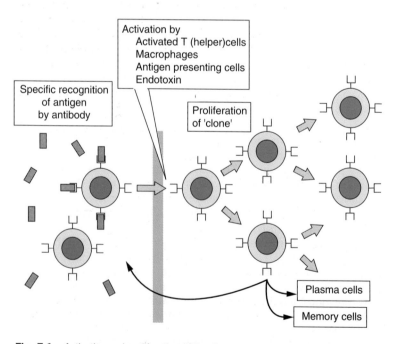

Fig. 7.1   Activation and proliferation of B cells.

Before it can do so, however, it must receive another set of complex signals; these signals come from the T lymphocytes or T cells.

T cells

T cells originate, like B cells, in the bone marrow but have spent some time sequestered in the thymus gland (Table 7.1). Having been programmed in that organ in contact with thymic epithelium they spend much of their subsequent life circulating around the body and passing through the lymphoid tissues. There are two main subsets of T cells:

- *Helper cells* are T cells which give the 'go-ahead' signals to B cells. They are also known as CD4 cells after the monoclonal antibody which was used to identify them. Not all antigens require helper cells, but their existence is due presumably to evolutionary pressure to make antibody production more efficient. Macrophages, antigen presenting cells, certain bacterial cell walls and endotoxins can also activate B-cell antibody production. T-helper (TH) cells are further divided into two subsets, TH-1 and TH-2, which depend on the type of lymphokines they can stimulate (p. 67).
- The other important subpopulation of T cells are known as *suppressor cells* (CD8 cells); they can prevent B cells from multiplying and making antibody. This can occur even though the B cells have reacted with an apparently effective antibody-worthy antigen. The suppression seems to occur when the T cells recognise part of the antigen as too closely resembling a constituent of host tissue. If T suppressor cells were deficient in numbers or effectiveness it would be predicted that antibodies would arise to host tissues (autoimmunity, p. 69). This situation may arise in a

Table 7.1   A comparison of the main properties of T and B lymphocytes

T cells	B cells
Re-circulating long-lived lymphocytes	Re-circulating short-lived lymphocytes
Formed in bone marrow	Formed in bone marrow
Programmed in thymus	Not programmed in thymus
Do not form plasma cells	Form plasma cells
Do not form immunoglobulins	Form immunoglobulins
Present in paracortical areas of lymph nodes	Present in cortex and germinal centres of lymph nodes
Help or suppress immunoglobulin formation by B cells	Respond to T-cell regulation
Responsible for cell-mediated immunity and hypersensitivity	Responsible for humoral (antibody mediated) immunity and hypersensitivity
Form lymphokines	Do not form lymphokines
Do not possess Fc and C3 receptors	Possess Fc and C3 receptors

number of diseases. Suppressor cells also play a major role in immunological tolerance.

The mechanism by which T cells recognise antigen is more complex than for B cells. It appears that antigen has to be processed by an antigen presenting cell such as a macrophage. In addition a second signal is required from a glycoprotein on the presenting cell which has been coded for by histocompatibility (HLA) genes within the major histocompatibility complex (MHC) on chromosome 6 (p. 75).

Primary and secondary response

After the arrival of antigen, 10–14 days elapse before antibody is detected in the blood; the so-called *primary response*. During the interval between introduction of antigen and the appearance of antibody there is a proliferation of the appropriate clone of B cells as described above. Some of the clone proceeds to the synthesis of the appropriate antibody. Other members of the clone of B cells develop the capacity to produce the antibody but remain in latent form as memory cells. If and when the host receives a second dose of antigen, the memory cells provide a clone of cells ready to synthesise antibody immediately. As a result, a second challenge is met by a more rapid and long-lasting antibody production (*secondary response*).

The process of antibody formation in response to bacterial or viral antigen is known as *active acquired immunity;* this may be a result of a natural infection or may be artificially induced by injecting dead organisms as in inoculation against typhoid fever, or those modified so as to be harmless (attenuated) as in the BCG vaccine against tuberculosis, or harmless organisms of similar antigenic composition as in smallpox vaccination.

Tolerance

Under some circumstances, a state of tolerance occurs whereby entry of an antigen to the lymphoid tissue leads not only to no antibody production, but to a state of unresponsiveness in which no amount of antigen succeeds in forming antibody. Tolerance is dependent upon T cells and can be thought upon as the converse of immunity. It occurs more readily in fetal or newborn animals than adults, is more readily demonstrated with weak than with powerful antigens, and can be achieved by giving either very high or very low doses of the antigen.

Tolerance is a survival mechanism for mammals in the sense that the fetus develops tolerance very readily. Since almost the only antigens which reach it are derived from its own or its mother's tissues, tolerance ensures that no lymphocyte clones appear with the ability to produce antibody against the individual's own tissues. This paralysis of response against one's own chemical constituents normally lasts a lifetime. If not, autoimmune disease may develop (p. 69).

Obviously, tolerance makes the fetus and newborn infant very vulnerable to infection since bacteria or viruses reaching it could be interpreted as self antigens as opposed to non-self. This situation is largely covered by the transfer of antibody (IgG) from mother to fetus across the placenta or by suckling. However, if the mother is herself a carrier of virus or bacteria, the fetus may become infected if placental infection occurs, as it does with rubella virus or the treponema which causes syphilis. Alternatively, a virus may be transmitted to the fetus from the mother (*vertical transmission*) and lead to a carrier state in the baby or remain in its cells in a latent form. Such successful transmission can be regarded as an example of a symbiote, e.g. a virus, using a host mechanism to ensure its own survival.

The mechanism of tolerance is still unclear but it can be induced in both B and T cells. Proposed modes of action include the induction of immature B cells leading to 'clonal abortion', overproduction of B cells causing 'clonal exhaustion' and inactivation of B cells by T cells causing 'clonal anergy'. Suppressor T cells may also be involved.

Diversity of specificity

The total number of antibody and T-cell receptor specificities which can be generated by the immune system is remarkably high and is accounted for by a process known as *gene rearrangement*. As B cells develop from their stem cells they undergo rearrangement of the genes which encode antibodies, thus generating the diversity of antibody specificity. A similar mechanism occurs by which T-cell receptors can express a large number of permutations of the variable region. B cells rearrange a heavy chain and a light chain gene giving rise to diverse antibody molecules; in T cells the alpha chains and beta chains are similarly rearranged. As illustrated in Figure 7.2, rearrangements occur in four gene regions—variable (V), diversity (D), joining (J) and constant (C)—which can produce large numbers of VDJC RNA molecules encoding for different proteins. Inaccuracies in the VDJC combination and somatic point mutations may occur, thus augmenting antibody variability and diversity.

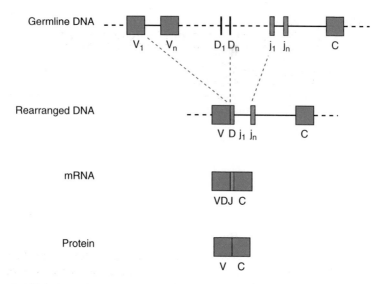

Fig. 7.2 Mechanism of antibody diversity. Examples: immunoglobulin and T-cell receptor. V = variable segment; D = diversity segment; J = joining segment; C = constant segment.

KEY POINTS

- Antibodies are produced by B lymphocytes in response to a specific antigen.
- The signal for B cells to proliferate is given by helper T cells, antigen presenting cells and other chemical mediators.
- Antibody production in response to antigen is responsible for the delayed primary response, 10–14 days afterwards, and the more rapid secondary response aided by memory cells.
- Tolerance is a survival mechanism whereby B-cell proliferation does not occur in response to host antigens.
- The diverse number of specificities of antibodies and T-cell receptors is due to a process known as gene rearrangement.
- T cells are long-lived cells responsible for cell mediated immunity and forming lymphokines.

8 Immunodeficiency and AIDS

Nature performs experiments which, although often terrible in their effects, help us in understanding the mechanisms and importance of phagocytosis, intracellular killing of bacteria and the control of microbiological symbiosis. These rare diseases have their counterpart in the lymphoid system and can be divided into *primary* or *secondary* *defects* of immunodeficiency.

Primary immunodeficiency syndromes

Primary immunodeficiency syndromes can affect either B or T cells separately or together, the consequences depending on which cell type is most affected (Table 8.1).

Table 8.1 Primary and secondary immunodeficiency

Type	Example	Infections
Primary immunodeficiency		
B-cell	X-linked agammaglobulineamia	Bacterial
T-cell	Thymic aplasia	Viral and fungal
Mixed B+T-cell	Wiskott–Aldrich	Viral, bacterial and
	Ataxia telangiectasia	fungal
	Severe combined immunodeficiency (SCID)	
Secondary immunodeficiency		
B-cell	Chronic lymphocytic leukaemia	Predominantly
	Myeloma	bacterial
	Drugs	
T-cell	AIDS	Predominantly
	Hodgkin's disease	viral and fungal

X-linked (Bruton's) agammaglobulinaemia is an example of primary B-cell deficiency, with plasma cells and germinal centres being sparse in the lymphoid tissues. Patients suffer from recurrent bacterial infections though viral infections are uncommon. Circulating levels of IgG, IgM and IgA are negligible, and currently treatment is with lifelong IgG injections.

Selective T-cell failure is even rarer and is sometimes due to a failure of the thymus to develop (thymic aplasia), a disorder known as the *Di George syndrome.* Children suffer from severe viral and fungal infections due to a lessened capacity for cellular immunity (p. 44) under the control of T cells.

Mixed forms of immunodeficiency may also occur, where a lack of both cellular and humoral immunity exists. In *severe combined immunodeficiency disease* (SCID), affected children have a rudimentary thymus and almost complete absence of lymphoid tissue throughout the body. They usually die at an early age of uncontrollable bacterial and viral infections. Other milder forms of mixed immunodeficiency also occur such as the X-linked *Wiskott–Aldrich syndrome,* which involves platelet and T- and B-cell defects, and the autosomal recessive disease *ataxia telangiectasia* with defects of cell-mediated and humoral immunity; these patients have an increased susceptibility to viral and bacterial infections as well as lymphoid neoplasias such as lymphoma.

Secondary immunodeficiency syndromes

Secondary immunodeficiency can be caused by a variety of factors, including malnutrition and drugs (Table 8.1). It also occurs naturally in infancy and old age. Neoplastic B- and T-cell proliferations such as lymphomas can also lead to a variety of immunodeficiency states. Infections can themselves lead to immunosuppression; an example is pneumococcal pneumonia leading to herpes simplex (cold sores). The most important infection leading to immunodeficiency is the newly recognised acquired immune deficiency syndrome (AIDS).

Acquired immune deficiency syndrome (AIDS)

Epidemiology   The first recognised cases of AIDS occurred in the late 1970s and early 1980s in America with reports of young homosexual males having *Pneumocystis carinii* pneumonia and Kaposi's sarcoma, a rare malignant endothelial tumour; they were also found to be immunocompromised. The virus now known to cause AIDS was discovered in 1983 and has been given various names, i.e. HTLV III, LAV, AIDS related virus, ARV. The accepted name is now human immunodeficiency virus (HIV) although variants of this have been isolated in Africa (HIV II); the significance of these other forms is at present unclear. The virus is transmitted mainly by sexual intercourse. Other methods of transmission are via blood or blood products, donated organs or semen, sharing of hypodermic needles and from mother to child in utero and at birth.

The origin of the virus is unknown but the disease is likely to have started life about 100 years previously in Central Africa as a mutation from a closely related virus of primates or other animals, i.e. Green Monkey virus or simian immune virus (SIV) and gradually spread to the USA via Haiti. The AIDS virus is very small and contains only sparse genetic information. It reproduces rapidly and is constantly changing and its genes mutating and evolving at a rate of 50 mutations per year. These characteristics make predictions and treatment difficult.

In certain parts of the world the disease has reached epidemic proportions. Estimates worldwide vary widely but it is believed that 20–30 million people will be affected by the year 2000, most of these in developing countries. In developed countries the majority of cases occur in homosexuals and intravenous drug users where the risk of infection is about 4% per year; in many cities in the USA it is the commonest cause of death in young males and a survey in 1992 found 0.3% of the US population affected. In parts of Africa, where cases may have pre-dated those in the USA, heterosexual transmission appears to be more important and large sections of the population are infected with the virus. The incidence of disease in developing countries is still increasing rapidly in heterosexuals, whereas in many western countries it is showing signs of plateauing in homosexual populations and increasing slowly in heterosexuals in a similar way to other sexually transmitted diseases.

Clinical features   Most of the clinical features of AIDS can be attributed to the profound immune deficiency which the virus provokes. The main target for the virus is a subset of T cells known as helper/inducer cells which carry a glycoprotein on their surface recognised by CD4 antibodies (p. 51). The HIV virus has a protein coat which binds specifically to the CD4 receptor and the virus is then taken up by these T cells. The virus replicates at frightening speed, producing 10 billion virions per day. The CD4 cells play an important role in the immune response, producing lymphokines and activating B cells. CD4 cells are affected in a number of ways, by direct viral cytotoxicity and by activation of cell cytotoxicity (ADCC).

The most obvious effect of this destruction of CD4 cells is the reduction in cell-mediated immunity leading to opportunistic infections such as *Pneumocystis carinii* pneumonia and candidiasis. Tumours reflecting a cell-mediated immune defect such as Kaposi's sarcoma and lymphomas also occur. With progression of the disease the patient succumbs to a multitude of fungal, viral and bacterial infections. The prognosis of AIDS once it is established, although improving, is poor, the mean survival time being around 12 months.

Typical HIV infection is usually asymptomatic but it can lead to a mild viral-type illness known as 'acute seroconversion'. Detectable antibodies are formed soon after infection; the patient then enters a long symptomless phase which on average lasts 2–8 years before developing the full clinical symptoms of AIDS described above. Progression to AIDS is, however, not universal and some studies suggest that up to 35% of HIV infected individuals may not develop the disease even after 10 years of follow-up. Why some HIV positive individuals develop AIDS sooner, and others later or not at all remains a mystery crucial to finding treatments.

AIDS is generally defined for epidemiological studies as the presence of one of 26 AIDS defining conditions, but this is not often clear cut. It has recently been proposed to alter the definition to a laboratory based one (when the number of CD4 cells are reduced below 200 per microlitre).

Treatment   The aim of treatment is to reduce the replication rate and levels of HIV and increase CD4 counts. Although some immunomodulatory agents such as zidovudine (AZT), a virus-specific enzyme inhibitor, have increased the length of survival in some patients, particularly when used in combination with other drugs such as nucleosides and nucleoside inhibitors, a curative treatment has yet to be found. Greater success appears likely in treating patients with early infection when the strains of virus are more homogenous. Large amounts of money are currently being spent on the development of various AIDS vaccines in the hope that this will halt the spread of the virus and the disease. Any vaccine needs to be group specific as the AIDS virus shows enormous heterogeneity and capacity for change. These vaccines are now being tested on humans.

KEY POINTS

- Immunodeficiency presents with abnormally increased susceptibility to infections.
- Primary immunodeficiencies are due to congenital defects which can affect:
  — T cells, leading to bacterial infection
  — B cells, leading to viral and fungal infections
  — both T and B cells.
- Secondary immunodeficiencies are due to leukaemias, drugs, infections or AIDS.
- The HIV virus causes AIDS by specifically destroying CD4 positive T cells leading to profound immunodeficiency and death from opportunistic infections and tumours.

9 | Hypersensitivity

Hypersensitivity or allergy can be defined as any immunological reaction which produces tissue damage in the reacting individual.

Students often find this concept hard to understand since the word immunological implies defence of the host tissues rather than their injury. They are not helped by the term hypersensitivity, which implies some kind of exaggerated response as the cause of illness or by words like allergy (other work) or anaphylaxis (reversed guarding). In fact, the immunological reactions which cause tissue damage are identical with those which destroy microorganisms.

The conceptual difficulties provoked by this paradox disappear when it is appreciated that, like other survival mechanisms, immunity can under certain circumstances work to the detriment of the host. These mechanisms evolve by natural selection and are favoured because they effectively evade a particular threat to survival. The fact that they also have disadvantages for the host will not prevent them being selected, provided that on balance they favour survival. If no immune mechanism existed, most mammals would die of bacterial or viral infections before they were old enough to reproduce themselves. Disease due to an attack by the immune mechanism on the host tissues, i.e. hypersensitivity, is far from negligible but is a small price to pay for survival of the species. The essential point to grasp is that hypersensitivity does not imply an abnormal or exaggerated immune response but merely such a response which happens to cause tissue damage in the host. All that is necessary is to accept natural selection as the imperfect force it is.

Disease due to hypersensitivity takes a number of forms, and four main types have been identified based on the nature of the immune reaction involved. Although it is now recognised that there is a degree of overlap in the immunological processes involved, these distinctions are clinically useful.

Type I (anaphylactic) hypersensitivity

Type I hypersensitivity is an immediate immune reaction, occurring within minutes of exposure to a particular antigen and involving *IgE* and *mast cells.*

It accounts for *asthma, hay fever, eczema* and *urticaria* and less commonly for a generalised reaction known as *anaphylaxis.* Type I reactions are due to one particular immunoglobulin, IgE, which has the special property of binding to cell surfaces, especially mast cells, by way of its Fc portion (p. 29).

Mast cells

Mast cells are found in large numbers in the vicinity of blood vessels. They contain lysosomal granules rich in preformed pharmacologically active chemicals such as histamine, heparin, proteolytic enzymes, chemotactic and activating factors, as well as substances formed on activation of mast cells, such as leukotrienes and prostaglandins. When released, these cause contraction of smooth muscle cells, e.g. in bronchial walls, and of vascular endothelial cells. As a result blood vessels become leaky, causing inflammation (p. 87) in the skin, nose or conjunctivae, and the bronchi become narrowed, causing asthma. These are local effects. If the antigen is introduced into the circulation, e.g. by injection of horse serum containing anti-tetanus antitoxin, there may be general circulatory collapse, pulmonary oedema and death. This is *anaphylaxis* or *anaphylactic shock.* Whether local or general, the effects of Type I hypersensitivity are attributable to pharmacological agents released mainly from mast cells.

IgE

IgE is formed by lymphoid tissue on initial contact with an antigen, frequently a common household contaminant like pollen, mites or animal fur, but sometimes foreign antiserum. If the IgE is specific it is often referred to as a *reagin.* When a second contact is made with the antigen, it combines specifically with the IgE it elicited previously, which is now coating mast cell membranes, and an explosive reaction ensues in which mast cells shed their lysosomal granules and release their potent chemical agents (Fig. 9.1). Complement does not play a major role and damage to the host cell membrane is associated with entry of calcium ions.

Type I hypersensitivity is characterised by a familial tendency with a variable pattern of inheritance. Those affected have high levels of circulating IgE and a stronger than average tendency to form IgE antibody in response to certain frequently encountered antigens.

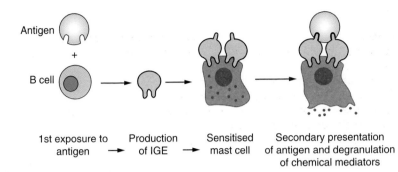

| 1st exposure to antigen | → | Production of IGE | → | Sensitised mast cell | Secondary presentation of antigen and degranulation of chemical mediators |

Fig. 9.1 Type I hypersensitivity.

The role of Type I hypersensitivity

The Type I immune reaction has survival value in that the contents of mast cells are lethal for various helminths which may infect the intestine. These worms cannot be dealt with by phagocytosis or complement-induced lysis so that the only immune mechanism likely to kill them is a Type I reaction leading to degranulation of mast cells. Another result of Type I reactions is the particular attraction of eosinophil granulocytes to the involved area. These may also help to kill extracellular parasites in association with specific antibody reactions—antibody-dependent cytotoxicity (ADDC, p. 47). They also inactivate mast cell products dangerous to the host.

Type II (cytotoxic) hypersensitivity

Type II (cytotoxic) hypersensitivity is characterised by *antibodies* reacting to *antigens which are an integral part of the surface of the host cells* (Fig. 9.2). These surfaces may be rendered antigenic by ways not yet understood but in some cases, at least, the appearance of antibodies is due to a drug or other chemical binding to the host tissues and thereby altering the chemical configuration the particular tissue presents to the antibody-forming apparatus of the body.

A chemical which makes an otherwise innocuous protein antigenic is called a *hapten*, and a number of useful drugs are known to have this unwelcome property.

Type II reactions involve the combination of antibody with the antigen at the cell surface and usually the fixation and activation of complement (Fig. 9.2). The commonest target tissues are the red blood corpuscles and the platelets. Activation of complement can also lead to lysis of the membrane of these cells by the so-called membrane attack complex (C5–9, p. 39). When red cells are involved a

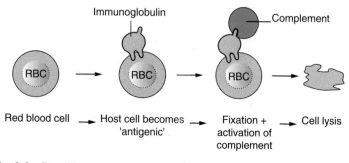

Fig. 9.2 Type II hypersensitivity.

haemolytic anaemia results (p. 246). One example of this is haemolytic disease of the newborn, a Type II reaction to the Rh blood group antigens on the fetal red cells. When platelets are involved, as in certain drug sensitivities, *bleeding* or *purpura* results since most of the body's platelets, which normally prevent spontaneous haemorrhage, may be destroyed. The antibody concerned in Type II reactions is usually IgG, but sometimes IgM.

Type III (toxic immune complex) hypersensitivity

Type III hypersensitivity reactions involve the formation of *immune complexes*. These form in the circulation or on vascular basement membranes and are composed of *antigen, immunoglobulin (IgG or IgM)* and *complement*, the latter being bound and activated by the conglomerate molecule of antigen and antibody (Fig. 9.3). Many different antigens initiate this train of events and a variety of diseases (*immune complex diseases*) result from them.

The classic example is known as *serum sickness* and follows the injection, often as a life saving measure, of serum containing antitoxin to diphtheria or tetanus. Type I reactions can also follow such an injection (see above). Their administration means giving the patient a large antigenic dose of horse immunoglobulins to which the patient forms his own antibodies. If the horse globulins are not eliminated quickly enough, they will combine in the circulation with the antibody (IgG or IgM) which the patient has formed in response to their presence.

Some of the complexes of horse protein and antibody will be removed and neutralised by phagocytosis. In other cases, however, the complexes will remain in circulation and be filtered from the blood and lodge in vulnerable parts of the circulation. The *glomeruli of the kidney* are a favourite site for their deposition as are the synovial *membranes of the joints*.

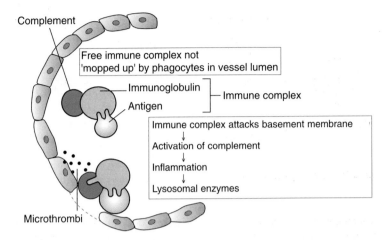

Fig. 9.3   Vascular damage in Type III hypersensitivity.

Many other antigens will induce the formation of these complexes including:

- bacteria (notably the streptococcus)
- the malaria parasite
- viruses
- the patient's own nucleoproteins
- drugs, either alone or as haptens linked to plasma protein.

The formation of soluble antigen/antibody complexes and their arrest within the walls of small blood vessels is an important mechanism in the causation of disease and seems to occur rather readily. Type III hypersensitivity is the major cause of *glomerulonephritis* (p. 239) and the underlying mechanism of a number of diseases, such as *systemic lupus erythematosus* (SLE) in which almost any system of the body can be affected.

All the pathological effects attributable to Type III hypersensitivity are due to the same simple event. The circulating antigen/antibody complex is arrested temporarily at some point on the surface of the endothelial cells lining the small blood vessels. It breaches the endothelial barrier but is held up in the basement membrane which separates these cells from the surrounding tissues (Fig. 9.3). The complex now activates the complement which it carried into the vessel wall or which it fixed after its arrival. Enzymes are activated in the complement system which attack the basement membrane and excite an inflammatory reaction which causes further damage (p. 87). Moreover, because of disruption in the normal smooth vessel lining, platelet thrombi are deposited leading to additional destruction. For these reasons, immune complex deposition often causes progressive and irreversible pathology.

A very wide range of exogenous and endogenous antigens seem to be capable of causing immune complex disease. Since many of these antigens are ubiquitous it is impossible to escape the awkward question of why only a small number of unfortunates succumb in this way. It has to be presumed that most people form complexes, e.g. with invading streptococcal antigens, but then succeed in eliminating them without suffering diseases such as immune complex glomerulonephritis.

The answer to the question is not yet clear, but evidence is accumulating that *complement* plays a key role in the elimination of immune complexes as well as in producing their inflammatory consequences.

In the three types of hypersensitivity just described, tissue damage begins between 15 minutes and 8 hours after antigen and antibody meet. They are therefore sometimes lumped together as *immediate hypersensitivity* (Table 9.1).

Type IV (delayed or cell-mediated) hypersensitivity

In Type IV hypersensitivity, a reaction requires the presence of *sensitised lymphocytes* and *antigen* and is not evident until 24–48 hours after a sensitised host is challenged, hence the term *delayed hypersensitivity*

Types I, II and III differ from Type IV hypersensitivity in another fundamental way, in that whereas the first three types are due to the presence of circulating antibody, Type IV reactions demand the presence of sensitised lymphocytes themselves. For this reason Type IV hypersensitivity is known also as *specific cell-mediated immunity* (or *allergy*), not to be confused with the more general term 'cellular immunity' which is used most often in relation to intracellular killing of bacteria by macrophages.

The importance of lymphocytes as opposed to antibody is best illustrated by transfer experiments. Immediate hypersensitivity, i.e. Types I, II and III, can be transferred passively by injecting immunoglobulin from a sensitised animal into a normal animal, but this does not work with Type IV hypersensitivity which can only be transferred passively by injections of lymphocytes from a sensitised animal.

Type IV reactions are of great importance in pathology. This type of hypersensitivity develops readily in response to microbiological antigens, notably tubercle bacilli. As a result delayed hypersensitivity plays a significant part in the tissue destruction seen in tuberculosis. Delayed hypersensitivity can also be provoked by other bacteria such as streptococci, the typhoid bacillus and the organism which causes

Table 9.1 A comparison of the three types of immediate hypersensitivity

	Type I	Type II	Type III
Description	Anaphylactic	Cytotoxic	Immune complex
Components	Antigen + IgE + mast cells	Antigenic host cell + antibody	Antigen, immunoglobulin + complement
Mechanism of damage	Mast cell degranulation releasing, e.g. histamine, eosinophil chemotactic factors, prostaglandins, thromboxanes, leukotrienes, PAF	Complement fixation + activation	Formation of immune complex exceeding the capacity of phagocytes. Activation of complement
Effect on host	Vasidilatation, increased vascular permeability, oedema, eosinophil attraction, bronchospasm	Cells lysed by phagocytes or by membrane attack complex	Vascular permeability and damage via microthrombi and lysosomal enzymes particularly in joints and kidneys
Host advantage	Allows antibodies, complement and phagocytes to enter tissues. Kills parasites	Kills bacteria	Attracts polymorphs to site of infection
Examples	Asthma, hay fever	Idiopathic thrombocytopenic purpura, haemolytic anaemia	Streptococcal glomerulonephritis, serum sickness

brucellosis, as well as viruses (e.g. measles, mumps), fungi and insect bites (due to antigens in insect saliva). Drugs and chemicals may cause Type IV hypersensitivity in the skin (*contact hypersensitivity*). In this instance the chemical acts as a hapten (p. 37) by combining with skin protein to produce an antigen. The result is a skin rash which may be severe enough to be disastrous to the patient.

The mechanism by which Type IV reactions cause tissue destruction is not completely understood. The basis is a reaction between the antigen, T-cell lymphocytes sensitised to the antigen and macrophages (Fig. 9.4).

Cytokines are the chemical mediators which enable this interaction and cell to cell communication to occur.

The cytokines produced by lymphocytes are called *lymphokines* and those from macrophages or monocytes, *monokines*. The basis of the reaction entails the antigen reacting with a sensitised T cell, thus stimulating the production of lymphokines which have a wide variety of activities (Table 9.2). Their main action is to:

1. attract macrophages to the site
2. keep them in situ
3. 'activate' them.

Once activated by macrophage activating factor the cells release lysosomal enzymes and monokines. Lysosomal enzymes released from

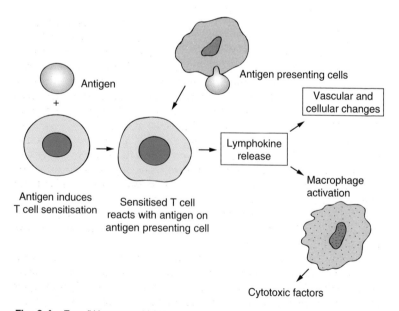

Fig. 9.4 Type IV hypersensitivity.

Table 9.2   Some actions of lymphokines

Target cell	Action	Example
Macrophages	Chemotaxis Arrest of movement Activation	Macrophage chemotactic factor Migration inhibitory factor Macrophage activation factor
Polymorpholeukocytes	Chemotaxis Arrest of movement Stimulation	Chemotactic factor Leukocyte inhibitory factor Eosinophil stimulating factor
Lymphocytes	Proliferation Clonal expression	Lymphocyte mitogenic factor Interleukin-2 (IL-2)
Other cells	Bone metabolism Marrow stimulation	Osteoclast activating factor Colony stimulating factors
Multiple	Defence, repair and metabolism	Tumour necrosis factor (TNF) Interleukin-1 (IL-1)

the macrophages cause *tissue destruction, inflammation* and *further entry of macrophages.* In this way, a small number of sensitised T cells can initiate a reaction involving a much greater number of non-sensitised cells and considerable damage to tissues. In addition, sensitised T cells produce a substance—interleukin-2 (IL-2)—which causes the proliferation of other T lymphocytes.

A common example of such a response is the *tuberculin* or *Mantoux reaction.* A small amount of protein antigen from dead tubercle bacilli is injected into the skin. If the patient has had previous contact with the bacillus a red swelling will appear in 24–48 hours and then slowly subside. Examination of the area under a microscope shows it to be made up of macrophages and lymphocytes, some of the latter cells being demonstrably sensitised to tuberculin. Although a measure of Type IV hypersensitivity, the Mantoux test is widely used to determine immunity or susceptibility to tuberculosis, since immunity and hypersensitivity go hand in hand. If children have a negative Mantoux reaction, i.e. have no evidence of having been sensitised by previous contact with tubercle bacilli, it is usual to immunise them with BCG, a harmless strain of tubercle bacilli.

There is at least one other cytotoxic mechanism which may operate in cell-mediated hypersensitivity: the lymphocyte which itself destroys cells by release of cytotoxic lymphokines.

It would be surprising if so powerful a response as specific cell-mediated immunity could have developed without having survival value for the host. In fact, the capacity of sensitised T lymphocytes after contact with antigen to arm macrophages is the basis of specific immunity to a wide variety of very dangerous microorganisms, notably those causing tuberculosis, leprosy and brucellosis. Only phagocytosis by macrophages can destroy these bacteria and it is their stimulation by specifically sensitised lymphocytes which gives them the extra power they need to do so.

Granulomatous hypersensitivity

A subtype of Type IV hypersensitivity is granulomatous hypersensitivity. In its commonest form it is simply the contribution made by the Type IV reaction to the accumulation of macrophages and their derivatives which occurs in infectious granulomas such as tuberculosis, tuberculoid leprosy and schistosomiasis.

A *granuloma* is a local accumulation of macrophages and cells derived from them and is the most important form of chronic inflammation (p. 105). In the infective granulomas listed above, delayed hypersensitivity contributes substantially to the infiltration and immobilisation of the participating macrophages and hence to the size and severity of the lesions.

The other type of granulomatous hypersensitivity is idiosyncratic in that, unlike the variety just described, only a proportion of individuals exposed to the antigen develop it. It is seen classically after exposure to certain rare metals, such as zirconium. It can be elicited by extremely small amounts of antigen and results in a granuloma which is slow to subside, unlike the tuberculin reaction which resolves in a week or two. This form of hypersensitivity may become increasingly important as uses are found for these rare metals in industry and in the home.

KEY POINTS

- Type I hypersensitivity is an immediate immune reaction caused when antigen combines with IgE to release mast cell contents.
- Type II hypersensitivity occurs when host cells become antigenic and provoke antibodies which activate complement and lyse the cells.
- Type III hypersensitivity is caused by the formation of immune complexes which lodge in the vascular basement membrane, activating complement and damaging tissues.
- Types I–III are often called 'immediate hypersensitivity'. Type IV is known as 'delayed hypersensitivity'.
- Type IV hypersensitivity does not involve antibody but requires the reaction between sensitised T cells, antigen and antigen presenting cells. The message for this comes from lymphokines which cause macrophage activation and vascular changes.

10 Autoimmune disease

It is obvious that the capacity of vertebrates to mount an immune reaction against foreign antigens may be as harmful to the host as to any bacteria or other would-be symbiote. For this reason a state of tolerance (discussed in Ch. 7) has evolved during the normal development of the fetus.

Autoimmunity is a state that occurs when the host loses its normal tolerance of self-antigens, resulting in tissue damage to the host.

Most of the end-stage damage caused by autoimmune disease is believed to be due to the formation of auto-antibodies. Autoimmunisation appears to happen quite frequently and does not necessarily indicate clinical disease, particularly in old age when the frequency of these antibodies tends to increase. When antibodies are detected at an early age or at high concentration they are more likely to be of clinical significance. Antibodies can be produced against a wide variety of host tissues which are regarded as 'antigenic' and can arise against intracellular components as well as cell surface proteins. If the antigen occurs in only one organ an *organ-specific autoimmune reaction* is said to occur; if the antigen is more widespread, such as nuclear DNA in the disease SLE, a more widespread or *multisystem autoimmunity* occurs.

Although some overlap occurs these two broad categories have different properties. In organ-specific autoimmunity the disease commonly affects endocrine organs and there is a tendency for an affected individual to have a number of organ-specific diseases (Table 10.1).

Type II hypersensitivity reactions (p. 61) are believed to be primarily responsible for the tissue damage; although Type IV reactions (p. 64) have been implicated in some diseases, their role is unclear.

Table 10.1   Examples of organ-specific autoimmune disease

Antigen	Effect	Example
Intrinsic factor	Blocks vitamin B_{12} absorption	Pernicious anaemia
Platelet	Lysis and destruction	Idiopathic thrombocytopenic purpura (ITP)
TSH receptor	Stimulates thyroid gland	Graves' disease
Thyroid cells and thyroglobulin	Depresses the thyroid gland	Hashimoto's thyroiditis
Epidermal basement membrane	Blistering of skin	Bullous pemphigoid
Islet cells	Reduces insulin production	Insulin-dependent diabetes
Basement membrane of lung and kidney	Immune complexes leading to lung and renal damage	Goodpasture's syndrome

Organ-specific autoimmunity

In organ-specific autoimmunity auto-antibodies can be directed against specific components within that organ or can be non-specific. Several disorders are closely related to the effects of the auto-antibodies produced. One of the earliest and best documented examples of organ-specific autoimmunity is *Hashimoto's thyroiditis* in which antibodies are formed to thyroid cells and to the thyroglobulin hormone produced by these cells. This usually results in destruction of the gland and clinical hypothyroidism, although a few patients can have an initial stimulatory phenomenon.

In *Graves' disease* an antibody of IgG class (called LATS) is formed to thyroid epithelium which mimics the action of thyroid stimulatory hormone (TSH) and, in contrast to most other autoimmune disorders, causes overfunction of the organ. *Myasthenia gravis* is a disorder where antibodies are produced against the acetylcholine receptors on striated muscle which results in reduced numbers of receptors and leads to a characteristic muscle weakness.

In other organ-specific diseases antibodies are produced which are non-specific, such as the smooth muscle antibodies formed in chronic active hepatitis, and anti-mitochondrial antibodies in biliary cirrhosis. These examples illustrate how in some cases a clear pathogenic link can be made between the antibody and the disorder and in others, particularly antibodies against intracellular components, there appears to be no clear mechanism to explain how the antibodies could result in the disease.

Multisystem autoimmunity

A good example of a non organ-specific autoimmune disease is *systemic lupus erythematosus* (SLE) which is characterised by the development of a number of auto-antibodies directed against nuclear antigens, the most notable being anti double-stranded DNA antibody. Lesions occur throughout the body in the skin, joints, kidneys, central nervous system, brain and muscle and are believed to be due to the deposition of immune complexes formed by Type III hypersensitivity, particularly in small blood vessels. Like the majority of autoimmune diseases it is much commoner in women than men (ratio of 9:1).

Rheumatoid arthritis is another multisystem autoimmune disease; it occurs in about 1% of the population and is three times commoner in women. It causes predominantly a chronic inflammatory swelling of joints, although as in SLE other non-articular sites may occasionally be involved. The majority of cases have an antibody in the blood called rheumatoid factor which is usually an IgM class antibody to the body's own IgG. Immune complexes form which lead to an inflammatory reaction in the joints. It is still unclear however whether the auto-antibody is actually involved in the pathological process or merely a marker. Of interest is the finding that many patients with rheumatoid arthritis have a minor glycosylation defect in their immunoglobulin which may be responsible for the formation of auto-antibodies. A certain percentage of cases of rheumatoid arthritis and to a lesser extent SLE have the clinical picture of the disease without having any detectable auto-antibodies. Conversely, more than 5% of the population have auto-antibodies and no disease. Nevertheless whatever their exact function, auto-antibodies in the blood are a useful diagnostic marker of the disease and can also have prognostic value as individuals with high titres tend to have a poorer outcome.

The mechanism of autoimmunity

The main question remains why autoimmunity occurs in the first place. We have discussed previously how the process of self-tolerance usually develops and prevents auto-antigens and their corresponding lymphocytes from interacting. For autoimmunity to occur these normal control mechanisms have to break down or be bypassed.

The formation of auto-antibodies themselves may not be the primary event in many diseases. The precise mechanisms remain unclear although there are several current hypotheses which involve an alteration in two fundamental processes (Table 10.2).

1. Depression of suppressor activity: the first and perhaps the traditional view is that a suppressor system is defective. T cells acquire the ability to recognise self-antigens in the thymus in early life and it was believed that they probably became suppressor T cells preventing

Table 10.2   Proposed mechanisms of autoimmunity

1. Depression of suppressor activity
2. Alteration in antigen presentation
   a. Class II HLA antigens
   b. Antigen stimulation at immune privileged sites
   c. Immunogenic drugs, e.g. methyldopa
   d. Antigen mimicry by environmental antigens
   e. Viral infections

B cells from producing auto-antibodies. In SLE and myasthenia gravis some evidence has been found of thymic dysfunction and the presence of defective suppressor activity, although it is unlikely that this defect alone is sufficient to cause the clinical disease.

2. Alteration in antigen presentation: currently the major abnormality is believed to lie in the way antigens are presented. This may occur in a number of different ways:

a. *Class II histocompatibility (HLA) molecules* are likely to be involved as certain target cells express Class II antigens on their surface which allow helper T cells to respond to antigens closely. As discussed in the next chapter, HLA antigens may resemble and therefore be mistaken for environmental antigens or else be linked to genes regulating the immune response. It appears that the expression of these Class II antigens can be induced by certain mediators.

b. *Abnormal antigenic stimulation* can arise when antigens in certain sites which have been hidden from the immune system (known as '*immunologically privileged sites*') become suddenly exposed following damage or trauma. Examples of this mechanism include injury to the testis, which can result in anti-spermatozoal antibodies and sterility, or injury to one eye which can cause auto-antibodies and blindness in the other eye.

c. Certain *drugs* can also make self-antigens more immunogenic and produce an antibody response. An example is the drug methyldopa which leads to antibodies against rhesus blood group antigens.

d. Host antigens can also be mimicked by *environmental antigens*, producing an anti-host reaction with a resulting bypass of the normal T-cell self tolerance. A good example of this is rheumatic fever in which auto-antibodies to heart tissue can be detected several weeks after a streptococcal throat infection in a small minority of individuals. The carbohydrate antigen on the streptococcal surface is mistaken for heart tissue by the host and auto-antibodies are formed bypassing the usual tolerance mechanisms.

e. *Viral infection* has been postulated for some time to be an aetiological factor in autoimmune disease; several autoimmune diseases of animals can be induced by inoculation with certain viruses.

Viruses form intimate relationships with host cells and can alter the way host antigen is presented, producing a strong immune response. If this initial defence only partially removes the virus by, say, removing the viral surface antigen, the intracellular virus may be immune to further attack and lead to viral persistence which could provoke a low grade autoimmunity reaction. HLA antigens may also be involved in the genetic tendency to persistent viral infections. Although infections early in life which persist and provoke subtle changes in the way host antigens are presented are a popular theory for many autoimmunity diseases, it is very difficult to prove. A big problem in autoimmune disease is separating the initial cause from the resulting changes that occur. It is now believed that for many diseases T-cell defects account for the initial changes in autoimmune disease, with the formation of antibodies being a rather late phenomenon by which the disorder is recognised and the gross tissue damage occurs. The suspected importance of T cells comes from animal experiments whereby autoimmune models have been treated successfully by the re-transfusion of immunised T cells from the animal. This offers some therapeutic opportunities, although the mechanisms are likely to remain unclear for some time.

Multifactorial autoimmunity

Most autoimmune diseases are multifactorial with a combination of genetic and environmental factors being responsible for the disease. A good example of the complex inter-relationships between genes and the environment is provided by *insulin-deficient diabetes mellitus (IDDM)*. Despite a number of recent discoveries the disease remains an enigma. There are two major types of diabetes: Type I insulin-deficient, and Type II insulin-resistant.

Diabetes is a common condition affecting 2% of the population. It can be defined as an absolute or relative deficiency of insulin causing defective carbohydrate utilisation with a raised whole blood glucose concentration in the fasting state of over 10 mmol/l or 2 hours after a 75 g oral glucose load. The term insulin-deficient diabetes (IDDM) means that the condition is associated with a demonstrable deficiency in the amount of insulin produced by the islet cells of the pancreas which is relieved by administration of insulin.

IDDM certainly has a moderate genetic component with a heritability of 20–40%. An environmental influence is also suggested by the fact that the disease is believed to be increasing in incidence. The disease is likely to be *polygenic* (p. 169), involving a number of genes at different loci. To date at least 6 main loci have been identified; the strongest associations have been in the HLA region (HLA-DQ and DR4). Other loci on different chromosomes are also involved including the insulin gene itself (INS) and genes nearby called the insulin gene minisatellite (IDDM2).

The presence of these HLA antigens correlates well with the presence of a variety of anti islet-cell antibodies found in 90% of affected patients within the first month of presentation. At least 80% of islet cells need to be destroyed before serious insulin deficiency occurs; this helps to explain the state of 'latent diabetes' which can exist for many years before the disease presents. The most commonly recognised auto-antibody associated with IDDM is the islet-cell cytoplasmic auto-antibody which has two main target antigens, the islet-cell glycolipid and the beta-cell enzyme glutamate decarboxylase. Other antibodies have been found against insulin, pro-insulin, and a variety of islet-cell proteins, the significance of which is unclear. Of interest is the fact that a protein from the Coxsackie virus (P2-C) resembles glutamate decarboxylase, suggesting that the virus could induce molecular mimicry and anti islet-cell antibodies.

Genes are only responsible for about 40% of susceptibility. A number of observations have indicated an effect of *diet* on the development of IDDM:

- Alteration of dietary proteins has induced diabetes in both rats and mice.
- Breast feeding of humans has been suggested as being protective.
- An increased frequency of antibodies to cow's milk protein has been reported in children with a recent onset of the disease.

Recent work has reported that in children antibodies can be detected which are directed against a specific segment of bovine serum albumin (found in cow's milk) and which cross-react with an inducible beta-cell protein in the pancreas, suggesting that the pathogenesis of the disease may be molecular mimicry.

If the incidence of diabetes is rising, it could be due to environmental factors such as the increasing use of cow's milk in feeding babies and infants or, alternatively, to an increasing frequency of the HLA antigens responsible for the susceptibility because they confer some other unknown selective advantage to the host.

KEY POINTS

- Autoimmune reactions lead to damage by Type II and Type III hypersensitivity reactions against host tissue.
- Autoimmune diseases can be organ-specific or generalised.
- They are more common in women.
- They are often recognised by the presence of auto-antibodies.
- The process is likely to be triggered by a defect in suppressor T cells or in the way antigens are presented which may involve the HLA system or viral infection.
- The pathogenesis of most autoimmune disease is multifactorial, involving a combination of genetic and environmental factors.

11 The HLA system and transplantation

The genetic basis for histocompatibility (tissue compatibility) is fundamental to our understanding of many normal and pathological immunological processes, such as:

- the basis of antigen presentation and recognition of self from non-self
- the way virtually all infected cells are eliminated
- acceptance or rejection of allografts
- genetic susceptibility to a variety of diseases.

The *major histocompatibility* (gene) *complex* (MHC) contains the genes responsible for histocompatibility antigens; in man it is situated on the short arm of chromosome 6 and is better known as the *HLA gene complex* (HLA standing for human leukocyte antigen).

All higher animals have such a system and an increasing complexity can be seen paralleling evolution. As its name implies, the MHC encodes histocompatibility antigens (transplantation antigens responsible for graft rejection) which are strongly expressed on the surface of white blood cells. However, they are found in one form or other on practically all nucleated cells of the body.

Loci

Within the HLA complex are a number of different genes, the position of each being referred to as a locus. These include the HLA-A, -B, -C loci, all expressing different cell surface antigens. In addition to these are several other genes encoding a number of the complement pathway components (Fig. 11.1).

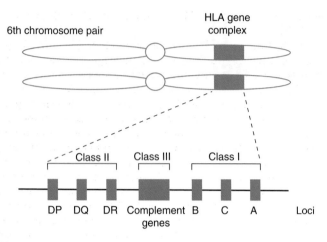

Fig. 11.1   The components of the HLA gene complex.

Alleles

One striking feature of the HLA system is that all of these genes are to varying degrees extremely polymorphic (i.e. they can take many different forms). The alternative forms of a gene are called *alleles* (p. 161). The A locus has at least 24 different possible allelic forms; thus an individual can be A1 or A2 or A3, or any other from the list of 24. As we have two chromosomes making up the sixth chromosome pair, each encoding an HLA region, we therefore have two A, B, C, etc. loci, one on each chromosome. It is therefore possible, for example, to be A1 on one chromosome and A2 or A3 or A11 on the other (*heterozygous* for the A locus). Alternatively it is possible to have the same antigen on both chromosomes, for example A1, A1 (*homozygous* for A). These principles apply to all of the other HLA loci. The B locus has in the region of 50 different alleles, the C locus 8, the DR locus 14, the DQ locus 4 and the DP locus 6. This list is ever-expanding as rarer allelic forms are discovered. For some antigens a small letter 'w' prefixes the number. This merely signifies that the antigen has yet to achieve official WHO recognition.

Haplotypes

If we examined an individual, his or her HLA type (known as tissue type) could be for example: A1, A3; B8, B7; C7; DR3, DR2; DQwl, DQwl; DPwl, DPw2. However in reality half of this information is encoded on one chromosome and half on the other. The information contained on one chromosome is known as an HLA *haplotype* (half type). Thus we all have two HLA haplotypes. If we know which antigen goes with which on the same haplotype we can rewrite the tissue type as A1, B8, Cw7, DR3, DQwl, DPw2/A3, B7, Cw7, DR2, DQwl, DPwl.

The allelic forms of an HLA locus are not found at equal frequency in a population. If we investigated a large random sample of individuals we would see that some antigens are common (e.g. A1 and B8 both have a frequency of about 20–25%), some less common (e.g. B27 with a frequency of about 8%) and others rarely seen (e.g. Aw33 and Bw63 at about 1% frequency). An antigen that is common in one population (e.g. A1 in caucasoids) may be absent or much rarer in another (A1 is much less common in African blacks). Some antigens are only usually found in certain populations, e.g. Bw46 in mongoloid populations. If we know what the frequencies of HLA antigens are in a population, we can calculate how often we should see certain combinations. For example, if A1 and B8 both have a frequency of 25% (1:4) we would predict that they should be found together at a frequency of 1:4 × 1:4 = 1:16. However, when we observe the number of times A1 is actually found with B8 instead of another locus antigen, we find that it occurs with more frequency than we expected.

Linkage disequilibrium is the term used to describe the phenomenon of disturbance between expected and observed frequencies of antigen combination and it is found between many alleles of different loci. For example HLA-A1 is in linkage disequilibrium (p. 188) with B8, A3 with B7, B44 with DR4. HLA genes are codominantly expressed. Thus an individual who is A1 and A29 will express equal amounts of these antigens on the cell surface.

The A, B and C antigens are often referred to as *'Class I'* antigens and they all have a similar structure, being composed of a glycosylated polypeptide chain bearing its unique antigenic specificity (e.g. A1 or A2 or A3, etc.). This chain is anchored at one end in the cell membrane and is associated with another chain known as β_2-microglobulin. β_2-Microglobulin has a constant structure, is identical for all Class I antigens, and is encoded for by a gene on chromosome 15. Class I antigens are identified by specific antisera which react with them. These are usually allo-antisera (from the same species), often coming from antenatal serum samples.

HLA-DR, DQ and DP antigens are known as *'Class II'* and have a more restricted tissue distribution than Class I. They are composed of two chains (an alpha and a beta chain) both of which are glycosylated and traverse the cell membrane. For DR antigens the antigenic site lies within the beta chain, and the alpha chain is common to all DR specificities. For DQ, both the alpha and the beta chains vary for each DQ allele.

Class II antigens are expressed on B lymphocytes and antigen presenting cells but not on normal T lymphocytes, which complicates testing for them using peripheral blood. A variety of procedures are used but many involve a purification step to remove T cells leaving a pure B-cell sample.

HLA types and susceptibility to disease

As mentioned briefly in the previous chapter, one of the most rapidly expanding areas of knowledge in medical research is that concerning the involvement of HLA in disease susceptibility. Originally it was shown that the MHC in the mouse controlled susceptibility or resistance to certain virally induced tumours. This prompted the investigation of HLA antigen in malignancies in humans, although the early results at best showed only weak associations (the first demonstration of HLA association was with *Hodgkin's lymphoma*). This was at a time when HLA typing was in its infancy.

Later, when a variety of non-malignant diseases were examined, some reproducible and clear examples of HLA antigen associations were seen. Perhaps the best known is that of HLA-B27 with *ankylosing spondylitis*. In this condition at least 90% of patients have been found to be B27 positive, compared to only about 8% of the normal population.

HLA and autoimmune disease

The number of diseases which have an HLA antigen association is very high and they can be classified into several broad areas (Table 11.1). The largest group of HLA associated diseases consists of those that have some immunological or autoimmune component to their pathogenesis. Examples include:

Table 11.1   Some HLA associations with disease

HLA antigens	Associations
Autoimmune	
DR4/DR1	Rheumatoid arthritis
DR3/DR4, DQ	Diabetes mellitus (insulin-deficient)
DR2	Multiple sclerosis
B8/DR3	Graves' disease (thyrotoxicosis)
	Coeliac disease
	Chronic active hepatitis
B27	Ankylosing spondylitis
	Reiter's disease
Non-autoimmune	
HLA-H	Idiopathic haemochromatosis
B35	Hodgkin's lymphoma
Bw47	21-hydroxylase deficiency
DR2	Narcolepsy

- multiple sclerosis—DR2
- rheumatoid arthritis—DR4 and DR1
- insulin-dependent diabetes—DQ and DR4.

Molecular analysis of the HLA gene has enabled us to appreciate the specificity of the HLA association with autoimmune disease. For example, in Caucasians it is the 2 HLA DR4 subtypes DRB1*0401 and DRB1*0404 that are associated with rheumatoid arthritis predisposition.

HLA and metabolic or neoplastic disease

Another group consists of those conditions which are not due to an immunological process but may involve a metabolic abnormality. These include congenital adrenal hyperplasia (21-hydroxylase deficiency) and idiopathic haemochromatosis. Both of these particular conditions behave as autosomal recessive disorders showing linkage to the HLA system. Haemochromatosis causes iron overload and is now believed to be due to a mutated Class I gene called HLA-H. It is important as it is the first HLA antigen useful in screening.

The remaining diseases associated with HLA are either of unknown pathogenesis, or tumours. Narcolepsy is an example of the former, where the association between DR2 and the disease is either absolute or very close to it. There are a few examples of associations between HLA and malignancies which include Hodgkin's lymphoma and bladder carcinoma. The prognosis of certain leukaemias has also been related to particular HLA types.

Very few conditions show anything like a 100% association with an HLA antigen. Narcolepsy is an interesting exception, and B27 has a very high frequency in ankylosing spondylitis. In the remaining majority of conditions the absence of complete association may be explained either by heterogeneity of the disease or by the possibility that the HLA antigen is acting merely as a marker for another disease-susceptibility gene absolutely associated with the disease and in linkage disequilibrium with the HLA marker. Alternatively, other genetic components (possibly non-HLA) together with environmental factors may be important in development of the disease.

Mechanism of HLA and disease

Several suggestions have been made to explain why HLA antigens are often associated with disease:

1. One is the theory that there is *molecular mimicry* or antigenic cross-reactivity between microbial and human tissue antigen, e.g. streptococcal antigen and heart myocardium. It has also been shown that cross-reactivity may exist between B27 and *Klebsiella pneumoniae*

in seronegative arthropathies. There are so many examples of HLA associated diseases it would seem to be unlikely that this hypothesis could explain more than a small number of associations. In addition, although most people are presumably exposed to the same environmental factors, only a small percentage of individuals expressing an antigen such as B27 develop ankylosing spondylitis.

2. HLA antigens may also act as receptors for *viruses*. Many viruses enter cells by first attaching to glycoproteins (HLA antigens are also glycoproteins). If this process were specific, i.e. if certain HLA antigen types bound a particular virus well, and others did not, it could provide an explanation for susceptibility or resistance to particular viral infections, possibly triggering other disease processes.

3. An alternative suggestion has been that of *immune response genes*. Experiments with certain MHC strains of mouse indicated that genes encoding within the Class II region controlled their ability to respond immunologically to particular antigens. The injection of synthetic (and thus absolutely pure) antigens induced reproducibly poor antibody responses in one strain and a good response in another. These were referred to as 'immune response genes'.

The HLA system may confer susceptibility via a *linked gene*. This appears to explain the relationship between certain HLA antigens and 21-hydroxylase deficiency. This mechanism may be responsible for other diseases, especially as a number of housekeeping genes have been found in the MHC which appear to be involved in the processing of antigens. It is also possible that molecules containing certain HLA antigens present a unique antigen to circulating T cells thus bypassing the usual self-tolerance mechanisms.

Class II antigens

A striking feature of HLA and disease studies is that the majority of associations seen are with Class II antigens (usually DR). We know that Class II antigens are necessary for the normal processes of both antigen presentation (p. 45) and the mediation of T helper or suppressor cell activity (p. 51). It is therefore possible that certain Class II antigens present some antigens (which may be degraded antigen and self HLA antigen) very well or alternatively others very badly. Similarly it is possible that certain Class II antigens may facilitate good or poor helper/suppressor activity for certain antigens. In some HLA associated conditions, it is possible that the 'autoimmune process' is just the normal elimination of virally infected cells but with a highly vigorous course of response due to the possession of a particular Class II antigen type.

Inappropriate expression of Class II antigens by tissues has been suggested as a means by which an autoimmune process may develop.

Class II antigens normally have a restricted tissue distribution. When cells are activated in some way or exposed to the action of γ-interferon (p. 46), they can be induced to express Class II antigen on their surface. A viral infection may result in a localised immune response whereby T cells release interferon and induce Class II antigen on other tissues. This inappropriate expression of Class II antigen together with organ-specific differentiation antigens may then result in this composite antigen (Class II and organ-specific antigen) being recognised as 'foreign'. The initiation of a response to this antigen (autoimmune response) would then lead to inflammation and potentiate this reaction, further inducing yet more Class II antigen expression. Whilst this is an interesting hypothesis, the transient expression of Class II antigens on tissue not normally expressing them may be a perfectly normal situation, and many common viral infections do not lead to those types of response.

Class I antigens

Although we have discussed HLA and disease it must be remembered that the primary function of the system is protective. It is known that Class I antigens are important in the recognition and elimination of virally infected cells. Cytotoxic T cells can only be raised which have the ability to recognise viral antigen in association with their own Class I antigens (p. 47). Such T cells will not recognise and kill virally infected cells from another individual with different Class I antigens. This phenomenon is known as *HLA restricted killing*.

The process of dual recognition of viral antigens and HLA antigens also serves the purpose of restricting the cytotoxic effects of T cells. Class II antigens on antigen presenting cells are recognised by helper T cells which interact with B cells to produce specific antibodies to the foreign antigen but also provide protection for the antigen presenting cell from cytotoxic T-cell attack. Discrimination between self and non-self HLA antigens serves as a recognition process between cells of the immune system, promoting interactions which are essential for all kinds of immune response. The high number of diverse polymorphisms present in HLA antigens enables considerable diversification of immune response in individuals of a population, preventing molecular mimicry in parasites and hampering epidemic spread of infection. In this way survival of at least some members of past populations in the face of plague or pestilence was ensured.

Transplantation and organ rejection

Skin may be grafted from one part of an individual's body to another part and thrive in its new location. The operation is performed routinely in the case of burns. However skin from one individual

Table 11.2   Major types of transplant rejection

Type of rejection	Time	Primary mechanism
Hyperacute	5–30 minutes	Type II hypersensitivity
Acute	4–30 days	Cell-mediated immunity, Type IV hypersensitivity
Chronic	> 3 months	Probably Type III antibody-mediated hypersensitivity

grafted to a different individual (an *allograft* or *homograft*) will die and be rejected within 10–14 days. The same is true of grafts of kidneys and other organs. Similarly grafts between different species are not usually possible. The variable levels of HLA antigen expression on different organs, i.e. high in kidney and low in heart and liver, may also affect the chances of rejection.

The failure of a graft is due to the recipient's immune system recognising the grafted tissues as foreign and attacking them as it would any other foreign pathogen. Indeed, a second transplant from the same donor is rejected even faster than the first (within a week), just as a secondary immune response to a bacterial antigen is faster than the primary response (p. 52). It has now been demonstrated that HLA matching is beneficial in kidney transplants, the closer the matching the higher the success rate. Organs from living donors are also preferable to cadaveric ones. In man, rejection can occur at different times and probably involves different mechanisms (Table 11.2).

Hyperacute rejection

Hyperacute rejection occurs within minutes of graft insertion and is an example of Type II hypersensitivity (p. 61). Rarely it can be delayed for up to several days due to a low titre antibody response, a process known as *accelerated rejection*.

Acute rejection

Acute rejection usually occurs one week after transplantation and is largely due to specific cell-mediated immunity akin to Type IV hypersensitivity (p. 64). The basic mechanism by which graft rejection occurs is outlined in Figure 11.2. HLA antigens on donor cells are expressed by circulating macrophages acting as antigen presenting cells. They return to lymph nodes where cytotoxic T cells and more macrophages are produced as well as specific antibodies against the graft. The role of the T lymphocytes is highlighted by the inability of animals to reject allografts if their thymus is removed immediately after birth.

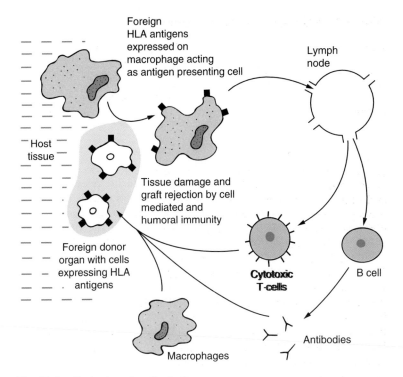

Fig. 11.2 Mechanism of graft rejection.

Chronic rejection

Chronic rejection can occur even in patients treated with immunosuppressive therapy. The rejection often takes place after several weeks or months and is probably due to the formation of circulating antibodies to the foreign antigens. Although some cell-mediated immunity is likely, this is mainly a Type III hypersensitivity reaction in which complexes of IgG or IgM and complement form on the walls of the kidney vessels and in the glomeruli. A repetitive cycle of vascular damage, platelet aggregation and more vascular destruction occurs and results in rejection of the kidney. It is possible that some of the antibody is produced locally within the graft bed by host lymphocytes. *Late rejection* can also occur several years after transplantation. The mechanism is believed to be HLA mediated and involves the hyperplasia and eventual occlusion of small and medium-sized renal vessels.

Antibody formation in grafts can occasionally be beneficial, the antibodies binding to HLA antigens and thus masking them from T-cell recognition—a process known as *graft enhancement* (Table 11.3).

Table 11.3   Factors influencing graft rejection

Good outcome	Poor outcome
Good HLA + ABO crossmatch	Infections
Tolerance induced by previous	Drug toxicity
transfusions	Disease recurrence
Immunosuppressants	

Prevention and treatment of rejection

With the use of ABO and HLA matching, hyperacute rejection is now thankfully rare. Immunosuppressive therapy is now usually used in all grafts other than autografts and includes *corticosteroids*, *azathioprine*, *cyclophosphamide*, and *lymphoid irradiation*. One of the most useful drugs however is *cyclosporin* which interferes with cell-mediated immunity against the graft by targeting primed T cells.

Chronic rejection is not reversible and usually requires removal of the transplant. This unfortunately remains a problem: although most renal grafts now survive one year, only 50% are viable after 5 years.

Graft versus host disease

Another somewhat different problem that arises in transplantation is graft versus host disease (GVHD). This is a major consideration in bone marrow transplantation, used in the treatment of certain leukaemias and aplastic anaemia. A graft versus host reaction occurs when a patient receives normal immunocompetent lymphoid cells from a non-identical donor and is unable to reject them. The donor cells may survive and, being immunologically competent, attack the recipient's cells which are regarded as being foreign. The tissue damage is mainly caused by mature cytotoxic T cells within the donor marrow, and efforts to deplete T cells beforehand—either with immunosuppressants (cyclosporin) or by cell separation with monoclonal antibodies—have had some success.

Clinically, GVHD can occur acutely within 60 days or chronically after 100 days following a marrow transplant. It affects primarily the skin and digestive tract but can also involve the lungs and liver. GVHD can rarely occur in sick patients given large blood transfusions. Although the condition is usually fatal it can be prevented by irradiating the blood before it is given.

Certain organs such as the liver appear to provoke rejection and GVHD less frequently than other tissues. There is some evidence that these organs become chimeric, being partly replaced with host cells, the donor cells being found at other distant sites in the host. For most transplants, however, it is of importance that donors and recipients are well (if not completely) HLA matched. The majority of successful bone marrow transplants are usually between HLA identical siblings. Although the success rate for transplants is increasing with the use of routine HLA typing and immunosuppressants such as cyclosporin, there remain a number of HLA identical marrow transplants which fail. Recent studies have suggested that these cases may be due to the presence in the donor of T-cell precursor cells that secrete cytokines such as interleukin-2. Pre-transplant analysis for such cells could reduce the failure rate still further.

KEY POINTS

- The HLA gene complex encodes cell surface antigens responsible for cell recognition and interaction.
- Class I antigens are expressed on all nucleated cells and Class II on B cells and antigen presenting cells.
- HLA antigens are associated with a number of diseases (particularly autoimmune diseases) through poorly understood mechanisms.
- The HLA system is protective to the host, providing genetic diversity and restriction of the damaging effects of cell-mediated immunity.
- Graft rejection is often due to HLA mismatch and often results from a variety of hypersensitivity reactions with T cells playing a crucial role.

12 Acute inflammation

Invertebrates, with no true circulatory system, respond to an irritant by surrounding it with specialised cells (haematocytes) which then ingest it. If the damage is very severe the invertebrate simply rejects the injured portion of its anatomy as a prelude to its regeneration. In higher forms of life, including man, the local reaction to injury is much more complex because of the evolution of the circulatory system and the disappearance of the kind of major regenerative powers possessed by the earthworm.

Inflammation (derived from the Latin word *inflammare*, to burn) is this local reaction to injury.

The name is apt because when the skin reacts in this way it is red, hot, swollen and tender (the four cardinal signs of inflammation described by Celsus in AD 35). Inflammation also causes loss of function, as first pointed out by Virchow and stressed by John Hunter with the common sense of the practical surgeon.

Although any tissue may suffer injury, inflammation is essentially the reaction to injury of the living microcirculation and its contents. Inflammation of an organ is commonly designated by adding the suffix *-itis*, as in appendicitis. Injury is most commonly bacterial infection, i.e. a breakdown of symbiosis such as to produce demonstrable tissue damage. However, excessive heat or cold, irritant chemicals or trauma or antigen/antibody reactions can lead to similar results. The microcirculation (that part which can be seen only with the aid of the light microscope) includes arterioles, venules, capillaries and lymphatics. Its contents comprise the fluid and cellular constituents of the blood (Fig. 12.1).

Inflammation may be *acute*, i.e. of short duration, or *chronic* (from the Greek for time), i.e. prolonged, depending on the nature of the injury; both have their characteristic pattern although in chronic inflammation there are usually preliminary and sometimes recurrent

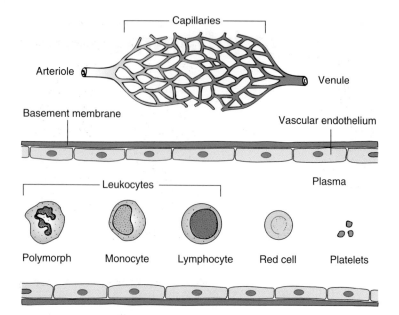

Fig. 12.1   The microcirculation and its contents.

acute phases. Chronic inflammation will be discussed in the next chapter.

Initial response to injury

The changes in the small blood vessels which constitute the initial tissue reaction of acute inflammation may last for only a few hours or for several days. The reaction can be seen in transparent structures such as the web of the frog's foot or by inserting a transparent perspex disc into the rabbit's ear. It is essentially a stereotyped sequence of events whatever the causative agent. Immediately after entry of the irritant stimulus there is a brief *constriction* of arterioles followed by their *prolonged dilatation*. This leads to *flushing* of the capillary network with blood and the opening up of dormant capillary channels. There is also *dilatation of venules and lymphatics* (Fig. 12.2).

The triple response to injury described by Lewis characterises these vascular changes:

1. Following the scraping of a blunt instrument across the skin, a momentary white line appears due to the contraction of arteriolar smooth muscle.
2. The flush due to capillary dilatation then follows, appearing as a dull red line, followed by an irregular red flare due to arteriolar dilatation.

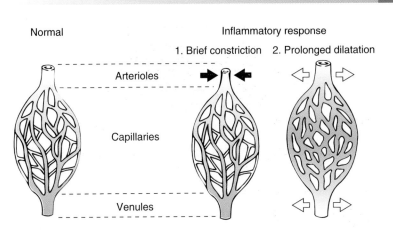

Fig. 12.2   The response of the microcirculation to local injury.

3. Finally a zone of oedema known as a wheal appears, produced by an exudate of fluid in the extravascular space.

The flow of blood is generally increased. The white cells, the leukocytes, leave the centre of the stream which they normally occupy to move to the periphery. They then form a layer against the inner surface of the cells which line the lumen of the blood vessels, the vascular endothelium, a process known as *margination*. This is a prelude to the migration of leukocytes through the vessel wall into the adjacent tissues (Fig. 12.3). At sites of inflammation these leukocytes can attach themselves to the vessel wall, a poorly understood process known as *pavementing*.

Increased vascular permeability

At the same time a crucial change occurs in the wall of the venules and capillaries. These vessels are normally freely permeable to water and small solutes but only slightly permeable to plasma proteins, i.e. albumin, the globulins and fibrinogen. In fact, it is the *oncotic pressure* of these retained molecules which counters the hydrostatic pressure of the blood. The oncotic pressure keeps water inside the vessels whereas the tangential thrust of the blood pressure pushes it out through the vessel wall like a positive pressure filter. In inflammation, *hydrostatic pressure* inside the vessel may rise, upsetting the balance and causing more water to leave the blood and enter the tissues. More important, the wall of the venule and capillary now loses its impermeability to protein. As a result, albumin, globulins and fibrinogen pour out through the wall into the tissues, which thus come to contain fluid with a composition similar to that of blood plasma (Fig. 12.4).

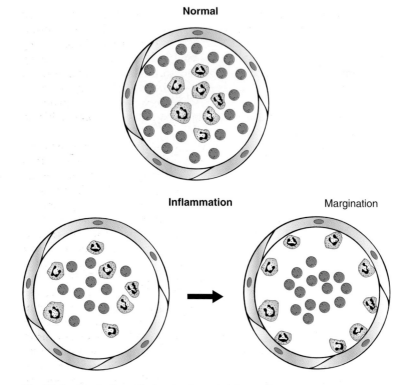

Fig. 12.3 Margination of leukocytes in acute inflammation.

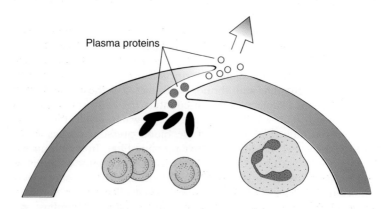

Fig. 12.4 Increased permeability of venule to plasma proteins. The proteins escape in inverse proportion to the molecular size (molecular sieving).

The swelling of the tissues is known as *oedema* and the fluid itself is the *fluid exudate*. The change in the properties of the vessel wall is called increased vascular permeability. It is demonstrated not only by the high plasma protein levels in the inflammatory oedema but also by observing experimentally the passage through the vessel wall of plasma albumin linked to a coloured azo dye such as trypan blue. Another experimental method is to introduce into the circulation a visible colloid, usually carbon, with a particle size comparable to molecules of plasma protein.

The protein which collects outside the vessels is gradually removed by way of the lymphatics. Since the proteins include immunoglobulins and complement, it is obvious that their presence will accelerate the destruction of any bacteria in the vicinity (p. 29). The fibrinogen in the exudate is converted to insoluble *fibrin* by the usual process of blood coagulation in which a terminal peptide is split off by a ubiquitous and readily activated protease called thrombin, the residue then polymerising (p. 225). Pathologists have long pondered over whether fibrin in exudates is of any value to the host, e.g. by acting as a mechanical barrier to the spread of bacteria. Although fibrin is a very prominent feature of many inflammatory exudates, its benefit to the host in these circumstances is still in doubt. However it may assist in phagocytosis of non-opsonised organisms, and in the control of bleeding it is essential for life itself (p. 225). Whether or not fibrin hampers bacterial spread, its effects in inflammation can be harmful to the host. It leads to knitting together of previously free surfaces such as the pericardium, with impairment of function; in diphtheria, where it forms a dense membrane in the throat, it frequently causes death by asphyxiation. For good or ill, however, its presence in exudates is simply a consequence of leakage of fibrinogen through permeable vessels and its inevitable subsequent conversion to fibrin.

It is plain that increased vascular permeability to protein causes great discomfort both to invading microorganisms and to the host. It tends to develop in a complex multiphasic way depending on the nature and severity of the injury. It may last for less than an hour or for several days, perhaps weeks, with leakage from both venules and capillaries. The electron microscope has shown that the protein escapes through gaps which appear between endothelial cells in the vessel wall, replacing the tight oblique intercellular junctions of the normal vessel. These newly formed channels are the escape route even in fenestrated vessels which, as in the gut, exhibit permanent discontinuities between endothelium. Similarly, the intracytoplasmic transport pathway which exists in endothelial cells appears to be almost entirely ignored in inflammation. Most of these facts have been established by the use of small marker molecules such as carbon or ferritin, and this technique shows such particles and presumably

Normal

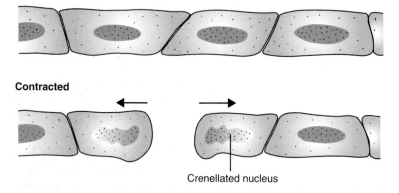

Contracted

Crenellated nucleus

Fig. 12.5 Contraction of vascular endothelium to allow escape of plasma protein.

plasma protein to be temporarily detained by the vascular basement membrane. Plasma proteins leave these vessels with an ease roughly proportional to their concentration in the blood and inversely proportional to the size of their molecule (molecular sieving, Fig. 12.4). Selective escape of plasma proteins could therefore result from gel filtration through the basement membrane or it could be due to differential concentration-dependent rates of bulk flow.

A major cause of the inter-endothelial gaps is active contraction of the endothelial cells due to the action of *chemical mediators* such as histamine. Only the endothelial cells of venules are affected; capillaries seem not to respond to these mediators, although they leak plasma protein after direct injury. In their response to mediators, the cells of the venular endothelium behave like smooth muscle. As they contract they shrink away from each other, thus allowing channels to form between them (Fig. 12.5). The contraction is accomplished by the intracytoplasmic network of microtubules and fibrils and involves the contractile protein actomyosin and the utilisation of energy. It is likely that the widely distributed substance cyclic AMP, together with the enzyme which forms it, adenyl cyclase, regulates this process.

In many types of injury, e.g. burns, significant leakage occurs as a result of structural disruption of the vessel wall. Such change affects both capillaries and venules. Direct damage of this sort also causes these vessels to leak by loosening the inter-endothelial junctions, a kind of unzipping effect.

In summary, increased vascular permeability can be due both to direct endothelial damage affecting both capillaries and venules, and to the action of chemical mediators causing endothelial contractions only in venules.

Chemotaxis

The emigration of white cells requires the leukocytes to expend energy and this demands that they be stimulated in some way. Injury seldom directly persuades leukocytes to adhere to vessels and migrate through their walls. This important effect is achieved by activation of a group of chemical mediators.

Leukocyte emigration can occur simply by an acceleration of the natural random amoeboid movement of the cells (*chemokinesis*) or by true *chemotaxis* which is the migration in a certain direction of the cells induced by a chemical influence at the site of damage.

In vitro experiments using time-lapse cinephotography and the Boyden chamber have enabled the chemotactic response of neutrophils to different chemical stimuli to be observed. The relative importance of chemotaxis in vivo is, however, unclear. Neutrophils may primarily arrive at a site by accelerated random chemokinesis where they are immobilised by specific factors.

Many substances cause leukocytes to show chemotaxis and increased movement. With a few exceptions, however, they all require the presence of fresh serum before they can exert their effect. The main obligatory factor in serum, although probably not the only one, is *complement*. This, as we have learned (p. 37), is a complex assortment of plasma proteins, constituting a cascade of enzyme reactions and playing an important role in the removal of bacteria. When suitably activated, complement generates peptides known as C3a and C5a which are chemotactic for white cells and which are split off from the third (C3) and fifth component (C5). The mode of action of C3 and C5 products on leukocytes is not known but enhanced mobility is almost certainly due to activity of the cytoplasmic microtubules involving the cooperation of cyclic AMP on the cell surface.

Many substances have been shown to be chemotactic for leukocytes. Among the most important in vitro are:

- prostaglandin E_2
- the C5a complement fragments
- leukotriene B_4
- the cytokines IL-1 and tumour necrosis factor (TNF).

However, their relative importance in vivo is still unclear.

The pattern of leukocyte infiltration varies with the nature and age of the inflammatory lesion. Neutrophil granulocytes are usually replaced progressively by monocytes with the passage of time; in some types of damage, due for example to helminths or Type I hypersensitivity, eosinophil granulocytes predominate. Monocyte predominance could be due simply to disappearance of the more short-lived granulocytes, since both cell types usually emigrate concurrently. It is probable, however, that complement, lymphokines or other serum factors generate substances which are more chemotactic for one type of leukocyte than another. Such semi-specific factors have been identified for neutrophils, eosinophils, monocytes and even for B lymphocytes, although the ability of lymphocytes to respond to chemotaxis is not universally accepted.

The cellular exudate

Increased blood flow, access of plasma proteins to extravascular tissues and mobilisation of phagocytes are the features of acute inflammation which have survival value for the host. It would be expected therefore that the exudation of fluid would rapidly be augmented by the arrival of phagocytes. Indeed, within half an hour of injury, leukocytes are seen to migrate from the blood into the tissues, doing so by inserting pseudopodic processes into the inter-endothelial junctions and then wriggling through the vessel wall by amoeboid motion, somehow getting across the basement membrane without obviously destroying it (Fig. 12.6). At this stage the leukocytes involved are neutrophil granulocytes but they are shortly joined by monocytes. Red cells and platelets also pass out of the vessel in the wake of the leukocytes or via inter-endothelial gaps. The

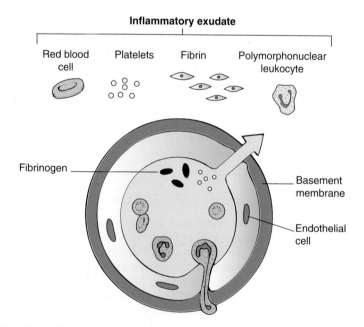

Fig. 12.6 Schema of vascular permeability, leukocyte emigration and formation of exudate in acute inflammation.

infiltration of these cells, especially the leukocytes, is known as the cellular exudate.

Mediators of inflammation

A mediator of inflammation is one of a group of chemicals which cause vasodilation, neutrophil migration and chemotaxis, and vascular permeability.

To qualify for the title of mediator of inflammation a substance should:

1. reproduce some or all of the inflammatory changes in low concentration
2. be demonstrable at the inflamed site at the appropriate time
3. when inhibited, e.g. by drugs, result in suppression of some or all of the inflammatory phenomena.

Needless to say, these criteria are seldom completely fulfilled.

Histamine

Although an increasing number of mediators are being proposed (Table 12.1), one of the best documented is *histamine*, which is widely distributed in body tissues and formed by histidine decarboxylase from the amino acid histidine. Histamine is released by all kinds of local injury and comes from degranulated mast cells as well as basophils, eosinophils and platelets. In very mild transient inflammation, such as the 'triple response' (flare, erythema and wheal), histamine together with a vasodilator axon reflex probably accounts for all the changes, and in other examples, e.g. vasomotor rhinitis (hay fever), accounts for the majority. In more severe inflammation, histamine is responsible only for the earliest changes, seen in the initial half hour or so. Local inactivation of adrenaline or noradrenaline may also play a role, since

Table 12.1 Postulated mediators of inflammation

Type of mediator	Example
Kinins	Bradykinin
Amines	Histamine
Complement fragments	C3a, C5a
Clotting system	Fibrin degradation products
Fibrinolytic system	Plasmin
Acidic lipids	Prostaglandins, leukotrienes
Lysosomal compound	Cationic proteins, proteases
Cytokines	IL-1, TNF
Phospholipids	Platelet activating factor (PAF)

the effect of these substances, if unopposed, would be to inhibit the inflammatory response. The role of histamine is easily demonstrated by giving doses of antihistamine drugs, which specifically antagonise the substance, or by depleting the body of its stores of histamine by injecting histamine-releasing substances. Histamine vasodilation is mediated by two types of receptors (H_1 and H_2), whereas only H_1 receptors are involved in vessel permeability.

The kinin system

It seems likely that mediators operate in sequence and that after the phase of histamine and adrenaline inactivation vascular changes are kept going by activation of the kinin system (Fig. 12.7).

Kinins are polypeptides composed of 8–10 amino acids. They are present in blood as inactive precursors, *kininogens*, converted to the active form by widely distributed plasma and tissue enzymes (*kininogenases*) and then rapidly inactivated by other enzymes called *kininases*. Activation is a complex process which shares some of the factors in the cascade pathway involved in blood clotting (p. 225). More specifically, initiation of the kinin cascade occurs as a result of

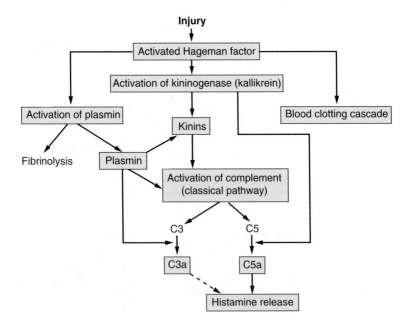

Fig. 12.7 The interaction of Hageman factor, proteases, kinins, complement, blood clotting, fibrinolysis and histamine release following local injury.

contact of *Hageman factor* (clotting factor XII) with negatively charged surfaces. These surfaces include the ubiquitous collagen, so activation is easily achieved.

The evidence for the participation of kinins in inflammation is somewhat tenuous since they are elusive substances, but depletion of bodily stores of the precursor by injection of cellulose sulphate does diminish the post-histamine phase of inflammatory oedema.

Eicosanoids

Another important group of mediators is the ubiquitous family of prostaglandins and leukotrienes derived from arachidonic acid and known as eicosanoids. This family consists of long chain compounds composed of polyunsaturated fatty acids (Fig. 12.8) synthesised in or on cells from arachidonic acid. There are two principal enzyme pathways of arachidonic acid oxygenation involved in the inflammatory process:

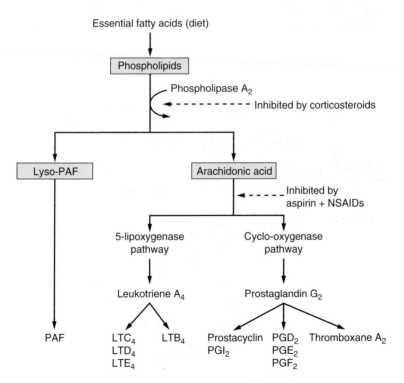

Fig. 12.8   The formation of inflammatory mediators from cell membrane phospholipid.

1. the *cyclo-oxygenase pathway* which produces prostaglandins and thromboxanes
2. the *5-lipoxygenase pathway* which produces leukotrienes.

The term prostaglandin was coined by early investigators who mistakenly believed the prostate gland to be the major source. Prostaglandins are not stored but are produced when stimulated by cell damage or during cell activation. In general the prostaglandins most commonly found in the body are:

- PGE_2
- PGF_2
- PGI_2 (prostacyclin).

These have a wide range of activity. PGE_2 and PGI_2 are potent vasodilators which relax bronchial smooth muscle and modulate the effects of other mediators such as histamine and kinin in increasing vascular permeability and producing pain. *Thromboxane A_2* is a powerful vasoconstrictor which also stimulates platelet aggregation. Some prostaglandins have effects directly opposed to others.

Prostaglandins, produced as they are on cell surfaces (especially mobile leukocytes) probably represent a widely distributed and self-contained regulatory system, capable of initiating, maintaining or suppressing inflammation according to circumstances. These opposing effects are probably achieved by way of the *cyclic AMP/adenyl cyclase system*. An excess of cyclic AMP restrains the contractibility and mobility of cells, possibly by stimulating the phosphorylation of the protein of the intracellular microtubules and fibrils.

The best evidence of the involvement of prostaglandins in inflammation is the finding that non-steroidal anti-inflammatory agents (NSAIDs), the aspirin-like drugs, exert their effect by inhibiting cyclo-oxygenase and thus prostaglandin formation. The recent finding that there may be a second cyclo-oxygenase enzyme system, induced by inflammatory stimuli, may explain some of the differing anti-inflammatory potencies and side effects of the aspirin-like drugs and possibly the effect of paracetamol which does not affect the classical cyclo-oxygenase pathway.

The *leukotrienes* were named because they were originally demonstrated in leukocytes and contained a triene system in their structure. They are formed via the 5-lipoxygenase pathway. Four main leukotrienes have so far been identified:

- LTB_4 is probably an important inflammatory mediator, being one of the most potent leukotactic substances known.
- LTC_4, LTD_4 and LTE_4 are a group of *peptidoleukotrienes* (formerly known as slow-reacting substance of anaphylaxis—SRS-A) which have an important role in asthma and allergic reactions: they cause

vascular permeability and are powerful spasmogens resulting in bronchial constriction. The peptidoleukotrienes are produced mainly in basophils and mast cells in response to chemical or immunological (mainly IgE) stimuli.

The production of leukotrienes is not affected by non-steroidal anti-inflammatory drugs, NSAIDs, which inhibit cyclo-oxygenases; 5-lipoxygenase inhibitors are currently being developed.

Glucocorticoids (steroids) appear to inhibit leukotrienes as well as prostaglandins and also inhibit the secondary cyclo-oxygenase system, which accounts for their powerful and broad range of anti-inflammatory properties. Steroids cause the synthesis of a peptide, lipocortin, which inhibits phospholipase A_2, so reducing the supply of arachidonic acid for metabolism.

Platelet activating factor

Platelet activating factor (PAF) is another recently discovered mediator which, like the eicosanoids, is derived from the action of phospholipase A_2 on phospholipids. It exists mainly as a stored precursor called lyso-PAF and was originally named because of its powerful platelet stimulating properties. It is a powerful promoter of vascular leakage as well as being a chemo-attractant and is unusual in that it can stimulate its own release. One of its major roles may be to initiate and potentiate the effect of other mediators.

PAF antagonists are now available and are clarifying its complex role in inflammation.

Complement

As well as its prominent role in chemotaxis, complement has other inflammatory properties (p. 38). Two peptides derived from the 3rd or 5th components, known as C3a and C5a (p. 39) respectively, cause inflammatory oedema when injected locally, e.g. into skin. They do so partly by direct action and partly by liberation from mast cells of histamine. This latter action is known as the *anaphylotoxin* effect. It is clear that C5a is the most powerful mediator of the two.

For C3a and C5a to be released it is first necessary for the complement cascade to be activated by the classical or alternate pathway (p. 39). C3 and C5 are then split by a variety of blood and tissue enzymes. The complement system interacts closely with another mediator of acute inflammation, the kinin system. Figure 12.7 shows the key role of the Hageman factor in activating both systems via the proteases plasmin and kallikrein. The additional links with blood clotting on the one hand and fibrinolysis on the other are not unexpected, since all these systems are essentially homeostatic in the face of injury and could be predicted to evolve together.

Other mediators of inflammation

An ever-increasing number of mediators of the vascular events of acute inflammation have been canvassed. These include a wide range of lysosomal enzymes and cytokines. In general, however, the substance acting on the microcirculation is either an amine (e.g. histamine), a peptide (e.g. kinins, complement fragments) or an acidic lipid (e.g. prostaglandins, leukotrienes).

Benefits and risks of the vascular changes in inflammation

The sequential appearance of mediators, each dependent on a complex cascade of enzyme reactions, seems an absurdly complicated way of dilating vessels and making them leak. However, bearing in mind the unvarying nature of the acute inflammatory response, even in widely different species, and the enormous variety of eliciting stimuli, the intervention of a final common pathway between injury and reaction seems a likely mechanism to have evolved.

Although the importance of antibodies and phagocytosis in destroying bacteria is obvious, the survival value of the vascular changes per se could be disputed. It has, however, been shown that small inoculations of bacteria which are killed within a few minutes before any phagocytes arrive at the area, survive and multiply if the early dilatation and increased permeability of vessels is prevented by injection of adrenaline. In other instances such as in lobar pneumonia, the inflammatory oedema, although diluting the effect of toxins, probably facilitates spread of the bacteria and may lead to death of the host. In other words, increased vascular flow and permeability bring antibody and other bactericidal agents to the scene but also accelerate the spread of those germs which survive. Similarly, increased lymph flow carries bacteria to the local lymph nodes which are well adapted for bacterial killing but which are also key junctions in any spread throughout the body (Table 12.2).

Table 12.2   Benefits and risks of the vascular changes in inflammation

Benefits to host
    Entry of antibodies and complement
    Toxin dilution
    Immune stimulation via the flow of antigens to lymph nodes
    Increase in nutrient and oxygen supply to phagocytes
    Fibrin formation may hinder growth and spread of infections

Harmful effects
    May increase risk of spread of infection
    Normal tissues destroyed by enzymes
    Swelling of tissues at certain sites, i.e. brain, meninges in meningitis or abscess or throat in epiglottitis

Inflammation and the nervous system

Although inflammation can occur in the absence of a nerve supply, it is now recognised that the sensory nervous system generates some of the manifestations of inflammation. A number of cases of rheumatoid arthritis have been reported in which the disease developed after a hemiplegia and spared the denervated areas. At the simplest level, the red flare that surrounds the skin reaction to mild trauma (the triple response) is abolished if the sensory or vasomotor nerves are blocked or cut. Axon reflexes produced after stimulation of primitive receptors (polymodal receptors) cause the release of *neuropeptides* from C-fibres in primary afferent neurons which initiate inflammatory changes. A number of neuropeptides are believed to play a role in inflammation including:

- substance P
- calcitonin-gene-related peptide
- somatostatin
- vasoactive intestinal peptide
- neurokinin A
- neurokinin B.

Of these, substance P is probably the major neuropeptide involved in the inflammatory reaction and evidence has been found of its local release in inflamed joints. Sympathetic efferent fibres are also likely to be involved as suggested by the inflammatory reactions that often occur in disorders which affect sympathetic function.

Hypnosis can persuade a subject with exactly similar areas of mild damage on each of his arms that one will produce an inflammatory reaction and the other not, and that one arm is painful and the other not. Interestingly, only the vascular changes are affected by hypnotic suggestion, leukocyte migration proceeding equally in the two arms.

The converse situation, where suggestion causes an inflammatory reaction to appear, is commonplace in patients with *Type I hypersensitivity* (p. 60). In these patients emotional factors may determine increased vascular permeability in the nose, eyes or skin. Emotion may possibly influence the onset or severity of inflammation in more serious diseases such as ulcerative colitis or psoriasis. All diseases in which emotional factors seem likely to play a major role are known as psychosomatic, but they should not be confused with unhappiness per se which may produce symptoms of organic disease without the physical stigmata (p. 348).

Generally speaking, emotion and suggestion affect only those pathological phenomena readily influenced by the autonomic nervous system. Thus vascular permeability may be restrained by neurogenic adrenaline release and result in vasoconstriction, or be exaggerated by depression of those same forces, whereas leukocyte migration factors could not be reached by them. Enthusiasm for the role of psychic factors in inflammatory diseases such as ulcerative colitis or peptic ulcer has waned somewhat. The consensus view at the moment is that tangible agents cause these conditions but that the patient's emotional state may raise or lower the level of the inflammatory response to them.

Pain

The heat, redness and swelling of acute inflammation are explained by vascular dilatation and increased vascular permeability. The pain is due partly to pressure on sensory nerve endings by the exuded fluid, especially if the space in which it can expand is limited, and partly to the release of bodily substances which stimulate these nerves. In fact all the chemical mediators—*histamine, serotonin, kinins* and *prostaglandins*—which are responsible for the vascular changes also cause pain, kinins being particularly effective, while histamine release may lead merely to itching as in urticaria. Prostaglandins may act by lowering the threshold of response to other pain-producing substances and potentiating the effect of other pain-producing factors. Other chemicals liberated by nervous stimuli or cell injury, e.g. *acetylcholine* or *potassium ions*, may also be painful.

The survival value to the host of pain is obvious since it tells him that the injured part must be favoured and rested and that appropriate action, especially retreat, should be considered. The reverse side of the coin is represented by the disability caused by pain itself.

In the context of survival it is important to realise that although pain is invoked by stimulation of sensory nerve endings, its appreciation is dependent on subjective factors. Soldiers receiving wounds in battle that would normally produce incapacitating pain will ignore the injury and even refuse morphine if by doing so their chances of survival are improved by remaining mobile and alert. Only when safety is reached will they experience real pain. Comparable wounds received in civilian life, e.g. in traffic accidents, will be experienced as severe pain almost immediately. Similarly athletes have higher pain tolerances. These observations show that the sensation of pain is determined ultimately in the higher centres of the brain and that it can be overridden by more urgent survival mechanisms such as the need for flight or self-defence. Since crippling wounds can be rendered painless by this expression of the brain's higher centres, it should not surprise us that hypnosis or autosuggestion should have a similar power over more trivial injuries. Recent studies in twins have shown that pain thresholds are also determined by upbringing rather than genes.

The discovery of the *endorphins*, endogenous pain-suppressing opiates produced in the brain, pituitary and adrenal and acting on the cerebrum, provides a pharmacological basis for these variations in the perception of pain. Endorphins also offer a possible explanation for the impressive local anaesthesia sometimes achieved by acupuncture if, as some believe, appropriate insertion of needles generates their release.

Sequelae of acute inflammation

In most cases the sequence of events described in this chapter will result in the resolution of the tissue injury with resulting repair mechanisms. Sometimes however this may not occur and suppuration or chronic inflammation may result (Fig. 12.9).

Suppuration

Suppuration may occur in the face of persistent infection or when an excess inflammatory exudate is produced. The life of a neutrophil granulocyte is measured in days and it seldom, if ever, survives the act of ingesting and killing microorganisms. In some cases it is obvious that the bacteria are more effective at killing the leukocytes than vice versa; if antibiotics are not administered this situation will lead eventually to the death of the patient.

Suppuration is an intermediate situation with two main components.

1. Very large numbers of granulocytes are summoned into the tissues, usually by the chemotactic influence of certain bacteria, notably *Staphylococcus aureus*.

2. The exuded leukocytes are killed in large numbers by the bacteria and their bodies liquefied by their own lysosomal enzymes to form a creamy viscous fluid rich in lipids, proteins and nucleic acids and known as *pus*.

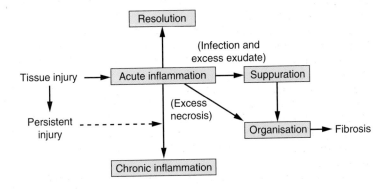

Fig. 12.9 Sequelae of acute inflammation.

The mass of bacteria, dead, dying and liquefied leukocytes and surviving inflamed tissue is termed an *abscess*. When present in skin, as it commonly is, it is called a *boil* or, if very large, a *carbuncle*. The painful abscess is the price we pay for survival since it is an inevitable result of confining certain dangerous bacteria to one part of the body rather than allowing them to disseminate. The natural history of an abscess is either to release its contents via rupture or else to undergo a process known as *organisation* and eventual fibrosis.

Organisation is the term used to describe the replacement of solid material (i.e. exudate, thrombus, necrotic debris) which usually has no self-regenerative powers by granulation tissue. A good example is when an episode of acute lobar pneumonia fails to resolve and the lung undergoes organisation and eventual fibrosis. These processes are outlined in more detail in Chapter 15.

The following chapter deals with the events that occur when inflammation persists as a chronic state.

KEY POINTS

- Acute inflammation is the initial reaction to injury and is characterised by:
  — redness
  — heat
  — swelling
  — pain
  — loss of function.
- The process involves:
  — constriction and prolonged dilatation of arterioles
  — increased vascular permeability
  — formation of a cellular exudate
  — emigration of neutrophil polymorphs.
- Involved in all these processes are chemical mediators which include:
  — kinins
  — eicosanoids
  — cytokines
  — the clotting, fibrinolytic and complement systems.
- Acute inflammation usually resolves but can lead to suppuration, organisation or chronic inflammation.

13 Chronic inflammation

When an inflammatory response lasts long enough to extend over a year or more it is termed 'chronic'. Sometimes the process is merely a succession of attacks of acute inflammation, and in these cases the patient suffers recurrent bouts of pain and fever; microscopical examination of the affected tissues shows changes not very different from those of non-recurrent acute inflammation, although there may be evidence of healing between attacks. Organs prone to this type of chronic inflammation are the gall bladder, kidney and large intestine. Chronic inflammation is often a sequela of suppurative inflammation and pus formation, i.e. osteomyelitis.

More commonly chronic inflammation differs from acute inflammation in that the cardinal signs of redness, heat and pain are often absent and in that the microscopical picture also is different, with dense masses of cells instead of oedema, fibrin and polymorphs.

Chronic inflammation can also be defined as an inflammatory process where macrophages, plasma cells and lymphocytes predominate, usually accompanied by a healing process.

The compact nature of these lesions led to the idea that they were some sort of tumour and to their being named *granulomas*, that is to say tumours of granular appearance. The discovery that some granulomas were caused by bacteria, e.g. tuberculosis, leprosy and syphilis, and the later discovery of the nature of the constituent cells of the granuloma revealed their inflammatory nature. Like other examples of inflammation, granulomas originate in a local reaction to injury of the microcirculation and its contents. The special character of granulomatous inflammation lies largely in the important role played by a particular circulating cell, the *monocyte*, and its derivative in tissues, the *macrophage*. The key to chronic inflammation lies in the biology of these cells.

Chronic inflammation is the basis of some of the most important diseases of man and animals:

- tuberculosis
- leprosy
- syphilis
- rheumatoid arthritis
- inflammatory bowel disease
- sarcoidosis
- a variety of tropical diseases
- industrial diseases such as pneumoconiosis.

Although the first three have generally declined in incidence in developed countries in recent years, they are still common problems in the rest of the world. Tuberculosis kills at least three million people annually and is increasing in some urban areas in western countries.

Inflammatory granulomas are characterised by massive infiltration with monocytes and their derivatives, and often by widespread death of host tissue with the formation of cavities or abscesses as in tuberculosis. Such destruction may be followed by permanent crippling as in rheumatoid arthritis, in which articular cartilage is irreversibly damaged, or by replacement with fibrous tissue as in silicosis.

The pathogenesis of chronic inflammation

At first sight it may seem that these chronic inflammatory diseases affecting different organs, due to different causes have nothing in common except their prolonged duration. In fact, however, the underlying pathological mechanisms are similar. Chronic inflammation is generally caused by stimuli which, while unable to destroy the host quickly, cannot themselves be easily dealt with. Large bacteria of complex chemical composition, destructive but lacking maximal toxicity, are the ideal pathogens for inducing such lesions.

The reason why certain bacteria are killed with such difficulty is unclear. The tubercle bacillus may be resistant due to the presence of mycolic acid and wax on its cell walls. Some parasites which cause chronic inflammation become coated with host antigens once inside the host's body. These 'wolves in sheep's clothing' must become as impervious to attack as the host's own cells. In other cases the ingested organisms may simply be resistant to the macrophage's armoury of bactericidal mechanisms or alternatively be shielded from them by sequestration in inaccessible parts of the cytoplasm. Even when dead the bacteria may leave indigestible chemical residues (usually the cell wall) which, because they are phagocytosed, demand a local presence of macrophages which thus constitute a focus of chronic inflammation.

Table 13.1   Classification of chronic inflammation

Type	Mechanism	Example
Primary		
Granulomatous	Material or pathogen resistant to digestion	Tuberculosis, silicosis
Autoimmune	Host tissue recognised as foreign	Rheumatoid arthritis, chronic active hepatitis
Secondary		
Following acute inflammation	Persistence of or repeated infection	Chronic cholecystitis, osteomyelitis

The other form of chronic inflammation occurs in the autoimmune diseases (p. 69) where the body recognises its own tissue as foreign and obviously has problems in eliminating it (Table 13.1).

Monocytes and macrophages

The best way to start to understand chronic inflammation and inflammatory granulomas is with the monocyte and its derivative, the macrophage. The monocyte comes from a precursor cell in the bone marrow, the promonocyte, and circulates in the blood. The trio of promonocyte, monocyte and macrophage makes up the *mononuclear phagocyte system* (p. 29).

An individual monocyte does not remain long in the circulation before migrating into the tissues. It does this even when there is no inflammation but the process is enormously accelerated after local injury. Once in the tissues it enlarges and develops and becomes known as a *macrophage*, a name coined by Metchnikoff in the 1890s. The word means 'big eater' and refers equally well to the size of the cell, its great capacity for phagocytosis and the large particles which it can engulf within its cytoplasm.

In invertebrates it is the haematocyte, the equivalent of the macrophage, which acts as almost the sole defence against irritant particles. It does so by phagocytosis followed by digestion of the particle within the cytoplasm, and it is precisely this programme which is followed by the mammalian macrophage in chronic inflammation. Chronic inflammation and the dominant role of the macrophage can therefore be viewed as an important survivor of an early phylogenetic era. The advantage of the macrophage over the other blood phagocytes, i.e. polymorphs, is its capacity to ingest bacteria and particles too large for other cells. Its other relevant property is the capacity to survive for days, weeks or months while within its cytoplasm lie bacteria, sometimes alive and even dividing. The toughness of the macrophage is due partly to its ability to resynthesise enzymes and intracellular structures lost during phagocytosis and digestion, a property which polymorphs do not possess.

It is these masses of macrophages, many containing endocytosed bacteria or other irritant particles capable of surviving this experience, which make up the bulk of chronic inflammatory granulomas. The retention by macrophages of irritants is an obvious example of symbiosis, and chronic inflammation is a phylogenetically old technique for stabilising a symbiotic relationship.

The cellular biology of the macrophage (Fig. 13.1) makes it particularly suitable to cope with alien particles which are especially difficult to kill or digest. Its wide expanse of cell membrane (plasmalemma) and active pseudopod formation facilitate pinocytosis and phagocytosis. The abundance of membrane favours the formation of intracellular phagocytic vesicles (phagosomes). The cell contains a large number and variety of lysosomes which fuse readily with the phagosomes to form secondary lysosomes in which bacteria are killed and digested. There is sufficient endoplasmic reticulum to resynthesise the lysosomal enzymes. Within the cytoplasm exist bactericidal systems which are usually effective, if not fully understood (p. 27). The cell is very hardy, capable of both division and long life, and can proceed with phagocytosis and intracellular digestion under conditions of low oxygen tension. It is able to respond to information passed to it from T lymphocytes by lymphokines (p. 67) which makes it even more effective. The effect of these chemical messages is to enlarge the cell and increase its ability to divide (*stimulation*) and to enhance its bactericidal capacity (*activation*). If unable to kill a

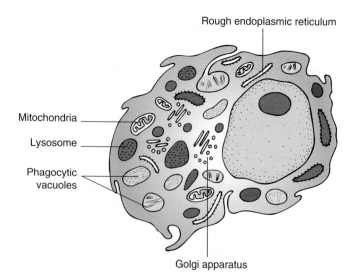

Fig. 13.1   Macrophage.

microorganism it can at least sequester it and thus prevent unimpeded spread. The macrophage destroys microorganisms and tissues impartially and is an effective scavenger. Even trivial short-lived injury may lead to the migration of monocytes into the tissues but they persist there only if the irritant is not eliminated.

The peculiar marriage of indestructible bacteria or other irritants with a macrophage reaction is preceded by an initial efflux of neutrophil polymorphs, but these are quickly and permanently replaced by macrophages. It seems likely that certain types of infection or injury activate factors in serum such as interleukin-1 that are particularly chemotactic to monocytes. The cells emigrate from blood vessels in the same way as polymorphs by inserting pseudopodia through the inter-endothelial junctions.

Once a collection of monocyte-derived macrophages is in the tissues in contact with the stubborn irritant, the host's survival demands that the macrophage accumulations persist as long as the irritant remains. In practice this accumulation is maintained in three ways (Fig. 13.2):

1. The first is by sustained migration from the circulation; if the granuloma is of constant size, this migration is balanced by a corresponding loss of cells by death or drainage to lymph nodes. The

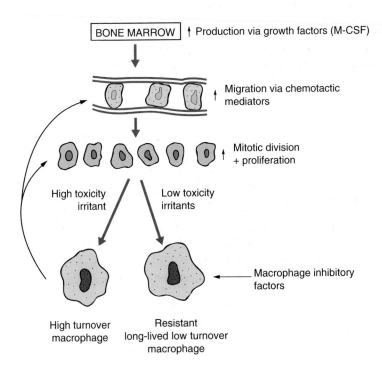

Fig. 13.2   Macrophage turnover in chronic inflammation.

continued emigration is due to the prolonged operation of factors chemotactic for monocytes. It is accompanied by some augmented release of monocytes from the bone marrow due to the action of factors such as M-CSF (p. 79). An exaggerated response in the shape of a monocytosis is seldom seen.

2. The second mechanism for maintaining a macrophage population in granulomas is mitotic division of the cells. Monocytes enlarge and tend to divide once, soon after leaving the circulation. Having settled down, they may undergo one or two further divisions but seldom more, before dying or retiring. This division is probably triggered by the local release of mitogenic cytokines derived from other macrophages or other types of cell. Analysis of the chromosomes of the proliferating macrophages reveals numerous abnormalities likely to limit their viability. It is this which probably restricts the number of successful mitoses that they can achieve.

3. The third strategy which has evolved is the immobilisation of macrophages at the site of inflammation so that they rarely die and rarely divide. As a result a stable population of storage cells is created which is dependent for its existence neither on recruitment from the circulation nor on mitotic proliferation.

In practice granulomas fall into two categories:

- those with much continued emigration and division, known as *high turnover granulomas*
- those with a stable population of long-lived macrophages, known as *low turnover granulomas* (Fig. 13.2).

Bacterial or fungal infections or inflammation due to irritants toxic to macrophages usually produce high turnover reactions. Irritants of low toxicity to macrophages, e.g. carbon particles, cause low turnover lesions.

Other cells present in granulomas

Epithelioid cells

By no means all the cells in an area of chronic inflammation have the appearance of macrophages. Some may be epithelioid cells, particularly numerous in tuberculosis and sarcoidosis, with foamy interlocking cytoplasm. These are macrophage derivatives, the cytoplasm of which seems specialised for secretion rather than phagocytosis. Epithelioid cells have only one tenth the phagocytic activity of macrophages but much more endoplasmic reticulum, Golgi apparatus, plasmalemma and exocytotic activity (Fig. 13.3). They seem particularly adapted for the extracellular secretion of *lysosomal enzymes* and other cytoplasmic proteins such as *lysozyme* as well as *angiotensin converting enzyme*.

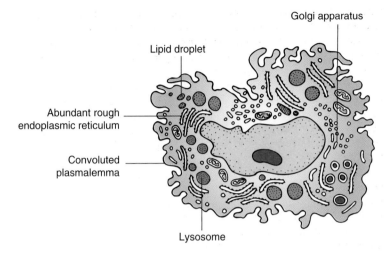

Fig. 13.3 Epithelioid cell.

Epithelioid cells arise from macrophages or monocytes by a special kind of maturation. The maturation takes a few days and is retarded if the parent macrophage undertakes phagocytosis, especially of indigestible particles. Epithelioid cells have a life of 1 to 3 weeks, and when they divide produce daughter cells with the features of young macrophages.

The presence of large numbers of epithelioid cells in diseases such as tuberculosis is probably due to the presence of macrophages which are immobilised but shielded from the necessity to phagocytose bacilli by a barrier of non-epithelioid macrophages. In other diseases rich in epithelioid cells, such as sarcoidosis, their presence may be due to lack of indigestible particles so that without having to undertake phagocytosis and digestion, macrophages can undergo epithelioid maturation at their leisure.

Multinucleate giant cells

Multinucleate giant cells are another feature of granulomas. They are formed by fusion of macrophages (Fig. 13.4) and are seen in chronic inflammation whenever fresh monocytes are in constant supply as in tuberculosis. Formation of multinucleate giant cells (macrophage polykaryons) seems to depend upon intimate contact of freshly migrated monocytes simultaneously with other monocytes or macrophages, and with material demanding endocytosis. This material may be particulate, e.g. bacteria or foreign bodies, or soluble, e.g. protein-rich exudate. It seems likely that a combination of high

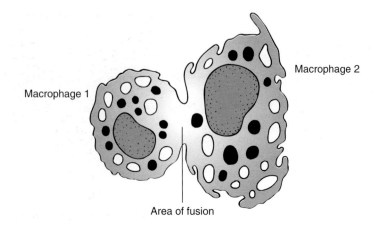

Macrophage 1

Macrophage 2

Area of fusion

Fig. 13.4   Macrophages fusing to form multinucleate giant cells.

cell density and simultaneous endocytosis of the same material by two or more macrophages is the fusion stimulus in giant cell formation (Fig. 13.5).

Classical pathology recognises foreign body and Langhans types of giant cells but the electron microscope shows the latter to be merely a more highly organised development of the former. Indeed, interference with movement of intracellular organelles by dosage with colchicine prevents the conversion of foreign body cells to Langhans cells.

Once the multinucleate cells are formed they grow by the additional fusion of macrophages. They also behave like other polykaryons in biology in that they undergo synchronous or nearly synchronous entry of nuclei into the mitotic cycle. In macrophage polykaryons this usually ends in pooling of chromosomes, many of which are defective, and the resultant formation of polyploid cells of very limited life span. Thus the division of macrophages which could have ended in uncontrolled growth is neatly curtailed. Figure 13.6 shows the various fates that can befall the inflammatory macrophage.

Role of the immune system

Other cell types are also present in chronic inflammation, in particular *lymphocytes* (both T and B cells; Fig. 13.7), *plasma cells* (Fig. 13.8), *eosinophils* and *fibroblasts*. The presence of lymphoid cells indicates some form of immunological activity and plasma cells mean that immunoglobulin is being formed. The different types of cells participating in inflammation are depicted in Figure 13.9.

There is a close relationship between lymphocytes and macrophages since the former are able to increase the activity of

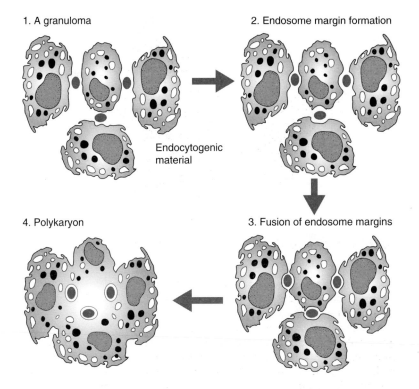

1. A granuloma

2. Endosome margin formation

Endocytogenic material

4. Polykaryon

3. Fusion of endosome margins

Fig. 13.5 The fusion of macrophages to form inflammatory giant cells as a result of simultaneous endocytosis of particles or colloids.

the latter by the secretion of chemical substances known as lymphokines (p. 67), particularly when cell-mediated immunity or Type IV hypersensitivity is present (p. 64). Sensitised lymphocytes in contact with the appropriate antigen will instruct macrophages (via lymphokines) to migrate to the inflamed area, i.e. the site of antigen deposition, and there to accumulate, die and divide. T cells are also capable of directly producing factors which act as inflammatory mediators (p. 95). The complex interactions between macrophages and T cells are depicted in Figure 13.10.

Chronic inflammatory diseases vary in the extent to which cell-mediated immunity is involved. In mycobacterial infections such as leprosy or TB, the clinical picture varies with the strength of the immune response. High immune resistance occurs in discrete self-healing focal pulmonary TB lesions (Ghon focus) with high numbers of lymphocytes produced in the presence of only sparse organisms, producing an epithelioid rich granuloma (Fig. 13.11). An example of

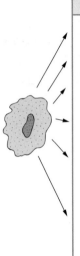

Fate	Cause
Death	Phagocytosis of toxic material
Migration from site	Disappearance of inflammatory stimulus
Division	(1) Entry into inflamed tissues (2) Exposure to mitogens
Conversion to long-lived form	Phagocytosis of non-toxic, indigestible material
Conversion to epithelioid cell	(1) Immobilisation without phagocytic activity (2) Immobilisation after successful phagocytic activity
Conversion to giant cell (macrophage polykaryon)	Co-existence of effete and young macrophages in close proximity, with simultaneous endocytosis.

Fig. 13.6   Fate of inflammatory macrophage.

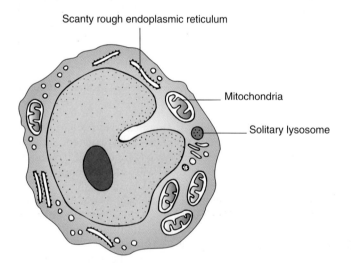

Scanty rough endoplasmic reticulum

Mitochondria

Solitary lysosome

Fig. 13.7   Small lymphocyte.

low resistance disease is diffuse miliary TB where even with overwhelming numbers of microorganisms only a feeble immune response is mounted; low numbers of lymphocytes are seen and the

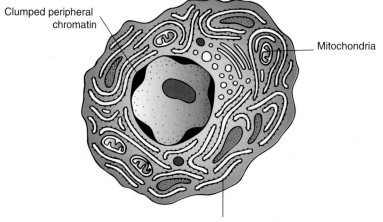

Clumped peripheral chromatin

Mitochondria

Extensive rough endoplasmic reticulum

Fig. 13.8   Plasma cell.

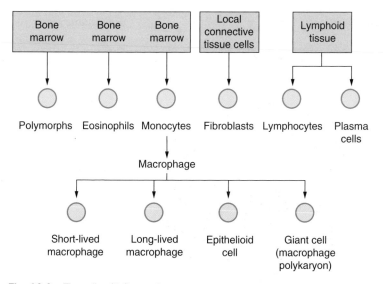

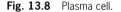

Fig. 13.9   The cells of inflammation.

patient often dies. In tuberculosis, lymphocyte-mediated immune responses play a complex dual role in that they probably aggravate the inflammatory reaction and cause local tissue necrosis (caseation) at the centre of the tubercle while also stimulating the macrophages to ingest and destroy the tubercle bacilli. Both facets of the immune

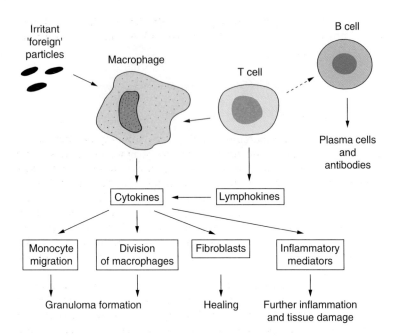

Fig. 13.10 The central role of the macrophage and T cell.

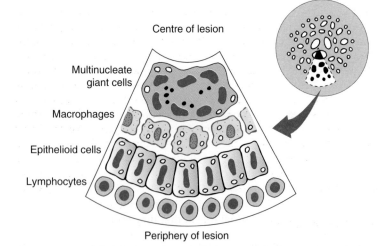

Fig. 13.11 Architecture of a chronic inflammatory granuloma.

response develop progressively in adult life so that childhood tuberculosis tends to be less destructive and also less localised than the adult disease.

Adverse effects of cell-mediated immunity

Macrophage damage

In diseases such as tuberculosis and leprosy the only defence of the host is the ability of the macrophage to phagocytose and kill the bacilli. However, we have the advantage over invertebrates in which a similar system operates, in that the macrophages are rendered more efficient by the development of lymphocyte-mediated immunity. Unfortunately, as already mentioned, this exaggerated response may do as much damage to the host as to the invading microorganism. Indeed much or most of the damage in tuberculosis and leprosy is the result of the erosive action of the digestive enzymes of the lysosomes within macrophages.

This is even more evident in granulomas such as rheumatoid arthritis or sarcoidosis where intensive research has failed to identify such an invader and only the infiltrating inflammatory cells can be blamed. It is widely believed that these macrophages too are reacting to an immunological stimulus which may be an exogenous agent, as yet unidentified, or a component of the patient's own tissue (p. 69). A number of other diseases are suspected to have a similar origin. Although lymphocytes may damage tissue cells by direct action it is more likely that they usually kill by instructing macrophages to do so.

Cell-mediated hypersensitivity is then specially associated with chronic inflammation. When hypersensitivity is absent the tissue destruction and continued emigration and division of macrophages in chronic inflammation is most likely to be due to leakage and secretion of *lysosomal enzymes* and other *cytoplasmic irritants* from the macrophage into the tissues. This escape of damaging substances is sometimes accelerated by phagocytic activity. It is the most likely explanation of diseases such as silicosis which are associated with uptake by macrophages over long periods of time of material which is both indigestible and toxic but not obviously immunogenic. Macrophages undertaking phagocytosis also release *cytokines* such as IL-1 which stimulate fibroblasts to divide and to make collagen, so the connection between chronic irritation, granuloma formation, tissue destruction and scarring, especially prominent in silicosis, seems to be complete.

Production of mucus

One other aspect of chronic irritation is of importance. This is the permanent increase in *secretion of viscid mucus* which occurs from the epithelial cells lining the bronchial tree when there is prolonged inhalation of irritants. A chronic excess of bronchial mucus is the pathological basis of chronic bronchitis, a disease which is a common cause of death in western countries. Of the inhaled irritants, cigarette smoke is probably the most important but atmospheric pollutants such as sulphur dioxide and smoke are also heavily implicated. Ironically, but predictably, chronic bronchitis, which was once called the 'English disease', is now a major cause of death in Hong Kong, Tokyo and São Paulo.

As pointed out earlier (p. 13) secretion of respiratory mucus is a useful defence, especially against inhaled bacteria. It is predictable that some means of increasing this secretion in the face of repeated irritation would have evolved by natural selection and the respiratory epithelium of patients with chronic bronchitis shows evidence of enlargement of the mucus secretory glands and increase in their number. Unfortunately this prolonged over-stimulation causes the air passages to become clogged with sticky secretion. As a result, instead of being preserved, lung function is eventually irretrievably damaged.

Amyloid

Amyloidosis is the deposition of amyloid proteins in blood vessels, liver, spleen, kidney, gastrointestinal tract and lymph nodes, or within the myocardium or respiratory tract.

It can arise as a primary disorder or secondarily as a complication of chronic inflammation. Amyloid acquired its name from the Greek because its staining properties with Congo red, giving an apple green colour with polarised light, wrongly suggested that it was of a starchy nature. Electron microscopy reveals 90% of amyloid to consist of fine non-branching rigid fibrils giving a highly characteristic appearance. A number of different precursor proteins can form amyloid fibrils, but these are nearly all bound to a constant glycoprotein, amyloid P component, and have a remarkably uniform ultrastructural appearance (see Table 13.2).

However, when amyloidosis occurs in association with chronic inflammation or infection (such as in leprosy, TB or syphilis) the fibrils, composed of amyloid A protein (AA), are thought to be derived from the acute phase reactant, serum amyloid A protein (SAA). Chronic infection used to be the major cause of amyloidosis; however, it is now more often seen as a result of chronic inflammation in diseases such as rheumatoid arthritis and Crohn's. Immune disorders such as Hodgkin's disease or myelomatosis also often lead to amyloidosis where the fibrils are derived from immunoglobulin light chains, and their constituent protein is designated AL (amyloid light chain). Amyloidosis also appears as a heredofamilial disorder in which the fibrils are often derived from genetic variants of

Table 13.2 Different forms of amyloid and disease

Fibril proteins	Cause	Example
AA (derived from SAA)	a) Chronic infection b) Chronic inflammation	TB, leprosy, osteomyelitis RA, Crohn's disease
Prealbumin	Hereditary	Familial amyloid neuropathy
B protein	a) APP gene on chromosome 21/ageing b) Trisomy 21	Alzheimer's senile dementia Down's syndrome
AL (derived from IG light chains)	Immune dysfunction	Myeloma, Hodgkin's disease
β_2-microglobulin	Dialysis	Chronic renal failure

prealbumin. Dialysis associated amyloid is increasingly being seen; this is due to increased plasma levels of β_2-microglobulin. Amyloidosis can occur as part of the ageing process, and the β protein forms the cerebral amyloid in Alzheimer's disease and Down's syndrome (p. 182). The protein is encoded for by the APP gene on chromosome 21. As many as 25% of elderly individuals produce the fibrils, and its deposition in the brain may play a role in senile dementia (p. 357). Quite why the fibril-forming degradation products should accumulate is unclear; once formed amyloid deposits rarely progress, but tend to increase in size inexorably, leading to a poor prognosis in the host with chronic renal failure being the commonest cause of death.

KEY POINTS

- Chronic inflammation is characterised by an inflammatory process where macrophages, plasma cells and lymphocytes predominate, usually accompanied by healing.
- Chronic inflammation can occur either after repeated attacks or persistence of acute inflammation, or where foreign organisms are resistant to digestion or where host tissue is attacked in autoimmunity.
- The key processes in chronic inflammation are usually due to the interaction between macrophages and T cells (involving Type IV hypersensitivity).
- Amyloidosis is a further complication of chronic inflammation and involves the deposition of protein fibrils locally or systemically.

14 The systemic response to injury

In pathology the word 'injury' embraces every form of tissue damage including bacterial or viral infection, chemical or thermal insult or mechanical destruction of body tissues by accident or by deliberate violence, the latter category including surgical operations. Even trivial injury produces a local reaction of the surviving tissues, i.e. inflammation (p. 87). More serious injury is accompanied also by a systemic reaction in which the cardiovascular system, the endocrine system and indeed the whole bodily metabolism are involved. The knowledge we possess of these responses has been accumulated mainly from research initiated in time of war when information was necessary to reduce battle casualties.

Injury as defined above is the main threat to those individuals young enough to hold the responsibility for reproducing the species. It is predictable therefore that the systemic reaction to injury as described in the pages which follow consists largely of compensatory mechanisms which must have been selected for by evolutionary pressures.

Reaction of the bone marrow

Red blood corpuscles

When blood is lost from the body (haemorrhage) in large amounts, either acutely, i.e. for a short period, or chronically, i.e. in smaller amounts over a long period, the red cell precursors in the bone marrow react appropriately. Red cell production *(erythropoiesis)* is regulated by a refined system involving a hormone, *erythropoietin*, partly produced in the kidney. When there is a need for more oxygen, e.g. at high altitudes, the marrow puts out more oxygen-binding haemoglobin by producing additional red blood corpuscles. After massive haemorrhage there is a transient drop in the number of circulating red cells but this deficiency is soon made good provided that adequate amounts of iron (part of the haemoglobin molecule) and other nutritional factors are available. In chronic blood loss, e.g. from a bleeding peptic ulcer or excessive menstrual bleeding, it is common for the dietary intake of iron to be inadequate and for an iron-deficiency type of *anaemia* (shortage of haemoglobin; p. 244) to result. There are of course a number of diseases, such as pernicious anaemia, affecting the red cell precursors in the bone marrow which are discussed later (p. 249). As regards the general reaction to injury the essential point is that a successful humoral feedback system regulates red cell production and returns it to normal levels, without overreacting. The main constraints in the adaptive process which prevent overreaction are:

- the high daily output of red cells
- the resultant very great demand on the essential ingredients in their manufacture, especially iron, which quickly becomes a limiting factor because any increase in its absorption from the diet is difficult to achieve and because the body's stores are small (Fig. 14.1).

Platelets

Obviously the major effect of injury on the bone marrow is to create a demand for replacement of blood cells lost by haemorrhage to the

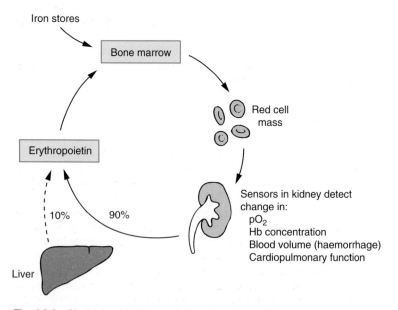

Fig. 14.1 Mechanisms for the regulation of red blood cells.

exterior or into damaged tissues. In the case of red cells this need is met by positive feedback mediated by erythropoietin. A similar mechanism operates in the case of platelets. Although the exact mechanism is poorly understood, platelet function is regulated by a number of *humoral haemopoietic growth factors* (IL-3, IL-6 and IL-11 and granulocyte-macrophage stimulating factor). Unlike the comparable erythropoiesis there is usually an overproduction of platelets by up to 50% over normal circulating values and this has its dangers since it may lead to undesirable effects such as thrombosis (p. 209).

Thrombocytopenia is a deficiency of platelets in the circulation which develops when the nature of the injury is such as to consume platelets faster than they can be replaced; it may be caused by:

- excess pooling
- excess destruction
- decreased production.

However this situation seldom occurs as a result merely of repeated haemorrhage so there is no direct parallel with red blood cells which become scarce under such circumstances due to shortage of iron. Platelet deficiency is usually due to:

1. disease of the bone marrow itself, or
2. antibodies which destroy these cells in the blood, as in Type II drug hypersensitivity (p. 61).

If, as in some diseases, however, there is generalised coagulation of blood inside vessels with massive incorporation of platelets in the clot (*disseminated intravascular coagulation*), persistent thrombocytopenia may result. This will lead to further bleeding since platelets are needed for normal haemostasis and a progressive failure of adaptation typical of pathology will result.

Neutrophil polymorphs (granulocytes)

Any form of local tissue injury leading to exudation of polymorphs is likely to be associated with an increase in the number of these cells circulating in the blood (*neutrophil leukocytosis, neutrophilia*). The largest neutrophilia is seen usually during bacterial inflammation. Sterile inflammation, such as occurs in infarcted heart muscle, has a similar but smaller effect on blood leukocytes. As an exception to the rule, a few examples of bacterial inflammation, notably typhoid fever, lead to a drop rather than a rise in numbers of circulating polymorphs. Virus-induced inflammation seldom causes a neutrophilia although there are exceptions such as poliomyelitis.

In general there is a good correlation between the number of polymorphs exuding into the inflamed tissue site and the size of the accompanying leukocytosis. This suggests at once that leukocytosis is the result of a positive feedback mechanism and indeed there is convincing evidence in man and animals that positive and negative feedback occurs. Positive feedback means that a deficiency of cells results in their increased production and negative feedback means that an excess of cells leads to a diminution in their production.

The kinetics of granulocytes are complicated because three compartments must be considered: the bone marrow, the blood and the tissues. In inflammation, in order to maintain a steady state there is a demand for mature neutrophils to replace those lost in the injured tissues (p. 94). This demand is met by maintaining the size of the total polymorph pool. As we have seen, feedback mechanisms in pathology tend to overreact and the response to leukocyte loss is no exception. As a result of the exaggerated reaction, the polymorph pool usually increases to well beyond its normal size so that there is an excessive number of neutrophil polymorphonuclear leukocytes in the circulation, i.e. neutrophil leukocytosis.

One result of this excess is that individual cells spend more time than usual in the blood stream (i.e. their half life or T_2 is raised) because the augmented entry of leukocytes into the total blood leukocyte pool from the bone marrow is faster than their disappearance into the inflamed site. Nevertheless the absolute number of leukocytes replaced each day by fresh leukocytes from the marrow (the polymorph turnover rate) is also raised.

The exaggerated increase in the size of the total blood polymorph pool is of course achieved by an additional output of leukocytes from the bone marrow. The extra output is due largely to a release of mature leukocytes earlier than would normally occur. In addition the cell cycle time of the leukocyte precursors, i.e. the time needed to divide and produce mature leukocytes, is probably shortened (Fig. 14.2). Under extreme conditions of leukocyte demand, immature forms escape into the blood but the more primitive leukocyte precursors only leave the bone marrow in primary disease of that organ such as leukaemia.

It is well known that various sorts of 'stress' such as physical exercise, fear, or even sitting an examination induce a leukocytosis of neutrophils. This is due to release of extra amounts of adrenaline and of corticosteroid hormones from the adrenal cortex, the process being controlled from the pituitary gland and the hypothalamus. The kinetics of this situation differ from tissue injury in that although the total blood polymorph pool is increased, the polymorph turnover rate remains normal because there is no increase in migration of leukocytes into the tissues. The granulocytosis of stress is due to release into the circulation of leukocytes sequestered along the walls of blood vessels throughout the body. This sequestration of 'marginated' granulocytes is normal and release of the cells leads to no change in the size of the bone marrow pool (Fig. 14.2).

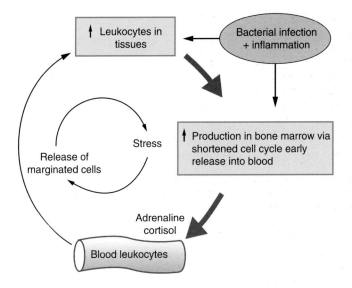

Fig. 14.2 Mechanisms of leukocytosis.

Monocytes

Although monocytes migrate freely into inflamed tissues, especially if the process is prolonged (chronic inflammation), an excess of monocytes in the circulation is unusual. Nevertheless, a positive feedback mechanism has been demonstrated in which loss of these cells into peritoneal exudates is balanced by augmented production and release from the bone marrow. The production rate of the monocyte precursor cell, the *promonocyte*, also shows a transient rise. The rate increases mainly because the DNA synthesis time, i.e. the 'S' phase of the mitotic cycle, is shortened in the bone marrow cells. There is much less effect on the later parts of the mitotic cycle. *Corticosteroids* prevent these effects of inflammation on the bone marrow monocytes and to some extent therefore act in a contrary fashion to their effects on polymorphonuclear leukocytes although the details of this difference are not yet clear.

The positive feedback for monocyte regulation probably operates through *interleukin-1* released from macrophages or one of the specific *colony stimulating factors* (M-CSF), which appear in the circulation in acute inflammation and which when injected into normal mice cause a threefold rise in blood monocytes with no effect on polymorphs or lymphocytes.

Lymphocytes

Changes in numbers of circulating lymphocytes are not of major importance in the reaction to injury. The numbers may rise in a variety of virus infections and fall when output of adrenocortical hormones is elevated. In one virus disease (infectious mononucleosis) abnormal lymphocytes appear in the blood stream and their recognition by the pathologist helps to establish the diagnosis. Lymphocyte kinetics are of course very complex since there are at least two major subpopulations and a number of compartments in which they exist for widely differing lengths of time.

Eosinophils

The eosinophil is a cousin of the neutrophil polymorphonuclear leukocyte with a similar life pattern. It originates in a bone marrow precursor cell, circulates in small numbers in the blood and enters the tissues freely. Its life span may be longer than that of the neutrophil polymorph. The eosinophil gets its name from the affinity of its lysosomal granules for eosin dyes but the significance of this staining is not known. The eosinophil appears in large numbers in a number of situations, predominantly *infestation with worms* and *atopy* (p. 61). Eosinophils probably cooperate with mast cells in the elimination from host tissues of certain worms and their mobilisation is probably assisted by sensitised lymphocytes exerting cell-mediated immunity (p. 64). *Eosinophilia* may also occur as a by-product of the mast cell degranulation which occurs in both worm infestation and in Type I hypersensitivity although the mechanism of the link is not yet clear. Indeed, the properties of the eosinophils and the nature of their participation in these events also remain obscure. In general the increase in circulation eosinophils parallels their appearance in large numbers in sites of inflammation.

Eosinophils are released from bone marrow under the influence of several growth factors including *IL-3, IL-5* and *GM-CSF,* and a number of specific *chemotactic factors* have been identified at suitable sites of inflammation (p. 93).

Haemopoietic growth factors

Steady state haemopoiesis is maintained by the proliferation and differentiation of pluripotential stem cells in bone marrow. This regulatory mechanism is adapted to deal with stresses such as blood loss and injury.

Haemopoietic growth factors are part of the *cytokine* family and are all glycoproteins which regulate the differentiation and proliferation of blood precursors via their action on receptors expressed at different levels of stem cell development.

We have already mentioned briefly the role of some of these factors; some have kept their original names i.e. *erythropoietin*, others are part of the *interleukin* family and the third group of cytokines are called *colony stimulating factors* (CSFs), the prefix standing for the major cell line stimulated by the factor. These include granulocyte macrophage (GM-CSF), granulocyte (G-CSF), and macrophage (M-CSF) colony stimulating factors and stem cell factor (SCF).

Haemopoietic growth factors are produced in a number of different cells including:

- macrophages
- monocytes
- activated T cells
- fibroblasts
- endothelial cells.

They can be broadly divided into two groups:

1. lineage-restricted factors such as erythropoietin or G-CSF which act on committed progenitors and affect specific cell types
2. multilineage factors such as GM-CSF and IL-3 which affect the production of many cell types (Fig. 14.3).

Although, with the exception of erythropoietin, their mechanisms of action are poorly understood and the costs of synthesis are high, these factors are becoming increasingly important in clinical practice to increase levels of circulating cells in severe disease situations. Erythropoietin is used as a therapy to reverse the anaemia of chronic renal failure and to a lesser extent anaemias due to chronic disease, i.e. rheumatoid arthritis. The other factors are now being used with increasing success in the treatment of post-chemotherapy neutropenia, bone marrow transplants, rare myelodysplastic syndromes and the neutropenia and thrombocytopenia of AIDS; they may also have a role in treating aplastic anaemias. Current trials indicate that maximum benefit with low levels of side effects are likely when combinations of these factors are used.

Fever

Regulation of body temperature

Fever is the elevation of the body temperature above normal. The normal body temperature is approximately 37°C measured by a thermometer inserted in the mouth, rectum or axilla.

Of all the general systemic accompaniments of injury fever is the most widely and readily observed. Precise regulation of body

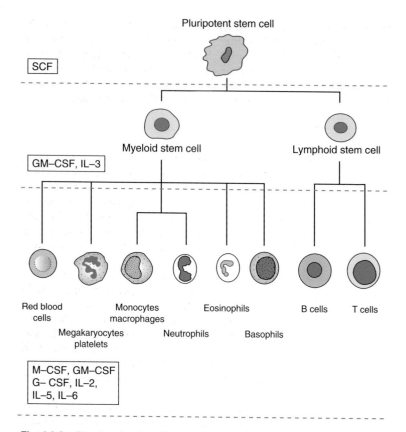

Fig. 14.3   The site of action of haemopoietic growth factors.

temperature is a vital element in physiological homeostasis and is controlled for the most part through the skin.

- When it is necessary to *lose heat*, e.g. because heat has been produced through exercise, the skin vessels dilate and blood flow and heat loss increase via radiation.
- If this is insufficient, the sweat glands are stimulated to lose heat by means of evaporation.
- Conversely, to *gain heat*, e.g. because of low environmental temperature, the skin vessels constrict; cutaneous blood flow and therefore heat loss via radiation are reduced.
- If it is necessary to *generate heat* there is repetitive contraction of muscle fibres causing shivering.

All these physiological phenomena are reproduced during fever, often in rapid succession, shivering under these circumstances being known as *rigors*. In pathology, however, the fever is due to the resetting of the part of the brain which controls body temperature, the *thermoregulatory centre* in the hypothalamus. Thus fever results from interference with the thermostat itself, whereas non-pathological temperature regulation is dependent on environmental temperature and the amount of heat generated by the body's metabolism.

Pyrogens

Fever can be deliberately induced in humans by injection of *pyrogens*, i.e. substances of biological origin such as bacterial extracts which cause fever. When this is done it is easy to show how contraction of skin vessels, reduction in skin blood flow (causing a feeling of coldness) and shivering precede a rise in body temperature. Often the increase is overdone and there is a response of sweating and vasodilatation (with a feeling of being hot) followed in a turn by a compensatory increase in heat loss.

The changes in blood flow are dependent on the vasomotor nerves and fever is prevented if these nerves no longer function, e.g. in patients with damage high up the spinal cord. In such cases the accompaniments of fever, notably headache, are also abolished. Thus it seems likely that headache is a result of the fever. Patients with non-functioning thermoregulatory centres do not become feverish if pyrogen is injected. Fever is therefore due to an action of fever-inducing substances on this brain centre and is brought about by the vasomotor nerves.

Animal experiments indicate that the site of the thermoregulatory centre is in the anterior hypothalamus and that it contains warm and cold receptors which are triggered as appropriate. During fever they work with normal sensitivity but the threshold at which they work is raised so that body heat is maintained at an abnormally high level (Fig. 14.4).

The commonest injury causing fever is of course bacterial or viral infection and for some time now it has been possible to obtain purified chemical pyrogens from dead bacteria. When obtained from Gram-negative organisms such as *E. coli* or *Salmonella abortus* (p. 18) these are known as *endotoxins* and consist of lipopolysaccharides. Many other bacterial species including Gram-positive cocci also yield pyrogens. However they are believed to cause fever by acting indirectly via a quite different group of peptides released from leukocytes and known as *endogenous pyrogen*.

It is now known that the major component of endogenous pyrogen is the cytokine *interleukin-1*, and to a lesser extent *tumour necrosis factor* (TNF). Normal leukocytes released from blood do not normally contain IL-1 or TNF, whereas those harvested from inflammatory exudates do, indicating that injury or activation makes the cells

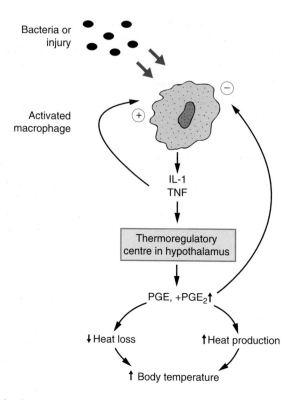

Fig. 14.4   The mechanism of fever.

synthesise the substance. It is now known that the primary sources of endogenous pyrogen are *monocytes* and *macrophages*, although it is produced by a number of more specialised *phagocytic cells* throughout the body. The injury-associated stimulus needed to synthesise IL-1 or TNF can be almost any infection, immunological reaction or inflammatory process. The mechanism consists of two parts:

1. *synthesis*, which is easily suppressed by inhibitors of respiration or protein synthesis
2. *release*, which is prevented with much more difficulty.

As well as IL-1 and TNF other bodily substances have been found to produce fever on injection. Certain steroid degradation products have this property, notably *aetiocholanolone* which causes release of IL-1. *Noradrenaline* causes fever in some mammalian species, especially when injected directly into the hypothalamus. Recently the potent antiviral agent *α-interferon* has been found to be pyrogenic as have interferon β and γ. Finally, the *prostaglandins*, notably PGE_1 and PGE_2, will induce fever on injection; their mode of action probably consists of raising the thermostatic set point in the hypothalamus. It is likely that IL-1 initiates fever by inducing an abrupt rise in the synthesis of these prostaglandins.

The role of prostaglandins explains the antipyretic action of drugs such as aspirin which are powerful inhibitors of prostaglandin release and synthesis but do not affect IL-1 release (p. 96). Glucocorticoids probably reduce temperature by interfering with cytokine synthesis as well as reducing arachidonic acid production centrally. The cause of the feeling of ill-being (*malaise*) which usually accompanies fever is uncertain. It may be a direct consequence of pyrexia or may result from an independent action of prostaglandins on some part of the brain. The regulation of temperature is a complex system involving positive feedback signals from IL-1 and TNF and negative feedback from PGE_2 (Fig. 14.4).

Tachycardia

A usual companion of fever is an increase in the heart rate, so that taking the pulse is usually combined with taking the temperature in the solemn bedside ritual of the doctor's visit. The increased heart rate (tachycardia) indicates an increased cardiac output which is very closely linked to a rise in body temperature. It is not certain how these two events are related, but it is known that if fever is prevented by damage to the nervous pathways in the spinal cord, cardiac output fails to rise. On the other hand, the two phenomena may occasionally be disassociated, as in typhoid fever when the temperature is raised but the pulse is slow.

Benefits of fever to the patient

Until recently there was little evidence of any benefit from fever to the patient. Fever and the immune response are now seen as part of the same defence mechanism, being linked by the same mediator. IL-1 activates T cells and it has recently been demonstrated that the B- and T-cell immune response against the pathogenic organism is greatly enhanced even by small increases of half a degree C in body temperature. Thus it appears that evolution has carefully conserved the fever response despite all the metabolic hazards to the patient; the use of antipyretics in patients with infectious diseases (where the fever is beneficial) may actually reduce the immune response and prolong the fever. Conversely, in disease states where the fever is inappropriate, such as cancers and lymphomas (i.e. Hodgkin's disease) and autoimmune diseases, the effects of fever may be harmful to the host producing malaise, muscle wasting and weight loss.

Plasma proteins

After injury and its associated local inflammatory reaction, characteristic changes occur in some of the plasma proteins. These changes are evident as increased blood concentrations of the plasma proteins concerned but actually represent alterations in liver cell metabolism, the organ from where they are produced.

The *acute phase response* is a non-specific phenomenon by which increased levels of proteins are released into the circulation in response to tissue injury and prostaglandin and cytokine release (Table 14.1).

One of the most consistent features is an elevation of the level of circulating fibrinogen and its increased synthesis by the liver. This probably represents an exaggerated positive feedback response to loss of fibrinogen in the exudate from inflamed blood vessels (p. 89) or in the course of haemorrhage. *Fibrinogen* is a high molecular weight protein and when large molecules appear in the plasma in excessive amounts the red corpuscles clump together to form rouleaux. This is seldom evident inside the body but if a sample of such blood is removed, prevented from clotting and allowed to sediment under gravity, the red cells will settle much faster than normal. This *erythrocyte sedimentation rate* is easily measured and forms a simple and useful bedside index of the presence and severity of inflammation, although it will be raised by excess of any high molecular weight

Table 14.1   The acute phase proteins

Function	Protein	Protective role
Coagulation and fibrinolysis	Fibrinogen Prothrombin Plasminogen Factor VII	Homeostasis
Complement components	C3, C4, C5, etc.	Lyse bacteria and debris
Transport	Haptoglobulin Caeruloplasmin Ferritin	Regulates amines and mops up free radicals
Proteinase inhibitors	α_1-antitrypsin	Limits tissue destruction by enzymes
Adherence proteins	C-reactive protein	Binds to bacteria and activates complement
Miscellaneous	Serum amyloid A (SAA) Fibronectin Lactoferrin	?Anti-inflammatory Binds to cell debris Binds iron: bacteriostatic

substance in the plasma, so that in a few rare instances it will be due to a primary abnormality of the plasma proteins.

Beside fibrinogen, other plasma proteins made in the liver also appear in excess in the blood after injury and are normally maintained at low levels. The best known of these is *C-reactive protein*, so called because it reacts with the carbohydrate of pneumococci and the polysaccharides of a wide variety of other bacteria and fungi. This substance is now a common and accurate test of the acute phase response and can activate the complement pathway but its appearance is something of a mystery. It has recently been found in the serum of normal fish—plaice to be more precise—in which it probably acts as an opsonin, aiding phagocytosis of microorganisms pathogenic for aquatic creatures. Its presence in man may well be a phylogenetic hangover.

The acute phase response in man is generally considered to be beneficial, helping to restore disturbed homeostasis by:

1. stopping bleeding
2. demarcation and resorption of necrotic tissue
3. lysis of foreign cells and bacteria
4. binding and removal of excessive amounts of proteases and exogenous substances
5. creating the right conditions for repair and healing.

The role of some of the acute phase proteins remains unclear. Some proteins, such as *serum amyloid A* (SAA), which can cause reactive amyloidosis (p. 118), may have modest anti-inflammatory activity, and others may have a role in neutralising superoxide radicals, i.e. *caeruloplasmin* (p. 32), thereby terminating and controlling inflammatory reactions. Others, such as *lactoferrin*, have complex actions; by binding to extracellular iron they cause a moderate iron deficiency which has defensive properties in that it produces a bacteriostatic environment.

In summary, injury leads to stimulation of the liver via a mediator, interleukin-1, which triggers the hepatocytes to produce the acute phase proteins including complement, coagulation proteins, transport proteins, protease inhibitors and adherence proteins. These generally have survival value for the host, although the benefit of some of the proteins may be demonstrable only in primitive invertebrates.

Endocrine response to injury

Injury of any sort, be it trauma, sepsis, burns or haemorrhage, leads to a well defined set of responses from the body. Such stresses characteristically lead to well coordinated neuroendocrine and circulatory responses. Some of these responses are anticipatory, involving the hypothalamic defence area, and may stimulate the release of ACTH, GH, prolactin, vasopressin and the sympatho-adrenomedullary axis. Upon injury, there is reinforcement of this neuroendocrine stress response by:

- afferent stimuli from nosiceptive areas
- baroreceptor and volume receptors (responding to blood loss)
- osmoreceptors and glucoreceptors (responding to changes in the composition of the blood).

These nervous and chemical stimuli activate the hypothalamus. Typically, there is activation of the hypothalamo-pituitary-adrenocortical axis, with the liberation of *hypothalamic corticotrophin releasing factor* (CRF) and *vasopressin*, both of which will liberate *ACTH* from the anterior pituitary. There is a concomitant release of *β-endorphin* from the pituitary, as well as *growth hormone* (GH), and *prolactin*.

ACTH

ACTH acts on the adrenal cortex with the synthesis and release of cortisol. This glucocorticoid hormone is essential in the overall response to stress, and appears to have a permissive rather than an active effect. Thus, in the absence of an adrenal cortex, injury may lead to death, but even small amounts of cortisol are usually sufficient to allow the usual adaptive responses enabling survival to occur.

Adrenaline and noradrenaline

In addition to the requirement for cortisol of adrenocortical origin, adrenaline of adrenomedullary origin is also released in response to stresses of various kinds. Adrenaline released from the adrenal medulla effects a number of important metabolic and cardiovascular adaptations, in addition to provoking a minor leukocytosis. Pain, trauma and a fall in circulating volume reflexly lead to the release of adrenaline from the adrenal medulla and noradrenaline from the sympathetic nerve endings. The latter acts predominantly as a neurotransmitter at the sympathetic neuroeffector junction causing vasoconstriction in certain vascular beds, and a more forceful cardiac contraction. There is likely to be a major interaction between circulating adrenaline and the noradrenaline at the neuroeffector junction. This arrangement is appropriate since diminished blood volume (hypovolaemia) is the common denominator of severe injury.

Metabolic response to injury

The pattern of response to many types of injury and in patients recovering from major surgery is relatively easy to define (Fig. 14.5),

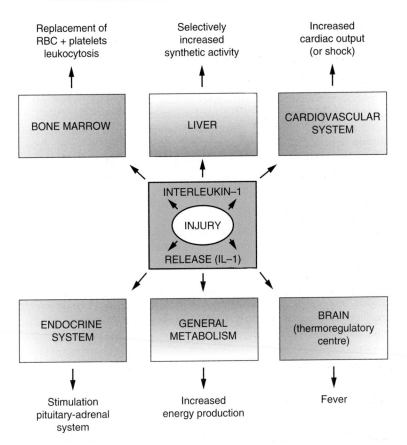

Fig. 14.5 The effects of tissue injury on various body systems.

though less so for sepsis, for which the hormonal and metabolic response waxes and wanes in intensity. The changes affect carbohydrate, lipid and protein metabolism, and fall into three categories, each seen at one characteristic stage after injury.

Initial (ebb) phase

In the initial, or ebb, phase there is increased breakdown of muscle glycogen to lactate and thence glucose, largely mediated by the actions of *adrenaline* and to a lesser extent *noradrenaline* secretion. Plasma levels of noradrenaline and adrenaline rise substantially above the threshold levels determined by experimental work as being necessary to produce metabolic changes. *Catecholamines* provoke lipolysis with the breakdown of triglycerides to glycerol and free fatty acids. High levels of catecholamines raise blood glucose and lactate through stimulation of liver and muscle glycogen breakdown. Higher levels still will inhibit insulin release. *Vasopressin* and *glucagon* release may facilitate the actions of the catecholamines. The action of vasopressin in stimulating glycogen breakdown as well as water retention is teleologically attractive, in that the mobilisation of water stored with glycogen could aid compensation for fluid loss. Cortisol, adrenaline and glucagon thus act synergistically to promote and sustain hepatic glucose production, and adrenaline promotes lipolysis. Thus, by these means, injury is quickly followed by mobilisation of readily utilised energy sources.

Shock (necrobiotic) phase

With severe injury and unsuccessful resuscitation, the patient may enter the shock or necrobiotic phase of metabolic change. Inadequate tissue perfusion leads to poor cellular oxygenation and a state of *acidosis*. A fall in body temperature may ensue. Glucose utilisation is increased under anaerobic conditions, and the accumulation of lactic acid is responsible for the acidosis. Under-perfusion of organs with inadequate oxygenation may lead to malfunction of several organs, such as the liver and kidneys.

Flow phase

With successful resuscitation, the patient enters the flow phase, characterised by:

- increase in metabolic rate
- elevation of core temperature
- increased excretion of urinary nitrogen

together with other markers suggestive of net muscle protein breakdown (urea, sulphur, phosphorus, potassium). There is also increased turnover of glucose, and *hyperglycaemia* may develop. The picture is essentially one of increased glucose utilisation and gluconeogenesis, using the labile protein stored in skeletal muscle as an energy store. Protein catabolism is particularly dramatic and is partly due to the failure of the homeostatic mechanisms which normally preserve muscle protein at the expense of fat. One such failure is the inappropriate secretion of insulin which helps block lipolysis. The enormous calorie requirement of severely injured patients is important clinically, as its balanced replacement will assist the recovery process.

Severe stress, such as that associated with *septicaemia*, is also associated with changes in the hypothalamo-pituitary-thyroid axis. In particular, serum T_3 and T_4 fall, with a peripheral conversion of T_3, into reverse T_3 production. Free T_4 is normal, as is the TSH secretion, and so biochemically the patient remains euthyroid. This condition has been described as the 'sick euthyroid syndrome'. Reverse T_3 is biologically inactive, and this manoeuvre is probably an anti-catabolic protective measure.

Electrolyte metabolism

Injury may be associated with particular loss of water and electrolytes, e.g. by *vomiting, diarrhoea, haemorrhage* or massive *exudation* of fluid into injured tissues. Quite apart from these possibilities, however, injury per se is accompanied by electrolyte changes, especially in sodium ions. The usual observation is of reduced sodium and enhanced potassium excretion in the urine, i.e. sodium retention. This is accompanied by a paradoxical fall in the plasma sodium concentration. Sodium retention may sometimes be due to secretion of antidiuretic hormone (ADH) from the pituitary or to aldosterone secretion from the adrenal cortex, both in response to hypovolaemia. There may also be enhanced resorption of sodium in the ascending limb of the loop of Henle due to diminished circulatory perfusion of the kidney, again consequent upon hypovolaemia (p. 236). The paradoxical fall in serum sodium concentration is usually attributed to its entry into tissue cells as a result of disturbance of cellular metabolism.

Regulation

We have seen how, by a number of changes in plasma proteins, bone marrow, body temperature, and other endocrinological, metabolic and immunological processes, the host responds to injury. This response to injury has the outstanding characteristic of being a generalised host reaction irrespective of the localised or systemic nature of the inciting disease. Until recently it was unclear how injuries, infections, immunological and inflammatory reactions were all able to elicit the wide variety of changes in the host. The substance elicited by all these stimuli is the chemical mediator interleukin-1 (IL-1) which deserves more detailed discussion.

Interleukin-1 (IL-1)

The term 'interleukin' was first proposed in 1979 as the name for the substance that allowed communication between leukocytes. Since then it has become apparent that it is not a single peptide but rather a family of multifunctional molecules acting on many different cell types which can be released by a variety of different cells.

An increasing number of different interleukins with different regulatory functions are being recognised: the likely main functions of these and the major cytokines are listed in Table 14.2.

Table 14.2   Principal functions of the interleukins and major cytokines

Cytokine	Biological effects
IL-1	Acute phase response, fever, T-cell and macrophage activation, stimulation of bone marrow
IL-2	Growth factor for B and T cells, activates cytotoxic lymphocytes, enhances NK cell function
IL-3	Proliferation of pluripotent stem cells in marrow
IL-4	Induces IgE synthesis, T-cell growth factor
IL-5	Eosinophil growth factor
IL-6	Differentiation of activated B cells
IL-7	Growth factor for immature B and T cells
IL-8	Neutrophil activator
IL-11	Megakaryocyte growth factor
Interferon (α, β, γ)	Interferes with viral replication
TNFα	Acute phase response, anti-tumour and leukocyte adherence
TNFβ	Increases release of IL-1, TNF, and other cytokines

The most important cytokine however is interleukin-1, which is really a family of three structurally related polypeptides. Gene cloning has shown that there are two different IL-1 genes (alpha and beta) which encode for two different proteins, and the cleavage of the parent molecule into a number of different-sized peptides may account for its wide variety of biological properties which may be both harmful and beneficial. As with most of the cytokines, they are not generally found in stored form in cells, and circulating monocytes do not usually contain IL-1 until they are activated to begin synthesis.

In addition to activating neutrophils and B and T cells, IL-1 also affects several non-leukocytic targets, such as the liver, pancreas, bone, muscle, fibroblasts and brain. An example of the effects of IL-1 on the host can be demonstrated by considering the effects of a local bacterial infection. Initially monocytes and macrophages become activated, either by the bacteria themselves or by their toxin; IL-1 is produced and acts as a local mediator of inflammation contributing to local oedema formation and leukocyte chemotaxis and increasing the power of leukocytes to kill the invading bacteria. As well as exerting local effects IL-1 enters the circulation and interacts with several distant target tissues: it initiates fever via its effect on the hypothalamus; in the bone marrow it stimulates neutrophil synthesis; in muscle it causes amino acid breakdown; and it increases the production of acute phase proteins in the liver. The principal actions of interleukin-1 are shown in Table 14.3.

The third component of the interleukin-1 family is the IL-1 receptor antagonist: this is structurally similar to the other two types

Table 14.3   The major actions of interleukin-1

1. *Inflammatory*
   a. Chemotactic for neutrophils, lymphocytes, and monocytes
   b. Increased collagen synthesis
   c. Increased collagenase and proteoglycanase synthesis
   d. PGE_2 production by skin and synovial fibroblasts
   e. Increased bone resorption via 'osteoclast activating factor'
   f. Stimulation of fibroblast β-interferon synthesis
   g. Stimulates degranulation and release of nitric oxide

2. *Immunological*
   a. T-cell activation: production of IL-2
   b. B-cell activation: acts as B-cell growth factor
   c. Lymphokine production increased: IL-2, IL-3, interferons

3. *Systemic*

a. CNS:	Fever
	Increased corticosteroid production
	Decreased appetite
	Increased slow-wave sleep
b. Metabolic:	Increased acute phase proteins
	Amino acid release
	Decreased albumin synthesis
	Reduced serum iron and zinc levels
c. Haematological:	Neutrophilia
	Lymphopenia
d. Vascular:	Increased adherence of leukocytes
	Increased PGI and PGE synthesis
	Increased platelet activating factor (PAF)

but has no biological activity apart from the ability to bind to IL-1 receptors without activating them and thus reducing the effect of IL-1. It is probably a natural defence mechanism of the body to reduce the adverse effects of this powerful cytokine in disease states.

IL-1 has been implicated in the pathogenesis of a large number of diverse diseases:

- septic shock
- rheumatoid arthritis
- inflammatory bowel disease
- myeloid leukaemia
- atherosclerosis
- insulin-dependent diabetes mellitus.

The relative balance of IL-1 to its receptor may be important in these conditions. Novel recombinant molecular technology has recently enabled IL-1 receptor antagonists to be developed for experimental and therapeutic use in these conditions, with some success. Use of the antagonist in septic shock has produced improvements in survival without any major alterations to homeostasis, suggesting that the major role of IL-1 is not in homeostasis but in regulating the response to injury.

Thus IL-1 appears to be a central mediator in the organisation of the body's defences against injury.

Tumour necrosis factor (TNF)

Another cytokine also produced by macrophages and monocytes is tumour necrosis factor (previously known as lymphotoxin and cachectin), which was originally named for its anti-tumour properties (p. 276). It appears to have a similar role and structure to IL-1, also having two genes coding for it, and is found throughout the body. It is likely that TNF and IL-1 represent a complementary controlling system for the host's response to injury, the interaction of the two mediators enabling precise regulation throughout the body. IL-1 activity is considerably enhanced in the presence of TNF and vice versa. As our understanding of the mechanisms of actions of cytokines increases, so will the range of therapeutic uses of these agents and their antagonists.

KEY POINTS

- In response to injury the bone marrow is stimulated by cytokines and colony stimulating factors to produce increased numbers of circulating cells.
- Fever is produced by the action of IL-1 on the anterior hypothalamus which alters the production of prostaglandins and resets the body temperature.
- Injury provokes the liver to release increased amounts of proteins into the circulation which have a wide range of protective functions for the host.
- Injury causes the release of hormones which alter the metabolic state of the body to enable it to defend itself more efficiently.
- The general response to injury is controlled by the action of a large group of hormone-like glycoproteins called cytokines, the most important of which is probably interleukin-1.
- IL-1 is implicated in the pathogenesis of a number of diseases and there is an exciting new area emerging in the therapeutic use of cytokines, antagonists and colony stimulating factors in a number of clinical situations.

15 Healing and repair

Healing is the basic response to destruction or loss of tissues insufficient to cause death, characterised by partial or complete regeneration and reconstruction of the part lost.

This process of complete regeneration is seen in most living organisms, all the way up to the lower vertebrates. The salamander will replace an amputated limb as readily as an earthworm its body segments. It is often stated that mammals have lost their regenerative capacity but this is only partially true. If a hole is punched right through a rabbit's ear, all the destroyed tissues will be replaced, including cartilage, skin, hair and glands. However, in no other mammal studied does the ear have this capacity. On the other hand, even in man some organs can regenerate as satisfactorily as the salamander's limb. Another frequent generalisation is that the more differentiated or specialised a tissue, the less its capacity to grow again. This pronouncement probably derives from the observation that brain cells, admittedly highly specialised, never regenerate, whereas simpler mesenchymal cells divide readily. Between these extremes, however, there are many exceptions and the general statement becomes invalid:

- Liver cells are certainly highly differentiated and have many specialised functions but they regenerate as fast as any other human tissue.
- Muscle cells, which are highly specialised only in being contractile, regenerate poorly.
- Lung tissue, which is fairly simple, is reluctant to grow again in adult life.
- Kidney tubule cells, less specialised than liver epithelium, regenerate poorly.

There must be reasons for these discrepancies but they remain unknown and do not conform to any general law or pattern yet apparent.

It is important to clarify the relationship between wounding, healing and regeneration. A *wound* implies structural damage with loss of tissue and most commonly refers to local destruction of the integument, i.e. the skin. Similarly, *healing* can refer to the restoration of any part but is most commonly used in relation to the body surface, so that wound healing generally implies reconstitution of the integrity of the skin. The major exception to this statement in human disease is the healing infarct (p. 215) especially in the cardiac muscle. In a cardiac infarct many muscle cells die but lack regenerative powers. However, there is an inflammatory reaction and the exudate and dead muscle cells become replaced by connective tissue and eventually converted to a dense scar by the process described in the next few pages.

The process of healing

Healing is generally considered as having two components:

1. *regeneration,* which is the replacement of lost cells by cells of the same type
2. *repair,* which is the process of synthesising connective tissue and its subsequent maturation into scar tissue.

Rarely, regeneration can occur independently of wound healing, as when special factors operate, e.g. in the lens of the salamander eye where the new lens is formed from the adjacent iris. Most other examples are really instances of organ *hyperplasia* due to increased stimulation, e.g. by hormones. On the other hand, experiments have made it clear that classical regeneration, as in the growth of new limbs in salamanders after amputation, depends on healing of the overlying skin wound. If this is prevented in some way, then the limb will not regenerate. The stimulus for the complex regrowth of the mesenchymal structures of the limb appears to come from the piled up epithelial cap of the healing skin, provided that it has an adequate nerve supply. The degree of innervation seems to be crucial and there have been several successes in inducing partial regeneration of limbs in frogs and lizards by augmenting the local nerve supply. In mammals, cyclical regrowth of male deer antlers after they are shed offers another example of complex regeneration and restoration of architecture dependent on healing of associated wounds in the integument.

The healing process as a whole is best thought of in the same way as acute inflammation, i.e. as a coordinated sequence of events.

When a wound occurs there is rupture of blood vessels with consequent escape of blood. If the body made no provision for this contingency the patient would bleed to death. Fortunately there are

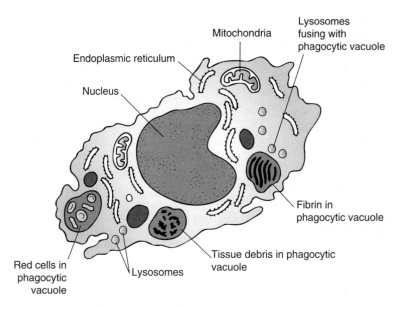

Lysosomes
fusing with
phagocytic vacuole

Mitochondria

Endoplasmic reticulum

Nucleus

Fibrin in
phagocytic vacuole

Tissue debris in phagocytic vacuole

Red cells in
phagocytic
vacuole

Lysosomes

Fig. 15.1 Drawing of the electron microscopic appearance of a macrophage after phagocytosis of fibrin, red cells and tissue debris.

efficient mechanisms for stopping bleeding within minutes (p. 225) but the wounded tissues fill up with partially solidified blood before haemostasis (the control of bleeding) is complete. The original tissue damage plus the presence of so much extravascular blood is sufficient to initiate inflammatory changes in the adjacent intact blood vessels and there is migration of leukocytes into the wound area. The stimulus for polymorph attraction is short-lived, as are the polymorphs themselves, so their appearance is fleeting. More important is the emigration of *monocytes*, directed by local formation of chemotactic factors (such as fibronectin) and the release of cytokines and growth factors (p. 93) from cells in the area of the wound. Once in the tissues, monocytes mature into *macrophages*, active phagocytes capable of ingesting and digesting large amounts of debris (Fig. 15.1), aided by the glycoprotein fibronectin. The accumulation of macrophages and the digestion of debris, sometimes known as the *demolition phase*, is the first requisite for repair of connective tissue and takes several days.

Epithelial regeneration

Epithelial regeneration takes place within 24 hours and is achieved by increased mitotic activity in the epithelium adjacent to the wound margin, especially in the deeper layers. The mitotic activity is seen no

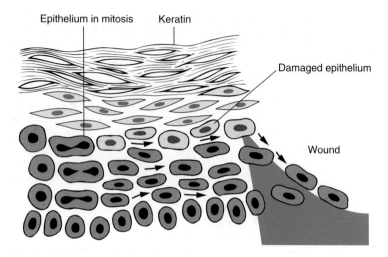

Fig. 15.2 Regenerating surface epithelium dividing and migrating to cover wound surface.

closer to the wound than four or five cells, since these four or five cells have either been damaged or are exposed to unfavourable environmental influences. As proliferation commences, epithelium glides out from the wound margins with a characteristic amoeboid motion (Fig. 15.2). The cells use the strands of fibrin and other extracellular matrix components such as fibronectin as 'guides' or 'conduits' in their journey. As the sheets of epithelium from different corners of the wound meet at the centre, the migration and mitosis cease, probably as a consequence of cell to cell signals known as *contact inhibition*. This flat sheet of epithelium cleaves a path between the dead and living tissues and advances rapidly so that by 48 hours the wound can be covered by a thin protective sheet.

Keratinisation begins quite early. Although hair follicles contribute to the development of new epithelium, it is unusual for hair follicles themselves to regenerate to any great extent, and the same is true of sweat and sebaceous glands.

Two processes then occur in parallel: production of connective tissue and neovascularisation.

Neovascularisation

Within a week there are clear signs that new blood vessels are growing into the wounded area. These appear first as solid cords of endothelial cells growing out as buds from the surviving capillaries at the wound edge (Fig. 15.3). The cells arise by mitotic activity in the endothelial cells of the parent vessel followed by their migration in the direction of the wound. The endothelial buds grow at about 0.1 to 0.6 mm per day. Mitotic division occurs also in the endothelium of the bud itself about 0.5 mm from the tip, and there is a strong tendency for buds to join each other to form loops and arcades (Fig. 15.3). The solid endothelial cords become canalised within hours and blood begins to flow in the lumen so formed (Fig. 15.4). The young vessels are leaky and are surrounded by plasma, red corpuscles and leukocytes that have escaped but they provide an essential prerequisite for regeneration of connective tissue, i.e. a blood supply. At first all the vessels are simply capillaries but soon some differentiate into arterioles and venules, in the former case by acquiring a coat of smooth muscle cells (Fig. 15.5). Newly formed arterioles acquire a vasomotor nerve supply sometimes as early as two weeks after wounding.

The process of changes to the connective tissue matrix and growth of new vessels is facilitated by the secretion from endothelial cells of localised connective tissue enzymes called *metalloproteinases*, principally *stromolysin* and *collagenase*. The result of these changes is the formation of a highly vascular *granulation tissue,* so called because the appearances are granular under the microscope. Soon an extensive remodelling process occurs, and many of the original capillary loops disappear through the shrivelling of redundant vessels, so that the blood supply of the wound becomes gradually reduced.

In parallel with the ingrowth of blood vessels, but quite separately, the *lymphatic endothelium* becomes re-established by a similar

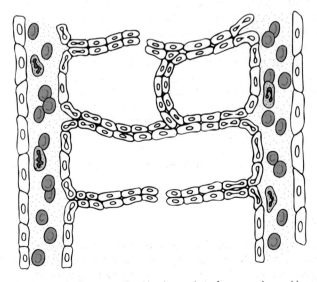

Fig. 15.3 Ingrowth of regenerating blood vessels to form arcades and loops.

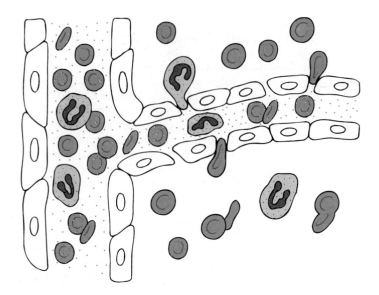

Fig. 15.4 New capillary bud develops a lumen.

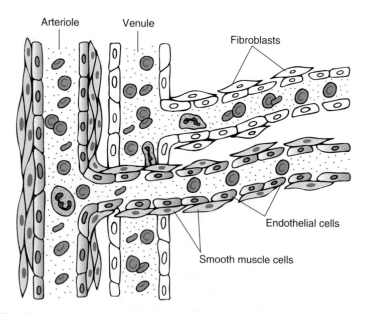

Fig. 15.5 Transformation of new vessels into arterioles and venules.

sequence of budding and joining. Lymphatic endothelium appears to have an unerring instinct for joining other lymphatic loops but avoiding blood channels.

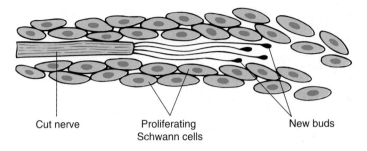

Cut nerve   Proliferating   New buds
Schwann cells

Fig. 15.6 Regeneration of damaged nerve.

Vasomotor nerves have already been mentioned but other *sensory and motor nerves* also regenerate, although more slowly. This occurs through the formation of sprouts which grow, at about 0.3 mm per day, from the central portion of the cut end, pushing through a guide channel formed by proliferating sheath (Schwann) cells and acquiring a myelin sheath in the process (Fig. 15.6).

Production of connective tissue

In parallel to the vascular changes is the production of the new connective tissue. The cell responsible for this is the *fibroblast* —the basic mesenchymal cell of adult tissue whose main property is the synthesis of collagen and mucopolysaccharides (Fig. 15.7). The

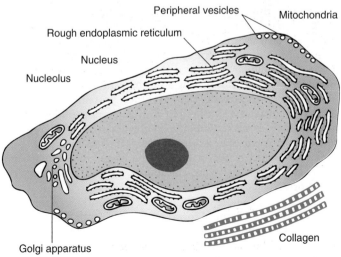

Peripheral vesicles   Mitochondria

Rough endoplasmic reticulum

Nucleus

Nucleolus

Golgi apparatus

Collagen

Fig. 15.7 Fibroblast.

osteoblast and chondrocyte, which form bone and cartilage respectively, are probably close cousins. The fibroblast is an elongated cell distinguished mainly by an impressive maze of rough endoplasmic reticulum lining wide cisternae in its cytoplasm. The electron microscope commonly reveals, closely related to the exterior of the cell, bundles of collagen with their characteristic regular transverse banding.

The fibroblast appears so promptly and in such large numbers in healing wounds that there has been much speculation as to its origin, but in general it is now accepted that fibroblasts are derived from preexisting local fibroblasts. Indeed the fibroblastic cells at the periphery of a wound can be seen to divide and migrate into the wound at the same time as the vascular buds and at a rate of about 0.2 mm/day. In the wound they continue to divide; about six days after their arrival the first collagen fibrils are recognisable, with their cross striations at intervals of 64 nm.

Collagen production

The way in which fibroblasts make collagen is well understood. *Collagen* is a protein which is assembled in the endoplasmic reticulum in the usual way, i.e. after the transcription of DNA into RNA and the translation of the nucleotide sequence into an amino acid sequence. At the initial stage of production the protein is known as *protocollagen* and contains an unusually high content of proline and of lysine. These residues are hydroxylated to become the amino acids hydroxyproline and hydroxylysine, which are characteristic of collagen. This post-translational modification is catalysed by enzymes such as proline hydroxylase. At this stage the hydroxylated collagen is still soluble, has acquired its characteristic triple helix form, and is called *procollagen* or *tropocollagen*. However, connective tissue collagen is insoluble and thus the cell has the problem of transferring soluble procollagen out into the extracellular matrix and yet simultaneously rendering it insoluble. This is performed by a mechanism extensively employed by the body in the production of other proteins such as fibrin (p. 226). Procollagen is synthesised with an extra peptide on the end whose presence confers solubility. At the moment of secretion, the enzyme procollagen peptidase cleaves off the end that confers solubility, whereupon the rest of the collagen molecule promptly polymerises to form the typical insoluble, immensely strong, cross-banded fibres.

A further point to note is that there are currently recognised to be at least 17 different chemical forms of collagen, with slightly different properties and found in different sites. Type I is the most common form, followed by Type II found in cartilage and Type III which is found in embryonic tissue and fresh wounds.

Matrix production

The other main constituent of connective tissue is the *mucopolysaccharide* (also known as glycosaminoglycan) *matrix* and this too is synthesised by the fibroblast. Its chemical composition is very variable and depends on the type of connective tissue. It links to proteins to form proteoglycans, fibronectin and collagen Type I and III, the essential components of the extracellular matrix. Over the next few weeks alignment and remodelling of collagen occurs such that the Type III is replaced by Type I. The tissue becomes progressively denser, with most healing wounds reaching their optimal strength of union within a few weeks unless the tissue loss is very great. The zone of new, dense connective tissue is known as *scar*.

The fibroblast has another property, that of contractility. To be more precise, this is a function of the *myofibroblast*, a modified fibroblast with ultrastructural and functional properties of both fibroblasts and smooth muscle cells. The ability of skin wounds to contract in size in the first week or so has long been a puzzle and it used to be thought that the contraction was due to the collagen fibres themselves. It has now been shown that it is the myofibroblast which is responsible for this useful reduction in the size of wounds.

The cells contract in response to as yet unknown stimuli but certainly by virtue of their cytoplasmic fibrils of actomyosin. As they do so they pull in the margins of the wound and thus reduce the size of the denuded area. The success of the restoration of the integrity of skin can be measured by recording the tensile strength of the wound, i.e. the degree of force needed to pull the two edges apart. As little as seven days may be needed to restore tensile strength to normal. The ability to withstand such force is due to the way the polymerised collagen fibres are deposited. Not only do they knit tightly into the adjacent connective tissue by interweaving of fibres but the strands also orientate themselves so as to lie along the lines of maximal stress.

Primary and secondary union

Repair of our body surface has inevitably acquired much emotional charge. If the process were less efficient the subject would no doubt be the source of even more anxiety. This emotive element is revealed by the use of terms such as 'healing by primary union or first intention', or by 'secondary union or second intention'. *Primary union* means the healing of a simple incised wound with close apposition of the cut edges. *Secondary union* means the healing of a wound where there is a substantial tissue defect that has gradually to be filled in and replaced by new connective tissue (Fig. 15.8).

It is important to realise that the terms 'first intention' and 'second intention' refer to exactly the same process, the difference lying simply

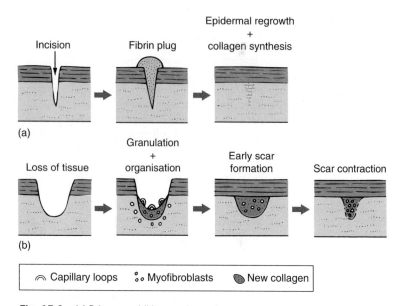

Fig. 15.8 (a) Primary and (b) secondary union.

in the amount of tissue that has been damaged and thus must be replaced. The events in both types of healing are the same, and under the microscope one can see all the features described above, the individual picture depending upon how far the response has proceeded towards completion. Generally, a number of young, thin-walled blood vessels are visible, apparently enmeshed in a pale staining jelly of mucopolysaccharide with variable numbers of fibroblasts, macrophages, granulocytes, red cells and collagen fibrils (Fig. 15.9).

Control of healing

The regeneration of epithelial layers is a highly coordinated and structured series of events taking place under complex control mechanisms that are incompletely understood. It is likely that it is mediated by a variety of chemical substances with both stimulatory and inhibitory influences, namely *growth factors* (p. 303). There is now evidence of the existence of a class of negative tissue regulators including:

- transforming growth factor
- fibroblast growth regulator
- anti-oncogene p53.

Considerably more evidence now exists for positively acting growth factors, and the best known that acts on epithelia is the peptide simply

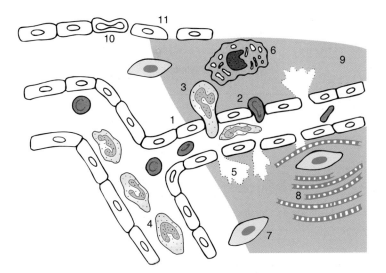

Fig. 15.9 The main features of a healing wound: 1. new vascular endothelium; 2. dropedesis of red cell; 3. emigration of leukocyte; 4. monocyte; 5. leakage of plasma; 6. macrophage; 7. fibroblast; 8. collagen; 9. mucopolysaccharide; 10. proliferating epithelium; 11. migrating epithelium.

termed *epidermal growth factor* (EGF) (Fig. 15.10). This material actively promotes mitotic division of skin epithelium in vivo and in tissue culture. It has the additional properties of promoting keratinisation of epithelium and accelerating migration of the cells across a surface, both of which would be useful in wound healing. It exists as a precursor complex with protein, from which it is released by the enzyme arginine esterase. This could be of significance since the same enzyme releases other biologically active peptides, e.g. kinins, relevant to tissue injury.

Epidermal growth factor appears to be but one of many growth factors which may act in concert in maintaining normal tissue architecture. Others with a postulated role in control of healing include platelet derived growth factor (PDGF) and TGF. Synergy and inhibition between these factors may form complex regulatory pathways for controlling epithelial cell proliferation and differentiation, both in normal development and in wound healing. It is conceivable that alterations in the control of such a mechanism may lead to pathological consequences and even be involved in neoplasia (see Ch. 26).

Regeneration in other organs

Growth factors exist for other types of tissue (e.g. nerves), and inhibitory growth factors have been proposed and have in some cases

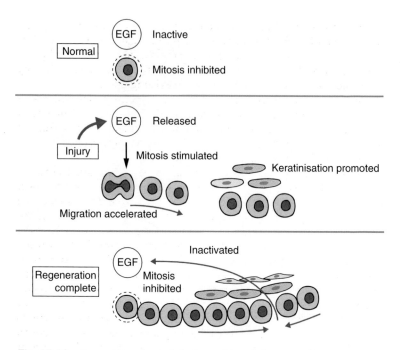

Fig. 15.10 How epidermal growth factor could control regeneration.

been identified, characterised and shown to be active in vitro and in vivo. However, the control of and interrelationships between such factors are still not known. It is more than likely that some disease processes are due to abnormalities of such control systems.

The liver

The capacity for liver regeneration was known to the ancient Greeks, since Prometheus was alleged to have had his liver eaten away every day by an eagle, yet it regenerated during the night! A similar experiment has been performed on rats: despite repeated subtotal hepatectomy, liver regeneration occurs. We understand little as yet about the control of this phenomenon.

Evidence of mitosis and selective cell death can be found in the normal liver. After the loss of liver cells by surgical extirpation or through chemical or biological damage, the process of liver cell division is greatly augmented. It is this cell proliferation which is responsible for the recovery of the organ's mass. Most of the mitotic activity takes place at the periphery of the hepatic lobule but is accompanied by migration of new cells to the centre of the lobule.

After partial surgical removal there is also regeneration of the portal tracts, including the branches of the portal vein therein, as well as hepatic artery radicles and bile ducts. There is preservation of architecture and the newly-formed lobules cannot be distinguished by their microscopic structure from the preexisting ones.

Well-organised regeneration of the liver is of importance in that it demonstrates that this capacity exists in highly developed organs of mammals and thus dismisses the simplistic generalisation about the inverse relationship between differentiation and phylogenetic level on one hand and regrowth potential on the other.

Liver hyperplasia in response to injury also has importance in human pathology because it is a prominent feature of the most important chronic liver disease, *cirrhosis*. The name derives from the Greek word for tawny, the colour (due to iron accumulation) of the afflicted liver. The essential features are a massive overgrowth of the fibrous stroma of the portal tracts, together with proliferation of the bile ducts, coupled with evidence of liver cell death or dysfunction, and above all with large areas of liver cell regeneration. The regenerated cells are commonly present in abnormal masses (regenerative nodules) lacking the normal architecture and probably with abnormal functional capacity. It is likely that cirrhosis represents a process of liver regeneration following injury, e.g. due to viruses, alcohol or other toxins, in which all the elements of the organ participate but in which the liver cells themselves regenerate inadequately because the injurious stimulus persists. The result is functional liver failure, with complications due to abnormal patterns of blood circulation through the organ (p. 241).

Differences in regeneration

One or two other examples of regeneration deserve mention. The inability of skin epithelium, with certain exceptions, to reform specialised appendages has already been noted. This incomplete adaptation does not apply to the mucous membrane of the stomach and intestine, which after surgical removal will reconstitute all the original cell types, including highly specialised secretory epithelium.

At the other end of the spectrum is the slow regeneration of the endothelium which lines large arteries such as the aorta. It may take months before a denuded area is fully lined by these cells, in sharp contrast to the exuberant proliferation of apparently identical capillary endothelium in regenerating connective tissue. Surgeons accelerate the reforming of the aortic lining after excision of a diseased segment by inserting artificial grafts. The synthetic material provides a framework for organised blood clot which contains capillary endothelium and it may be these cells that supply a new source of aortic endothelium. The alveoli of the lungs are lined by fairly simple cell types but regeneration after excision or damage is minimal. The explanations for the discrepancies in regenerative powers are still poorly understood but may reflect differential sensitivity to growth factors.

Healing of bones

Fractured bones heal in much the same way as subcutaneous tissue. The broken area fills with blood clot which is removed by mononuclear phagocytes (macrophages) (Fig. 15.11). Blood vessels grow into the area followed by migrating *osteoblasts*. These are a specialised form of cell, probably akin to the fibroblast, derived by proliferation of osteoblasts on the periosteum, the membrane covering the bone surface. The osteoblasts secrete collagen and mucopolysaccharides, known collectively in this context as *osteoid* (Fig. 15.12). Minerals are deposited in this material as apatite complexes of calcium, phosphate and magnesium.

The mass of calcified tissue is known as provisional *callus*. It is quickly remodelled by phagocytic giant cells known as *osteoclasts*, which are probably a bone marrow derived cell similar to mononuclear phagocytes. At the same time the bone is reconstructed to recover its final form complete with Haversian canals and related structures.

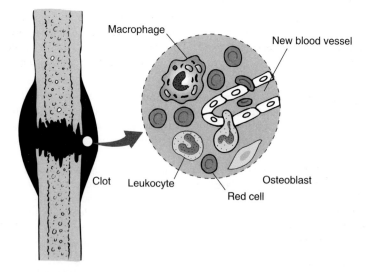

Fig. 15.11   Early events in healing of a fracture.

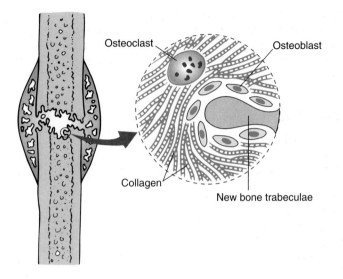

Fig. 15.12   Later events in healing of a fracture.

Factors influencing wound healing

Generally speaking wound healing is an efficient process whose progress is hard to arrest. There are factors, however, which can interfere with almost any stage (Table 15.1):

1. If the scavenging phase is disturbed, then healing will be slow. The most common cause is persistent active *inflammation*, for example from bacterial infection. This provides new exudate faster than the macrophages can remove it, or may replace macrophages

Table 15.1   Factors influencing wound healing

Local
Inadequate blood supply
Infection
Early movement
Foreign bodies or tissue
Irradiation

Systemic
Malnutrition (protein)
Vitamin C deficiency
Zinc deficiency
Corticosteroids
Jaundice

with polymorphonuclear phagocytes. It may also damage the macrophages by the action of bacterial toxins, or interfere with the phagocytosis of debris by blocking the phagocytic receptor sites on the surface with immunoglobulin plus bacterial antigen (p. 28).

2. A good blood supply is essential for wound healing since the actively metabolising site needs oxygen and substrates to provide it with energy, and new blood vessels must reach it from a patent adjacent microcirculation. As an example, elderly patients with *poor arterial circulation* develop poorly healing ulcers of the feet after only minor trauma.

3. *Excess movement* of the damaged wound site will obviously impede the remodelling process and in healing bones is a particularly serious handicap to good union.

4. *Foreign materials* such as sutures can also slow healing by causing mild inflammation and increasing the risk of infection.

5. *Chemical factors* may interfere with wound healing. Lack of ascorbic acid (vitamin C) prevents hydroxylation of proline and thus makes it impossible to synthesise mature cross-linked collagen. The active principle, β-amino propionitrile, causes inhibition of collagen cross-linking by blocking the cross-linking enzyme lysyl oxidase.

6. Simple malnutrition does not prevent wound healing, but *protein deficiency* in particular may seriously slow it. There is evidence that some trace elements, notably zinc, may be required in high amounts for optimal healing, perhaps because of its role as a co-factor in DNA and RNA polymerase.

7. *Corticosteroids* are thought to slow healing but because of their wide range of effects the mechanisms are unclear.

8. Finally, *jaundice* may inhibit wound healing. It is not clear whether this is a direct consequence of bilirubin or a reflection of disordered liver metabolism.

KEY POINTS

- Healing is a coordinated series of events in response to an injury resulting in repair and regeneration.
- The degree of regeneration varies greatly between organs of the body (e.g. brain and liver).
- The principal phases of healing are:
  — demolition (whereby debris is cleared)
  — epidermal proliferation
  — angiogenesis
  — production of extracellular matrix
  — formation of scar tissue.
- Both stimulatory and inhibitory growth factors control the process.
- A number of local and systemic factors influence rates of healing.

16 Basic genetic mechanisms

The first genes on earth probably appeared three thousand years ago. All human cells have variations of the same set of genes or *genome*, consisting of approximately 100 000 genes made up of 3 billion base pairs. Genes code for proteins but similar products can be made by expressing a variety of different proteins.

There is far more DNA than needed to make proteins. About 95% of the genome is believed to be non-functional and made up mainly of short apparently meaningless repeat sequences which are of uncertain purpose. We share 98.4% of our genetic material with chimpanzees and have many similar genes to fruit flies, which shows how far we have evolved.

Nucleotides and DNA

Deoxyribonucleic acid (DNA) is composed of chains of nucleotides, each nucleotide being made up of:

- a deoxyribose sugar
- a phosphate molecule
- a nitrogenous base.

The deoxyribose sugars and phosphate molecules link together to form a backbone.

The nitrogenous bases, of which there are four in DNA—*adenine, thymine, guanine* and *cytosine*—pair specifically with each other: adenine with thymine, and guanine with cytosine. The DNA molecule is therefore composed of two strands of nucleotides which are held together by hydrogen bonds and form a double helix (Fig. 16.1).

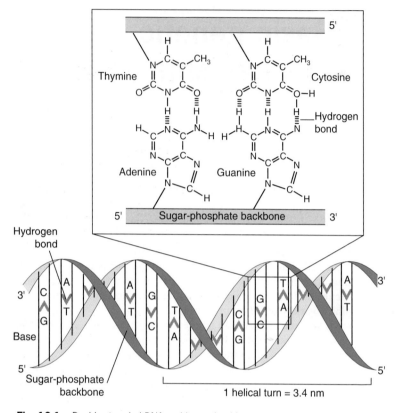

Fig. 16.1   Double-stranded DNA and its nucleotide structure.

Protein synthesis

A *gene* is a highly variable length of DNA which codes for a specific protein. It consists of subunits called *codons* which contain a sequence of three bases. There are 64 possible codon combinations corresponding to 20 common amino acids. Some amino acids are therefore coded by more than one codon, while other codons are stop and start markers of protein synthesis. Most genes from nucleated (i.e. eukaryotic) cells have coding sequences, which are called *exons*, interrupted by non-coding sequences called *introns*.

The first step in protein synthesis is *DNA transcription*: a single strand of ribonucleic acid (RNA) called *messenger RNA* (mRNA) is made from one of the DNA strands, which acts as a template. RNA is similar to DNA except that it is single stranded and contains *uracil* in place of thymine. Introns are then excised from the messenger RNA and the exons are spliced together (Fig. 16.2).

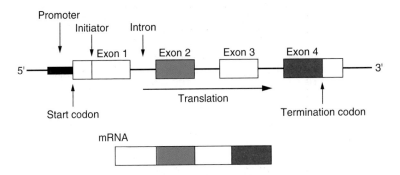

Fig. 16.2 Simplified structure of a gene and its mRNA product. Upstream of the gene is a promoter DNA sequence through which, by specific binding with regulating proteins, the translation of the gene is controlled. Start and termination codes mark the limits of the gene, bounded by untranslated sequences. The encoding portion of the gene is divided into exons, four in this example, interspersed with introns which do not appear in the mRNA product.

Transfer RNA (tRNA) is a complex about 80 nucleotides long. It carries specific amino acids and the anti-codon corresponding to a three-base coding region. For example, the anti-codon for GUG (i.e. CAC) is present on the tRNA carrying valine (Table 16.1).

A *ribosome* (a large protein synthesising machine) is required to order the tRNA molecules on the mRNA. It is a complex of more than 50 different proteins associated with several structural RNA molecules. The tRNA molecules position themselves on the ribosome and, as the ribosome moves along the mRNA molecule translating the nucleotide sequence into an amino acid sequence, the tRNA molecules add amino acids to the growing end of the polypeptide chain.

Transcription factors and gene regulation

Transcription is the production of a primary RNA transcript from the DNA of a particular gene and is the first stage of gene expression. It is the primary target of gene regulation, enabling the production of different proteins in different tissues.

There are many steps in the pathway leading from DNA to protein at which gene expression can be regulated. These are:

- transcriptional control (when and how frequently a gene is transcribed)
- RNA processing control
- RNA transport control to the cytoplasm
- RNA translational control by ribosomes
- mRNA degradation control.

Table 16.1 The genetic code. Nucleotides code in sets of three, or triplets, for individual amino acids. The triplets or codons are shown as they appear in DNA (T = thymine, C = cytosine, A = adenine, G = guanine). In mRNA, T is replaced by U (uracil). The code is degenerate, i.e. there can be more than one codon per amino acid. The genetic code is read from left to right, i.e. TTC = Phe (phenylalanine); TCC = Ser (serine); CCT = Pro (proline)

First nucleotide	Second nucleotide				Third nucleotide
[5']	T	C	A	G	[3']
T	Phe	Ser	Tyr	Cys	T
T	Phe	Ser	Tyr	Cys	C
T	Leu	Ser	STOP	STOP	A
T	Leu	Ser	STOP	Trp	G
C	Leu	Pro	His	Arg	T
C	Leu	Pro	His	Arg	C
C	Leu	Pro	Gln	Arg	A
C	Leu	Pro	Gln	Arg	G
A	Ile	Thr	Asn	Ser	T
A	Ile	Thr	Asn	Ser	C
A	Ile	Thr	Lys	Arg	A
A	Met	Thr	Lys	Arg	G
G	Val	Ala	Asp	Gly	T
G	Val	Ala	Asp	Gly	C
G	Val	Ala	Glu	Gly	A
G	Val	Ala	Glu	Gly	G

Amino acids are Phe = phenylalanine; Ser = serine; Tyr = tyrosine; Cys = cysteine; Trp = tryptophan; Leu = leucine; Pro = proline; His = histidine; Gln = glutamine; Arg = arginine; Ile = isoleucine; Met = methionine; Thr = threonine; Asn = asparagine; Lys = lysine; Val = valine; Ala = alanine; Asp = aspartic acid; Glu = glutamic acid; Gly = glycine.

Transcription is dependent upon specific gene regulatory proteins called *transcription factors*. These bind to particular DNA sequences in gene regulatory regions and control their transcription, thereby regulating the activity of a gene and its response to particular stimuli in different tissues and allowing tissue-specific gene expression. Modulation is achieved either by regulating the synthesis of the particular transcription factor, or by ensuring that an active form of the transcription factor is produced only in response to a specific signal.

An example of this mechanism is provided by the oct-2 transcription factor. This factor is involved in stimulation of immunoglobulin gene expression in B cells and is not expressed in cells that do not express immunoglobulin genes. The transcription factor nuclear factor κB (NFκB) is present in an inactive form in most cells because it is complexed to an inhibitory protein. In mature B cells the inhibitory protein is removed, enabling the transcription factor to move into the nucleus, where it can activate immunoglobulin gene expression. The combination of transcription factor synthesis and activity regulation therefore allows transcription factors to regulate the expression of numerous different genes and different cell types.

Genes and chromosomes

A gene contains an average of 30 000 base pairs, although this can vary from a few hundred to over a million base pairs. These form sequences of codons that contain some of the information required to construct a living organism (Table 16.2).

Genes are sited at specific chromosomal loci and there may be variations of the gene (called *alleles*, p. 76).

When maternal and paternal alleles are identical an individual is *homozygous* for that allele; if the individual inherits different alleles at that locus, he or she is *heterozygous*. There is therefore a 50% chance that a particular allele will be inherited from a heterozygous parent, and if both parents are heterozygous there is a 25% chance that the child will be homozygous.

The genes for specific proteins are located on different chromosomes, for example:

- Rhesus blood group genes, chromosome 1
- HLA Class I and II and complement genes, chromosome 6
- erythropoietin, chromosome 7
- β, γ and δ chains of haemoglobin, chromosome 11
- α_1-antitrypsin, chromosome 14
- haptoglobin, chromosome 16.

A *chromosome* is a continuous branch of DNA containing about 130 million base pairs, of which only about 5% is used to code for about 30 expressed genes. The DNA is tightly coiled and combined with a

Table 16.2 Approximate sizes of different subsamples of human DNA

Whole genome	*3 billion base pairs (2 metres long extended)*
Each chromosome	130 million base pairs on average (range 26–248 million containing 3000 genes)
Chromosome fragment detectable by light microscopy	5 million base pairs (contains ≈30 genes)
Each gene	30 000 base pairs (range 5–100 000 base pairs)

protein. Histones are commonly found in chromosomal proteins and when complexed with the nuclear DNA of eukaryotic cells are known as *chromatin*. Stained chromosomes have dark bands which are specific for each chromosome.

Chromosomes can be visualised at mitosis and during metaphase, and consist of two *chromatids* joined at a *centromere*. In healthy humans there are 46 diploid chromosomes (i.e. 23 pairs).

The study and detection of chromosomal abnormalities has been greatly improved by the use of *banding techniques* in a field known as cytogenetics. These are special stains which pick out the chromosome very clearly. Band staining can be achieved with Giemsa (G), chloroquine (C), reverse staining (R) or chromatin staining (C). Each stain delineates different regions and bands on the chromosome so it is necessary to specify which was used. Using all possible permutations, up to 10 000 bands can be detected on human chromosomes if special techniques are used which 'stretch' the chromosome. A new technique in cytogenetics is fluorescence in situ hybridisation (FIST) which allows small deletions to be detected. As a result of these advances, many new chromosomal syndromes have been described in the past few years. Most of the new defects can be localised quite specifically; for example, deletion of band 2 in region 14 of the long arm of chromosome 13 in retinoblastoma, a malignant tumour of childhood. This is written 13q14.2. If the short arm of the chromosome is affected the letter p is substituted for q. In the future there will be no clear division between cytogenetics and molecular genetics.

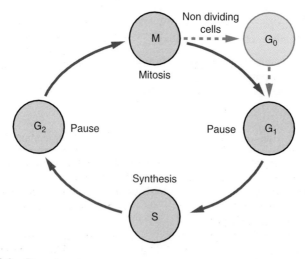

Fig. 16.3 The cell cycle.

Cell division

The reproductive cycle of a eukaryotic cell is divided into five phases (Fig. 16.3):

- G_1 (gap 1)
- S (DNA synthesis)
- G_2 (gap 2)
- M (mitosis)
- G_0 (optional resting phase).

The cell cycle requires activating signals: these are soluble cytoplasmic factors which when stimulatory are known as cyclins and are functional in different phases of the cycle. Inhibitory signals come from tumour suppressor genes (e.g. p53) and cyclin dependent kinase inhibitors.

Control of cell division

Growth factors

Cell division in multicellular organisms is very well regulated; this is achieved by protein growth factors which direct the proliferation of different cell types and generally act as local chemical mediators regulating cell population densities. Examples of protein growth factors are:

- platelet derived growth factors (PDGF)
- epidermal growth factor (EGF)
- transforming growth factor (TGF, p. 305).

Cell division stops after mitosis if growth factors and matrix adhesion are lacking. The cells then enter the quiescent phase G_0. If a cell passes G_0 there is a point of no return in G_1 phase, after which it will enter S, G_2 and M phases irrespective of the presence of growth factors or matrix adhesion.

Mitosis and meiosis

For the purposes of this chapter there are two types of cell: *somatic* or *body cells,* and *germ cells (gametes),* i.e. ova and sperm. The information needed to reproduce a replica of a somatic cell is contained in the chromosomes of its nucleus. These can be studied by arresting the cell in the metaphase stage of mitotic division. The chromosome can be stained by a variety of techniques, photographed and arranged in order of size and shape.

In every cell (except gametes) there are 46 chromosomes, each composed of one molecule of double-stranded DNA. There are two sex (XX female or XY male) and 44 autosomal (i.e. non-sex) chromosomes, numbered from the largest (1) to the smallest (22). In the female each ovum contains one of the two X chromosomes, whereas in the male each spermatozoon contains either an X or a Y chromosome.

Somatic cell division involves *mitosis*, and the production of two new cells occurs when the chromosomes separate longitudinally.

In gamete production cell division involves *meiosis*: the diploid number of 46 chromosomes is reduced to the haploid number of 23 with each gamete having an assortment of maternally and paternally derived genes. At fertilisation parental gametes are fused, resulting in a diploid number of chromosomes.

Molecular biology and genetic disease

In 1980 the first human genes were cloned and sequenced and since then remarkable progress has been made in unravelling the molecular biology of single gene disorders. Any gene that is worth studying can now be isolated; the idea of a complete map of the human genome, which would have been ridiculed a few years ago, is becoming a reality and is likely to be completed by 2005.

Gene analysis

The analysis of a single gene within the enormous quantity of genetic material in a cell depends on first shortening and purifying the long strand of human DNA isolated from tissues or peripheral blood lymphocytes into reproducible sections. The isolated DNA is treated with a *restriction enzyme*, a naturally occurring endonuclease which cleaves DNA at specific sites determined by the base sequences. This generates *restriction fragments* which can be separated by electrophoresis. These fragments are made into single strands and fixed to a nitrocellulose sheet by a process known as Southern blotting (named after a scientist, not the compass point). The sequences of these fragments are then identified by means of 'gene' or 'DNA' *probes* which are single-stranded copies of a sequence of DNA, having been cloned in bacteriophages or plasmids and labelled with a radioisotope. The radioisotope probe is added and hybridises with the fragment that contains a complementary sequence. This produces a radioactive band which can be recognised on an autoradiograph.

DNA polymorphisms

Only a small proportion of total genomic DNA codes for proteins; the intervening DNA is subject to point mutations and natural variation. One base change per 100 nucleotides occurs and results in differences

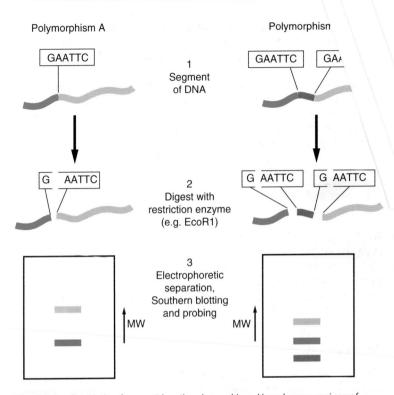

Fig. 16.4 Restriction fragment length polymorphism. Homologous regions of anonymous DNA from two individuals are shown. The polymorphic variations can be detected as follows: *Step 1*. The DNA is isolated. *Step 2*. The DNA is incubated with a restriction enzyme (EcoR1 in this example) that specifically recognises and splits DNA at sites only where there is a GAATTC base sequence. One such site exists in polymorphism A; an additional site is present in polymorphism B. *Step 3*. The enzymatically digested DNA fragments are loaded onto a gel and separated in an electric field according to their molecular sizes. After absorption onto a sheet of nitrocellulose filter paper (Southern blot), the location of the fragments of the polymorphic region can be visualised by probing with a radioactive complementary DNA strand. (MW = molecular weight)

in the chromosome pair; each change produces different restriction fragments when cut by the enzyme from each of the chromosome pair and is known as a *restriction fragment length polymorphism* (RFLP; Fig. 16.4). Identification of the RFLP (as present or absent), which is not usually of functional importance, allows the tracking of transmission of a single chromosome region through a family and enables linkage studies of *single gene disorders* to be performed. There are two other types of DNA polymorphism. Variable number tandem repeats (VNTRs) are different length fragments caused by insertion of a variable number of repeat units of base pairs. There is often a number of variants at each site. The third type, single sequence repeats (SSRs), are very small and vary in the number of, say, CA repeats. Amplification produces fragments of variable size.

There are many molecular techniques used for genetic analysis, for example:

- Northern blotting: a similar technique used by molecular investigators for RNA analysis
- Western blotting: cell protein analysis used by protein chemists
- polymerase chain reaction (PCR; Fig. 16.5) which allows multiple amplifications of a DNA fragment using DNA polymerase, primers and free nucleotides; it is now an essential step in nearly all genetic analyses
- polymorphism or mutation detection, using single strand conformation polymorphism (SSCP), denaturing gradient gel electrophoresis (DGGE), both of which involve electrophoresis, or

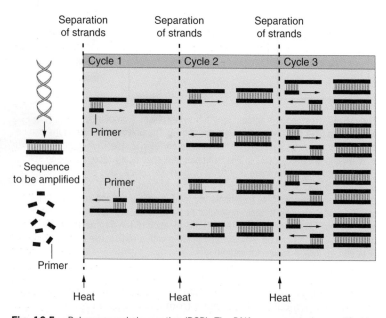

Fig. 16.5   Polymerase chain reaction (PCR). The DNA sequence to be amplified is selected by short synthetic oligonucleotide primers which correspond to the sequences flanking the target DNA. Excess primers and a heat stable polymerase are added and the mixture heated to separate the primers and the DNA. The mix is allowed to cool (annealing temperature), the primers bind and the polymerase elongates the primers on either strand, thus generating two new identical double-stranded DNA molecules. Each cycle doubles the number of copies of the original DNA fragment.

chemical cleavage of mismatch method (CCM) using chemical enzymes
- biallelic marker detection of random mutations in base pairs (single nucleotide polymorphisms—SNPs) throughout the genome; up to 3 million of these mutations exist, and markers to detect them are being developed
- gene chips, allowing rapid detection of large numbers of SNP gene markers without gels or electrophoresis using simple chemical reactions.

The main strategies for discovering genes involved in common polygenic diseases (functional genetics) are:

1. direct sequencing of genes expressed on the diseased tissues, known as expressed sequence tags (ESTs)
2. positional cloning, whereby gene markers evenly spaced over the genome are used to link a region to a disease where the protein is unknown
3. candidate genes—polymorphisms of known genes which are tested for their association or linkage with a disease.

The clinical samples most often used for gene discovery are large multigeneration families or large numbers of sibling pairs with the disease or trait of interest.

The clinical implication of genetic analysis

In many rarer diseases where a single major gene is responsible, the gene producing the defect is now known, even though the disease mechanism may be poorly understood. This has enabled prenatal and clinical diagnosis to be performed in incurable diseases such as cystic fibrosis, Huntington's chorea, muscular dystrophy and the haemoglobinopathies. The list of diseases in which genetic analysis is becoming possible is ever increasing.

For diseases showing *polygenic inheritance* (known also as complex trait diseases), a large number of different genes may be found to contribute to disease susceptibility, however the extent of each gene's contribution may vary, so that at least 20 genes are presently believed to regulate blood cholesterol levels—variation at two loci, apo-E and apo-B, may contribute 40% of the total genetic variance. Potentially, therefore, the genetic prediction of risk of coronary heart disease and other complex trait diseases may become possible.

Other common diseases such as asthma, diabetes, hypertension, depression, psoriasis, schizophrenia, obesity, osteoporosis and osteoarthritis have been recently recognised to be under genetic influence. They are all likely to be influenced by a number of different genes which it is hoped will be identified in the next decade as rapid leaps in technology occur.

KEY POINTS

- The genome consists of 3 billion base pairs made up of about 100 000 genes.
- Genes are lengths of DNA which code for specific proteins. Genes for specific proteins are located on different chromosomes.
- Their production of proteins is regulated by specific proteins called transcription factors and involves messenger RNA.
- There is a natural variation in 1% of the base pairs which allows polymorphisms to occur (RFLPs, VNTRs or SSRs); these are useful for identifying genes associated with disease.
- When identical alleles of a gene are inherited from both parents an individual is homozygous for that allele; if the parents differ for that allele the individual is heterozygous.
- Genes or variations in them can be isolated and analysed by various methods to enable diagnosis pre- or postnatally, to detect linkage with a disease and also to understand new physiological processes.
- By 2005, most human genes will be identified and a physical map of the genome will be complete. The challenge then will be to identify the function of the genes.

17 | Genetic abnormality

Introduction

A *congenital disease* is one with which the patient is born, and an *inherited disease* is one which is due to factors in the genetic material received from the parents. Both terms are often used loosely or synonymously but an inherited disease might not become apparent until middle age and is not therefore truly congenital. The subject is awesome in scope because, quite apart from obvious inherited defects (and these are numerous enough), even infectious diseases such as tuberculosis may exhibit inherited susceptibility as may conditions as diverse as cancer (p. 277), osteoporosis or cardiac infarction (p. 196). Thus, although an increasing number of chronic diseases are now known to be under genetic influence, the bulk of this chapter will concern itself with diseases in which inherited factors are the sole or major determining element.

A detailed logical classification of genetic abnormality is not yet possible. For the purposes of this chapter, therefore, it is proposed to consider such diseases as falling into one of three categories as follows:

1. abnormalities of genes
2. abnormalities of chromosomes
3. polygenic inheritance and abnormalities occurring after fertilisation.

This classification is based not so much on aetiology as on pathogenesis since a variety of factors known or unknown could activate any of these mechanisms.

Genetic disease may result from an abnormality of a single gene (e.g. thalassaemia or cystic fibrosis) or chromosome (e.g. Turner's syndrome). More commonly, however, it results from a combination of genetic and environmental factors.

Teratology

Before discussing this important topic it is necessary briefly to review current knowledge of inheritance and intrauterine development. This involves two separate subjects: the transmission of genetic information (genetics) and the control of growth and differentiation in the developing embryo (embryology). The pathological counterpart of embryology is teratology, the scientific study of congenital malformations. Since morphological defects present at birth may be monogenic, polygenic or environmental (see p. 184), teratology can involve study of all these mechanisms. Abnormal development of the embryo after successful fertilisation and implantation is, however, a major cause of such illness. Unfortunately, compared with the mass of information on genetics, there is still a great deal of ignorance concerning the environmental factors controlling growth and development of the fetus.

A number of substances are known to cause anatomical deformities in the newborn, often of one particular part of the body. Such agents are known as *teratogens* and fall into three classes:

1. viruses
2. irradiation
3. chemicals.

Irradiation

Irradiation—mainly X-rays, gamma rays or beta particles—may act chiefly by causing faulty chromosomal separation or an increased mutation rate (p. 299). Certainly the survivors of the Hiroshima atomic bomb explosion produced a higher proportion of deformed babies and for this reason pregnant women are subjected to radiography as infrequently as possible.

Viruses

Most viruses do not pass the placental barrier. The most important exception is *rubella* (German measles) which is liable to produce serious defects if the mother becomes infected in the early months of pregnancy. The fetus itself becomes infected and may suffer mental subnormality, cardiac malformations, blindness or deafness. In the case of deafness, at least, there is good evidence that its appearance depends upon a polygenic type of inherited predisposition as outlined above. In other words even the rubella virus needs a genetically susceptible fetus if it is to produce damage.

Cytomegalic inclusion virus is apt to cause fetal infection in utero by placental growth. Such infection usually leads to stillbirth but survivors may show defective cerebral development.

Genetic factors may also affect the fetus during pregnancy in other ways, for example:

- Phenylketonuria is associated with phenylalanine birth defects, such as mental retardation, hypopigmented skin and hair and eczema.
- Rhesus incompatibility causes erythroblastosis (p. 247).

Chemicals

Chemical teratogens have aroused much interest because of the disastrous effects of *thalidomide*, an otherwise useful sedative. Pregnant women taking this substance produced a high proportion of children with badly deformed arms or legs. Chemical teratogens show high species specificity and thalidomide has only weak effects on the offspring of rats, mice and rabbits.

Some teratogens have known destructive effects on the developing cells of the various anatomical systems of the fetus. In this category are cytotoxic drugs, e.g. cyclophosphamide used to destroy rapidly dividing cancer cells, and also, paradoxically, cancer-inducing compounds such as dimethylnitrosamine.

There is a long list of chemicals which have been found to cause general or specific anatomical malformations in various species, but information relating directly to man is scanty. A variety of *environmental pollutants* have been suggested, e.g. arsenic, cadmium, mercury, indium and lead. Excess of vitamin A has been proposed as a cause of brain malformation, as have mouldy potatoes. Because of these uncertainties it is standard practice not to give new drugs to pregnant women.

There is increasing evidence that the *lack of certain vitamins* may affect the fetus. Maternal multivitamin and folic acid supplementation is associated with a reduction in the incidence of live births with spina bifida and anencephaly.

Disease can result from an interaction between genetic and environmental factors in other ways. Inherited genetic mutations may cause *idiosyncratic clinical reactions* in response to:

- drugs (e.g. hydralazine)
- cigarette smoking (e.g. α_1-antitrypsin deficiency and emphysema)
- sunlight (xeroderma pigmentosum and malignancy)
- milk (e.g. galactosaemia).

Single gene abnormalities

The steps considered in the previous chapter lead to the formation of gametes which may produce normal offspring or may yield children with an inherited defect due to faulty genetic or chromosomal behaviour. Defective fertilisation of the gamete or faulty implantation in the uterus of the fertilised ovum may abort the conception but are unlikely to lead to congenital disease. In inherited disease the system fails at a point where the DNA molecule replicates itself during cell division by acquiring new bases from the nuclear sap to form new base pairs. If mistakes occur, faulty base pairing results and leads to mutation. Figure 17.1 shows the normal process of DNA replication as it occurs in dividing cells. The process has been likened to the formation of two new zip fasteners from one. As new bases arrive, the original paired strands of DNA peel away from each other carrying the newly attached bases with them. Mutation can occur at the level of individual genes (point mutation) or can involve whole chromosomes. In both cases it usually happens when the DNA strand is dividing and can occur spontaneously or be induced by ionising radiation or chemicals.

There are a number of mechanisms for single gene mutation, for example:

• the gene may be deleted (e.g. the gene for α-globin giving rise to alpha thalassaemia)
• there may be a single base change due to nucleotide insertion, deletion or rearrangement in either the intron or exon regions, as occurs in sickle cell anaemia and other haemoglobinopathies
• sometimes genes fuse.

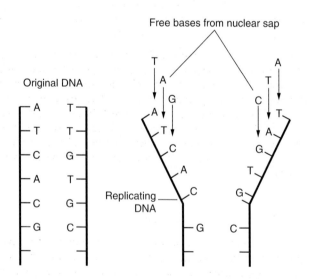

Fig. 17.1   One way in which single gene abnormalities originate. At the time of mitotic DNA replication in the germ cell, if new bases from the nuclear sap pair up in the wrong order, the new DNA is not an accurate copy of the original and a point mutation occurs.

Single gene disorders cause abnormalities for a variety of reasons including:

- an absence of protein end-product (e.g. aminoacidopathies)
- a tendency to cause chromosome breakage and a predisposition to malignancy (e.g. Fanconi's anaemia, ataxia telangiectasia, Bloom's syndrome and xeroderma pigmentosum).

Inheritance and single gene disorders

Single gene abnormalities are inherited as dominant, recessive or sex linked.

Autosomal dominant disorders are those diseases that are manifest in the heterozygous state. Only one abnormal gene (i.e. mutant allele) is present and the corresponding partner allele on the homologous chromosome is normal.

These conditions can be traced in family trees and are inherited according to the principles of Mendelian genetics. This means that they are due to point mutations in single genes and are called monogenic. From the viewpoint of the geneticist they come in three types: *dominant, intermediate (co-dominant)* or *recessive*. From the viewpoint of the pathologist they are manifest in two ways:

1. as anatomical defects, obvious grossly at birth
2. as abnormalities, functional or structural or both, which become apparent during childhood or adult life.

In the latter group are the classic inborn errors of metabolism in which the abnormality, however wide-reaching its effects, can often be traced to lack of a single enzyme. Also in this group is the much studied disease of *haemophilia*, caused by deficiency of a particular protein. Another disease in the group, which because of the painting by Velasquez is as famous as haemophilia, is *achondroplasia*, a characteristic growth defect. In achondroplasia, as in other genetically determined anatomical disorders, the gene defect causes structural abnormalities.

Single protein and enzyme deficiences

When a single protein or enzyme is demonstrably deficient, as in haemophilia or phenylketonuria, an error in coding has occurred involving a single gene or *cistron*, since this is the genetic unit responsible for a single protein. In fact, the error may be restricted to one codon since only one amino acid in the protein may be wrongly placed, as it is in the abnormal haemoglobin which when inherited causes the disease of sickle cell anaemia.

To the molecular and cellular biologist, the interest of genetic disease lies in the particular segments of the DNA strands which are wrongly assembled so that they code for an abnormal protein. As we have noted earlier, these errors occur during the replication of the DNA strands (chromosomes), are due to faulty pairing of bases and are known as *mutations*. Mutations can be caused by irradiation, or by chemicals or drugs or can occur spontaneously. Some genes are especially liable to spontaneous mutation. These unstable cistrons include those responsible for two diseases already mentioned, haemophilia and achondroplasia.

The *inborn errors of metabolism*, of which there are several thousand known examples, are each due to a genetically determined deficiency of one particular enzyme. The enzyme may be present in the mitochondria, endoplasmic reticulum or lysosomes, and no aspect of metabolism is spared. One of the most important consequences of these metabolic defects is *mental subnormality*, the brain cells being especially susceptible to damage from abnormal chemical metabolites. Mental impairment can develop from very different causes ranging from the abnormal accumulation of intracellular lipids due to lack of a lysosomal enzyme, sphingomyelinase (Niemann–Pick disease), to the accumulation of a toxic metabolite of phenylalanine due to lack of phenylalanine hydroxylase (phenylketonuria). These metabolic errors affect the child at a crucial stage of its development; if it can be tided over by feeding artificial diets free of the substrate, e.g. phenylalanine, which yields the toxic products, it may in adult life be found to have enough of the appropriate enzyme to live normally.

The examples of genetic disease so far quoted are easy enough to understand on the basis of errors of coding in specific cistrons or codons. However, there are conditions which are passed on from one generation to the next in classical Mendelian fashion but in which it is more difficult to imagine the mode of action of the faulty gene. There is for example the disease of anonychia in which there is a variable degree of malformation of the hands or nails. If the development of individual parts of the body were controlled directly by individual genes, there should be many other examples of comparable malformations inherited by Mendelian laws, but there are not. It may be, therefore, that in anonychia there is deficiency of a particular bodily protein or enzyme, the lack of which is critical only as regards the hands and nails. Similarly, some forms of cancer are transmitted by genetic faults, e.g. neuroblastoma or polyposis coli, and there are rare families in which thickening of the soles of the feet and cancer of the oesophagus are inherited in classical Mendelian fashion. It is difficult to make such pedigrees fit the accepted facts of gene action, but not impossible, since a single protein or enzyme could be imagined which restrains uncontrolled growth of certain cells or which inactivates certain cancer-inducing genes (p. 277).

The known *genetic abnormalities of the haemoglobin gene* provide a rich spectrum of disease mechanisms. This gene seems especially vulnerable and there are many diseases associated with abnormal haemoglobin. The best known is sickle cell anaemia in which, although only one amino acid is wrongly placed, fatal haemolytic anaemia may result due to crystallisation of haemoglobin and disruption of red blood corpuscles (p. 248). Understanding of the haemoglobinopathies represents a triumph of modern science. Thalassaemia, in particular, where there is an imbalance of production of globin protein and/or abnormal globin molecules are produced, can now be explained at the molecular level. There are many other types of haemolytic anaemia which are due to deficiencies of various respiratory enzymes in the red cell, e.g. glucose-6-phosphate dehydrogenase.

Carbohydrate metabolism genes

There are a variety of *disorders of carbohydrate metabolism* caused by deficiency of a single sugar metabolising enzyme, e.g. galactose-1-phosphate uridyltransferase which causes the disease galactosaemia, resulting in mental subnormality and death. Glycogen may be stored in vast amounts in the liver or spleen because of the lack of one of eight glycogen metabolising enzymes. There are similar *storage diseases of lipids*, e.g. Gaucher's disease due to genetically determined deficiency of glucosylcerebroside hydrolase (glucocerebrosidase).

The *porphyrin metabolising enzymes* may be absent with catastrophic results (George III is reputed to have suffered from one disease in this category and the loss of the American colonies has been blamed on his porphyria).

Amino acid metabolising enzymes may be deficient, e.g. tyrosinase leading to the albino state (melanin pigment cannot be formed) or phenylalanine hydroxylase causing phenylketonuria and mental defect as already mentioned.

Purine or pyrimidine metabolism may be disturbed, e.g. due to lack of xanthine oxidase, leading to xanthinuria so that stones form in the kidney. Gout is another inherited and much more common disorder of purine metabolism which leads to painful deposition of urate crystals in certain joints. This list is very far from complete but should give some idea of the scope of the subject even though many of these diseases are extremely rare.

Dominant inheritance

In this situation every individual carrying the abnormal gene suffers from the disease and pedigrees have a vertical mode of inheritance. Most serious genetic diseases are not dominant for the simple reason that a serious dominant genetic defect would soon extinguish itself from the population unless loss of a gene through death or infertility of the affected individual were balanced by a corresponding high mutation rate.

This is the state of affairs in *achondroplasia*, which is due to defective metabolism in bone epiphyses. The mutation rate of this dominant gene recently found to be part of the fibroblast growth factor on chromosome 4 has been measured and found to be 1:20 000. This means that once in every 20 000 replications the normal gene mutates. Since every individual has two such genes, one of each of the chromosome pair, he or she has two chances of suffering mutation, so that one child in 10 000 suffers from achondroplasia due to mutation in a parental gene. The achondroplastic population appears to be fairly constant in size, in spite of the fact that up to 80% die during childhood, which means that the rate of elimination due to the lowered average reproductive rate of those carrying the gene is balanced by the high mutation rate. In fact, the mutation rate can be calculated by equating it to the average effective fertility of affected persons as compared with normals. Dominant genes are controlled by the mutation rate for that gene. If reproduction is nil the gene can only be perpetuated by a very high mutation rate.

A dominant gene can be regarded as a defect, a single dose of which is able to produce disease. Thus most affected persons are *heterozygous*, i.e. one of the pair of genes is normal and the other is the abnormal mutant. There are rare cases in which an achondroplastic is found to be *homozygous* for the trait, i.e. both genes are abnormal, which means that an achondroplastic gene was received from both parents. This double dose of defective genetic material produces an achondroplastic not obviously different from a heterozygous achondroplastic. In the case of other dominant abnormal genes this is not the case. Thus those homozygous for brachydactyly (short fingers) have severe, widespread skeletal defects, whereas the heterozygotes merely have short fingers.

Recessive inheritance

A genetic abnormality is inherited recessively if it expresses itself only when present on both members of the affected chromosome pair of the individual concerned (Fig. 17.2). In other words a double dose of the abnormal gene is required to produce the disease. A single dose, i.e. one abnormal gene, produces no effect because it is dominated and suppressed by the corresponding normal gene on the other chromosome. This is the only difference between dominant and recessive genes but their distribution in the population is very different. In Britain the incidence of autosomal recessive inheritance is 2.5 per 100 live births. Pedigrees display a horizontal pattern of transmission.

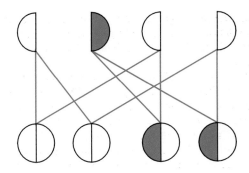

Fig. 17.2   Mendelian inheritance of disease. The semi-circles represent the parental gametes. The dark gametes carry the abnormal gene. The full circles represent the offspring. In this illustration one parent is heterozygous for the abnormal gene; the other parent is normal. Half the offspring will have the abnormal gene: if it is recessive, they will not develop the disease; if it is dominant, they will do so.

For any particular abnormal gene, heterozygotes are much more common than homozygotes (Fig. 17.3). Thus *albinism* (due to a defect in genetic coding for tyrosinase) affects about 1 in 10 000 people. Any given person stands a 1 in a 100 chance of receiving the abnormal gene on one of the relevant chromosome pair and a 1 in 100 chance of receiving it on the other chromosome of the pair, which is therefore a 1 in 50 chance of receiving it on one or other chromosome. This means that 1 person in 50 will be heterozygous for albinism. However, the chance of receiving two albinism genes, one from each parent, is 1 in 100 × 1 in 100, i.e. 1 in 10 000, which is the risk of being an albino.

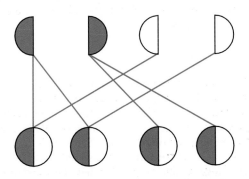

Fig. 17.3   In this example, one parent is homozygous for the above gene and one parent is normal—all offspring carry the affected gene and will be affected if dominant, or carriers if recessive.

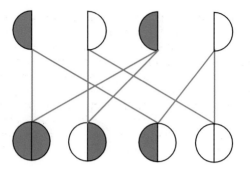

Fig. 17.4 In this example, both parents are heterozygous. Three children out of four will inherit the gene; one of them will be homozygous and develop the disease even if it is recessive.

When we see that a frequency of heterozygotes of 1 in 50 is necessary to produce 1 in 10 000 affected individuals, we realise how common are the genes of recessively inherited diseases compared with the diseases themselves, and how easily an abnormal recessive gene can be passed on undetected through several generations. Affected individuals usually arise from the mating of unaffected parents each of whom, however, is heterozygous for the condition. They will produce one affected (homozygous) child for every three unaffected (heterozygous) children. Since an individual carrying a defective gene is more likely to encounter that gene within his own family than in the general population, consanguineous marriages, e.g. between first cousins, have a greater than average chance of producing a homozygous, i.e. affected, child (Fig. 17.4). Consanguineous marriage does not influence the dominant gene inheritance of diseases such as achondroplasia where a single dose of defective gene material is sufficient. There are no known Y-linked disorders.

Sex-linked inheritance

If a mutant gene happens to be sited on the X or Y chromosomes the chance of an individual being affected will depend upon his or her sex. In practice, the X chromosome is usually involved because it contains about 80 possible mutant genes, including *haemophilia, colour blindness* and *muscular dystrophy* (Table 17.1). The male has only one X chromosome, so dominance and recessivity do not arise since there is no corresponding gene (allele) on the other chromosome to suppress or be suppressed, the other half of the chromosome pair being the Y chromosome. Hence, if a male carries the mutant gene he will exhibit the disease. If a female carries the mutant gene, she may or may not be affected depending on whether the gene is dominant or recessive and whether she is homozygous or heterozygous, i.e. whether she has inherited a single or double dose of aberrant genetic material. Thus, all males who inherit the haemophilia gene on their single X chromosome (1 in 10 000 males) will have haemophilia, but female haemophiliacs will be those who inherit the gene on both their X chromosomes, an exceedingly rare event. In other words, although haemophilia is carried on the female chromosome, practically all haemophiliacs are male. The chances of a female being a haemophiliac are 1 in 100 million, i.e. 1 in 10 000 × 1 in 10 000.

Table 17.1 Mode of inheritance of some genetic diseases

Dominant
Achondroplasia
Polyposis coli
Huntington's chorea
Epiloia
Porphyria variegata
Retinal aplasia
Anonychia
Congenital cataract
Marfan's syndrome

Recessive
Fibrocystic disease of the pancreas
Phenylketonuria
Albinism
Galactosaemia
Muscular dystrophy (late onset type)
Cretinism
Lipid storage diseases
Carbohydrate storage diseases
Glucose-6-phosphate dehydrogenase deficiency
Most other inborn errors of metabolism

Intermediate
Thalassaemia major/minor
Sickle cell anaemia/trait

Sex linked (X chromosome)
Haemophilia
Muscular dystrophy (Duchenne type)
Colour blindness
Chronic granulomatous disease

Sex linked (Y chromosome)
Hairy ears

Intermediate inheritance

We have seen that rare individuals who are homozygous for some dominant genes have a more severe form of disease than the more usual heterozygotes. Conversely, some heterozygotes with recessive genes show a milder form of the disturbance than is displayed by those with both defective genes, i.e. the homozygotes. This incomplete expression in heterozygotes is known as intermediate or co-dominant inheritance and is of importance in tracing carriers of a defective gene.

There are several important examples of intermediate inheritance in human pathology. The gene of *phenylketonuria* is revealed in carriers, i.e. heterozygotes not suffering from the disease, by biochemical tests which show impaired breakdown of phenylalanine. The same is true of *galactosaemia*. In *sickle cell anaemia*, disease-free heterozygotes carrying only one sickle cell gene exhibit the so-called sickle cell trait. This means that their red cells are healthy in normal circumstances but become fragile if exposed to a high CO_2 concentration in a test tube. A somewhat similar situation exists in another genetically determined haemolytic anaemia known as *thalassaemia*. The heterozygotes are said to have thalassaemia minor, and the homozygotes, thalassaemia major.

Chromosomal abnormalities

Chromosomal abnormalities may be caused by:

1. abnormal chromosome numbers
2. abnormal chromosome structures.

Genes are molecules of DNA, and genetic defects occur therefore at the molecular level. Chromosomes are strands of genetic material large enough to be seen with the light microscope and chromosomal abnormalities are by definition visible by light microscopy.

Defects of single genes may cause fatal disease, so it is not surprising that chromosomal aberrations involving hundreds or thousands of genes are usually incompatible with life. The only situation in which an entire chromosome may be absent and the individual survive is in females who lack one of their X chromosomes (see below). Major deficiency of even part of a somatic chromosome is rarely compatible with survival and occurs only in some very uncommon disorders of childhood.

These remarks of course apply to situations in which the chromosomal abnormality is present in all the cells of the body. Particular cell populations, especially malignant tumours (p. 262) or inflammatory macrophages (Fig. 17.5), may show gross disturbances of chromosome pattern, but if the tumour is eradicated and the macrophages eliminated the patient's survival will not be affected.

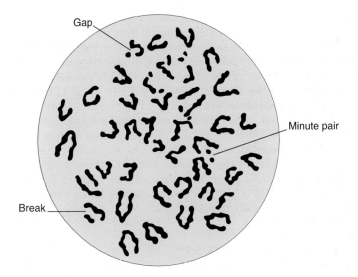

Gap

Minute pair

Break

Fig. 17.5   Gross chromosomal abnormalities in an inflammatory macrophage.

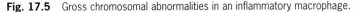

With the exceptions mentioned, chromosomal mutations as defined above—i.e. visible by light microscopy, affecting all somatic cells and compatible with life—occur usually in the form of an additional whole chromosome.

Chromosomes are studied by allowing cells from bone marrow or skin to divide in culture, arresting mitosis in metaphase and then inducing the chromosomes to spread out. The maps obtained in this way are known as *karyotypes* and the chromosomes classified and numbered in order of size with chromosome 1 being the largest (p. 161).

Chromosomal abnormalities are much more common than genetic mutations. About 4% of newly conceived human fetuses have chromosomal aberrations, and of these abnormal conceptuses about 90% will be aborted in the early months of pregnancy. Of abortions occurring spontaneously early in pregnancy 20–40% exhibit, and presumably result from, incorrect chromosomal patterns. Absence of one X chromosome is a common cause of non-viability, especially in male fetuses.

Abnormal chromosome numbers

Abnormal chromosome numbers can result when a chromosome fails to separate either in meiosis or mitosis. When this happens one daughter cell receives two copies of the chromosome and the other cell receives no copies. This is called *non-dysjunction*; if it occurs during meiosis, either the ovum or the sperm will have an extra chromosome. Any resulting fetus will then be either trisomic (i.e. having three instead of two copies of the chromosome) or monosomic (i.e. having one copy instead of two copies of the chromosome). Both autosomes and sex chromosomes may be affected. Only trisomies 13, 18 and 21 survive to birth and only individuals with trisomy 21 survive into adulthood.

If non-dysjunction occurs during mitosis and just after two gametes have fused, two cell lines will be produced, each with a different chromosome complement. This is known as *mosaicism*.

Rarely, multiples of the haploid number of chromosomes occur. *Aneuploid* individuals have multiples of the haploid number of chromosomes (i.e. 23): a *triploid* has 69 chromosomes; a *tetraploid* has 92. Such fetuses usually miscarry early.

Abnormal chromosome structures

Abnormal chromosome structures may result from *deletions, duplications, inversions* and *translocations.*

- A deletion of Y chromosome gives rise to Turner's syndrome.
- A duplication (i.e. there are two copies of a portion of the chromosome) occurs in Charcot–Marie–Tooth disease, which results from a duplication of a region of chromosome 17.
- An inversion describes a reversal of a segment within the chromosome.
- A translocation occurs when two chromosomes regions join together where they should not. This may involve chromosome 21 and cause Down's syndrome.

Incidence of detectable chromosome abnormalities

The incidence of detectable chromosome abnormalities (Table 17.2) is approximately 0.7% (about 1 in 140). Of these around 40% are sex chromosome abnormalities, 20% are autosomal trisomies (mostly Down's syndrome) and the rest are chromosomal rearrangements.

The mitochondrial genome

The mitochondria have their own genome, comprising circular DNA molecules of approximately 500 base pairs which have a high natural mutation rate. There are no introns. Mitochondrial DNA encodes:

- transfer RNA
- ribosomal RNA
- polypeptides of the respiratory chain enzymes.

Table 17.2   Disorders associated with chromosome abnormalities

Chromosome	Disorder
1	Gaucher's disease
4	Huntington's chorea
5	Familial adenomatous polyposis
6	Haemochromatosis
7	Cystic fibrosis
9	Friedrich's ataxia
11	Beta thalassaemia
12	Phenylketonuria
13	Wilson's disease
14	α_1-antitrypsin deficiency
16	Adult polycystic kidney disease
17	Pompe's disease
18	Familial amyloidosis
19	Dystrophia myotonica
21	Down's syndrome
22	Chronic myeloid leukaemia

The energy generated by the oxidation/reduction reactions of the respiratory chain is stored in an electrochemical gradient coupled to ATP synthesis from ADP.

Sperm contain few mitochondria, so all mitochondria contain DNA inherited uniquely from the mother. Mitochondrial DNA is therefore a useful tool for studying evolutionary and migratory patterns over centuries.

Management of genetic disorders

Genetic disorders are best managed if possible by prevention, but prenatal diagnosis and screening at birth allow early diagnosis and the provision of appropriate therapy.

Prevention

Genetic counselling allows couples to evaluate their offspring's risk of developing a genetic disorder and to be advised about preventing transmission of the disorder to future generations. From the molecular point of view, this may be straightforward when considering Down's syndrome and phenylketonuria, but more complex when considering X-linked disorders where carrier detection tests are necessary.

Prenatal diagnosis

Single gene defects, neural tube defects and major physiological defects can sometimes be diagnosed prenatally by obtaining samples of fetal tissue or by visualising the fetus, usually with ultrasound.

There are a number of common genetic disorders in which molecular techniques can now be used to help make a diagnosis (Table 17.3). When there are large defects in genes (e.g. in alpha thalassaemia and most Duchenne/Becker muscular dystrophies), detection is usually possible by Southern blotting. PCR using allele-specific oligonucleotides may be used to detect conditions such as cystic fibrosis and α_1-antitrypsin deficiency.

Screening at birth

Genetic disorders that can be diagnosed by screening include haemoglobinopathies (e.g. sickle cell anaemia), hypothyroidism and phenylketonuria. Screening at birth allows appropriate treatment of an individual with a genetic disorder before the disorder becomes clinically apparent.

Congenital malformations

The most common congenital diseases are anatomical malformations affecting the heart and great vessels, the gastrointestinal and urinary tracts and the skeletal and central nervous systems. Unfortunately less is known about the causation of these deformities than about the conditions already dealt with, most of which are of less importance in clinical medicine. The overall incidence of congenital malformations in Great Britain is about 16 per 1000 total births.

It is generally accepted that very few cases of congenital anatomical defects exhibit the classic Mendelian ratios that would be demonstrable if single gene inheritance were involved. In addition a small minority form part of the clinical pattern associated with

Table 17.3   Genetic disorders for which prenatal diagnosis is possible

Thalassaemia alpha, beta
Haemophilia A, B
Cystic fibrosis
Fragile X syndrome
Myotonic dystrophy
Huntington's disease
Tay–Sachs disease
α_1-antitrypsin
Retinoblastoma

particular chromosomal abnormalities, e.g. congenital heart disease in trisomy 21 or cleft palate in trisomy 13 (p. 182). On the other hand there is an accumulation of evidence to indicate that in a surprisingly high number of cases of such anatomical anomalies a definite but less obvious familial tendency is apparent. This tendency is of the type that geneticists associate with polygenic inheritance discussed in the next chapter.

KEY POINTS

- Genetic disease may result from an abnormality of a single gene or chromosome. More commonly it results from a combination of multiple genetic and environmental factors.
- Single gene abnormalities are inherited as dominant, recessive or sex linked.
- Chromosomal abnormalities may be due to:
  — abnormal chromosome numbers, resulting when a chromosome fails to separate either in meiosis or mitosis
  — abnormal chromosome structures, resulting from deletions, duplications, inversions and translocations.
- Genetic disorders may be managed by prevention or by prenatal diagnosis and screening at birth to allow the provision of appropriate therapy.
- Congenital malformations show familial aggregation and may result from a combination of polygenic inheritance and environmental factors.

18 Polygenic disease and natural selection

Polygenic inheritance as a contributory factor in disease

Thus far we have only considered diseases which are wholly determined by specific mutant genes. There is, however, good evidence that many other diseases, caused by a multiplicity of factors, have a familial component. Both genetic and environmental factors contribute to the aetiology of many common disorders; examples include essential hypertension, rheumatoid arthritis, coronary heart disease, obesity, osteoporosis, osteoarthritis and diabetes mellitus. In multifactorial genetic diseases, multiple genes interact with multiple environmental factors and this produces *familial aggregation*.

Essential hypertension is an important and common disease in which the arterial blood pressure is abnormally high for no apparent reason. The level of blood pressure in the population follows the usual Gaussian distribution pattern with most people having normal blood pressure, some having lower than average pressure and some having higher than average pressure. This last group is said to have essential hypertension; although some individuals may remain symptom free, many others will suffer fatal consequences such as cerebral haemorrhage or heart failure. For any given level of blood pressure there is a tendency for first degree relatives, i.e. parents, offspring and siblings, to resemble each other with respect to blood pressure. This tendency is of a similar order for all first degree relatives as they share on average 50% of their genes and the genetic element in determining blood pressure is therefore not of Mendelian type. It is important to note that familial clustering can be due to shared environmental factors as much as genes. Thus fat children may have fat parents due to shared dietary habits or shared genes. The best way to separate these factors is through twin studies, where identical (monozygotic) twins who share 100% of their genes are compared with non-identical (dizygotic) twin pairs who share 50% of genes.

Twin studies have shown higher rates of similarity in identical twins for many diseases for which there is no evidence of transmission by a single gene. These include heart disease, obesity, arthritis, peptic ulcers and schizophrenia.

In *cancer*, single gene inheritance occurs only in one or two specific instances, e.g. neuroblastoma and polyposis coli. In most cases, however, where a familial trend can be shown at all it is polygenic. Twin studies have shown that the risk of getting any form of cancer is approximately doubled if your identical twin has cancer compared to a non-identical twin. 5% of breast cancer is inherited and linked to two candidate genes (see p. 286). Polygenic inheritance means that some individuals inherit a general genetic package which predisposes them to certain illnesses and renders them susceptible to certain environmental influences, mostly of unknown nature. The concept is supported by statistical observations such as that people with blood group O are 40% more likely to develop a duodenal ulcer than those with other blood groups. Blood group and tissue transplantation antigens are inherited in Mendelian fashion but seem sometimes to act as markers for the polygenic transmission of susceptibility to certain diseases. The HLA system is a specific example of this (p. 75). The incidence of all important congenital malformations is likely to be polygenic as rates are higher in first degree relatives and increased further in families with two or more affected relatives and with severe rather than mild disease. The likelihood or liability of disease follows a normal or Gaussian distribution.

The mechanisms of polygenic inheritance

Polygenic inheritance appears to be due to the additive effect of a large number of genes of small effect, whereas the effects of single gene inheritance are due to the action of a single gene of large effect. However small-effect polygenes, like strong single genes, segregate at meiosis, display dominance and recessivity and are transmitted in linked blocks. Inheritance of these blocks of weak genes appears to be a major factor in the cause of many, if not most, congenital anatomical malformations. Other factors involved are the extent to which these inherited abnormal genes are diluted by normal gene blocks and the influence of environmental agents.

Some disorders are associated with classical genetic markers such as blood groups or tissue types, for example:

- peptic ulceration and blood group O
- ankylosing spondylitis and HLA-B27.

Genetic markers may be associated with specific diseases because of *linkage disequilibrium* (p. 77). If there is linkage disequilibrium the genetic marker is closely linked to a disease locus, hence they are found together more than would be predicted. Sometimes the genetic marker may be identifying an allele predisposing an individual to develop the disease, such as a predisposition to infection.

All this data fits well with the central concept of polygenic inheritance in which there is a gradation of total liability to the disease which becomes manifest when a certain threshold is passed.

Environmental influences and polygenic inheritance

Environment is well recognised to influence the operation of polygenic inheritance, common examples being inherited resistance to tuberculosis in relation to risk of infection, and inherited height in relation to nutrition. Newer examples are becoming apparent in cardiovascular disease where gene effects on lipoproteins only seem to operate at certain levels of obesity or in the presence or absence of alcohol. Gene–gene interactions are also likely to be important.

The survival value of disease-causing genetic mutation

So far in this book we have encountered several examples of pathology arising as a by-product of an evolutionary survival mechanism. The basis of genetic disease is harmful mutation which then persists in the population. This persistence may seem hard to understand because affected individuals should be slowly eliminated by natural selection. It is important to realise, however, that the human race is apparently committed to continuing evolution and that this can only be achieved by the process of mutation that we have described. Obviously therefore some of these mutations will be harmful and others beneficial.

With regard to persistence of harmful genes, we have to realise that we do not always see the whole picture. The *sickle cell trait* is extremely common in some parts of the world, notably Africa, where 20–30% of the population may have the gene. Such prevalence suggests a survival advantage in heterozygotes which outweighs the death rate from sickle cell anaemia in homozygotes. In fact, the abnormal gene confers a great deal of protection against malaria, since the abnormal red cells do not support the malarial parasite as efficiently as normal corpuscles. As malaria is one of the most common causes of death in children and people of reproductive age in these regions, the sickle cell gene has strong survival value and persists through natural selection. When the Africans move to countries where malaria is not endemic, the gene loses its value and slowly disappears as a result of natural selection eliminating the homozygotes. This process is going on in the black population of the USA and provides an example of Darwinism in action.

An interesting although less well documented example of the survival value of disease-causing genetic mutation is the decreased susceptibility to tuberculosis associated with the lysosomal storage diseases that have their epicentre in Eastern Europe: these include Gaucher's, Tay–Sachs and Niemann–Pick disease. Why genes should exist for other traits is often unclear. Recently it has been found that genes are responsible for the timing of the menopause which is related to an increase in the rate of heart disease and osteoporosis. Humans are the only animals with a menopause and it has been proposed that the menopause was an essential part of evolution, allowing 'grandmothers' to evolve who could assist in moving children from one cave to another to find food.

The process of mutation

When a mutation first occurs, the mutant gene is at first neither dominant nor recessive. If the change is favourable for the species concerned, dominance will develop due to natural selection favouring a weak corresponding gene on the other chromosome of the pair (the allele, in genetic terminology). If the mutation is unfavourable when fully expressed it will become recessive due to natural selection promoting a strong suppressive unmutated gene on the other chromosome. It follows from this that once a gene has become dominant, provided it does not prevent reproduction, it is no longer subject to the pressures of natural selection, whereas a recessive gene is always at risk of disappearing. We have seen why some common recessive genes such as that of sickle cell anaemia persist but in other cases, for example cystic fibrosis of the pancreas, there is no apparent reason. Achondroplasia (dominant) and haemophilia (recessive) seem to remain in the population because of the very high spontaneous mutation rate of the genes concerned.

KEY POINTS

- Many diseases have a polygenic inheritance; individuals inherit a genetic package which predisposes them to certain illnesses and renders them susceptible to certain environmental influences.
- Genetic mutations which cause overt disease in homozygotes may be perpetuated in the population because they confer a survival advantage on heterozygotes.
- If a mutation is favourable for the species concerned, dominance will develop. If the mutation is unfavourable when fully expressed it will become recessive.
- Both genetic and environmental factors contribute to the aetiology of many common disorders.

19 Atheroma

Atheroma (from a Greek word meaning porridge) is an arterial disease, the complications of which kill more people in the western world than any other disease, including cancer. It is the major cause of heart attacks and strokes and is an important factor in the deterioration of senility. It is the major complication of diabetes mellitus. Atheroma can affect all arteries above 2 mm in diameter but is most important in the aorta, cerebral, coronary, mesenteric and femoral arteries.

To understand atheroma it is first necessary to review the normal architecture of the large and medium sized arteries (Fig. 19.1).

1. The lumen of these vessels is lined by a single layer of flattened cells, the *endothelium*. They form the inner boundary of a narrow layer called the intima whose outer boundary is the internal elastic lamina.

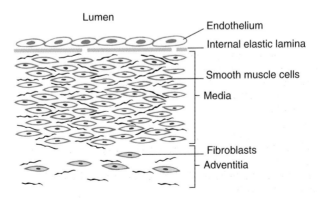

Fig. 19.1 Cross section of normal coronary artery.

Normally the intima is composed of a few smooth muscle cells, collagen fibres and glucosaminoglycans (proteoglycans, mucopolysaccharides, ground substance). The internal elastic lamina is an incomplete layer of fibres of elastin, a protein secreted by the arterial smooth muscle cells.

2. Beyond the internal elastic lamina is the *media*, which is composed of smooth muscle cells separated by small amounts of collagen, elastin and glucosaminoglycans. There are no fibroblasts in the intima or media of mammalian arteries.

3. The *adventitia* is the outermost coat, separated from the media by a loose elastin barrier, the external elastic lamina. The adventitia consists of fibroblasts, collagen and glucosaminoglycans. In larger arteries it is supplied by small blood vessels, the vasa vasorum.

The essential pathological change which distinguishes an atheromatous artery from a normal vessel is the accumulation in the intima of collagen and the lipid material which has given the disease its name. This lipid consists mainly of *cholesterol* and *cholesterol esters* and *triglycerides*. It is associated with large amounts of collagen and glucosaminoglycans and with greatly increased numbers of smooth muscle cells. Some of the lipid is in the cytoplasm of these cells, some within macrophages and some is extracellular. The combination of lipid, fibrous tissue and cells has led to the use of the term *atherosclerosis* as a synonym for atheroma, although Scottish pathologists have objected to it on the etymological ground that it means 'hard porridge', a concept which they find unacceptable.

ARTERIOSCLEROSIS AND ATHEROSCLEROSIS

Arteriosclerosis is thickening and hardening of the arterial wall of larger arteries causing coronary artery disease, aortic aneurysm and arterial disease of the lower extremities and cerebral vascular disease. It is a major cause of death.

Atherosclerosis is one type of arteriosclerosis. There are also other types of arteriosclerosis, e.g. focal calcific arteriosclerosis. Disorders associated with the early development of arteriosclerosis are shown in Table 19.1.

Atherosclerosis is a patchy nodular type of arteriosclerosis. The atheroma forms in stages as:

• early initial lesions and fatty streaks
• intermediate lesions
• fibrous plaques
• complicated lesions.

The initial fatty streaks and intermediate lesions are focal, small and non-obstructive.

Table 19.1 Disorders associated with early arteriosclerosis

Atherosclerosis
Diabetes mellitus
Hypertension
Familial hypercholesterolaemia
Familial combined hyperlipidaemia
Familial dysbetalipoproteinaemia
Familial hypoalphalipoproteinaemia
Hypothyroidism
Cholesterol ester storage disease
Systemic lupus erythematosus
Homocysteinaemia

Non-atheromatous arteriosclerosis
Diabetes mellitus
Chronic renal insufficiency
Chronic vitamin D intoxication
Pseudoxanthoma elasticum
Idiopathic arterial calcification in infancy
Aortic valvular calcification in the elderly
Werner's syndrome

Initial lesions   These are detected chemically or microscopically as lipid deposits in intimal macrophages. They are thought to evolve into lesions associated with clinical disease as they are located in regions of the arterial tree susceptible to atherosclerosis. They may start early in life and have been found in children.

Fatty streaks   These are visible to the naked eye on the endothelial surface of the aorta and coronary arteries. They are small, non-obstructive and contain lipid-filled smooth muscle cells and macrophages and fibrous tissue. They may be stained by fat-soluble dyes. The lipid is mostly cholesterol oleate and is mainly intracellular. Progression of fatty streaks to advanced lesions depends on haemodynamic forces and plasma levels of atherogenic lipoproteins.

Fibrous plaques   These are elevated areas of intimal thickening and are characteristic of advancing atherosclerosis. They first appear in the abdominal aorta, coronary arteries and carotid arteries around the third decade. They progress with age, appearing in men before women and in the aorta before the coronary arteries.

Morphology   The lesion is firm, elevated and dome shaped with an opaque glistening surface that bulges into the lumen. There is a central core of extracellular lipid with cholesterol crystals and necrotic cell debris covered by a fibromuscular layer or cap which contains smooth muscle cells, macrophages and collagen. The lipid is mainly cholesterol ester but the principal esterified fatty acid is linoleic rather than oleic.

Complicated lesions These are calcified fibrous plaques containing necrotic cells, with thrombosis and possibly ulceration. They are frequently associated with clinical symptoms. Increasing necrosis causes the arterial wall to weaken and the intima may rupture causing an aneurysm and haemorrhage.

Arterial emboli result when fragments of the plaque dislodge into the lumen. Gradual occlusion may occur as the plaque thickens causing stenosis and hence impairment of organ function.

Location of lesions

There is an irregular distribution with different vessels being involved at different ages and to varying degrees. Earliest and most severely affected is the abdominal aorta. There is also significant involvement at the level of the coronary and intercostal arteries, in the aortic arch and at the bifurcation of the iliac arteries.

The lower limb This is affected more than the upper limb, and the incidence decreases peripherally. Plaques and thrombosis are commonly found:

- in the femoral artery
- in Hunter's canal
- in the popliteal artery just above the knee joint
- in the anterior and posterior tibial arteries, possibly causing occlusion
- posteriorly, where the tibial artery travels around the internal malleolus, and anteriorly where it is superficial and becomes the dorsalis pedis artery.

The peritoneal artery may become the main blood supply to the extremity as it often escapes involvement.

Coronary arteries Lesions are commonly found in the main stem, a short distance beyond the ostia, usually in the epicardial portions of the vessels. Intramural coronary arteries may be spared. Once the process is present, all the intima of the extramural portions of the vessel is involved. It is rare to find a single tiny plaque occluding an otherwise normal coronary artery. The unique haemodynamic forces within coronary arteries may influence the location of involvement.

Cervical and cerebral arteries The carotid, basilar and vertebral arteries are common sites of involvement, especially the bifurcation of the carotid artery.

The causes of atheroma

Advancing age and high standards of nutrition are associated factors in the aetiology of atheroma. In western countries, in people over 60 years old, atheroma is always demonstrable and usually extensive so that disease can be said to be the norm. The exceptions are provided mainly by those suffering from prolonged malnutrition or wasting diseases.

Because of the normality of atheroma above a certain age, attention has been directed to factors inducing atheroma at an unusually early age or to a particularly severe degree. Evidence of premature or unduly severe atheroma comes mainly from the onset of the complications of atheroma, especially cardiac infarcts.

Risk factors of atherosclerosis

Lipoproteins Prospective community-based epidemiological studies have implicated increasing plasma cholesterol concentration as an important risk factor for coronary heart disease (CHD). This association is mainly determined by *low density lipoprotein* (LDL), which is the major atherogenic particle. High density lipoprotein is also strongly and independently related to the risk of coronary disease, but the relationship is inverse. High levels of HDL appear to protect against the development of CHD, while low levels are an important risk factor. The relationship between the risk of CHD and increasing *plasma triglyceride* remains to be resolved, but remnant particles are strongly linked with an increased risk. Obesity results in insulin resistance in peripheral tissues leading to hyperinsulinaemia. This causes the liver to produce triglyceride rich lipoproteins leading to elevated plasma triglyceride and cholesterol levels. Diet is an important factor: total daily calories and intake of saturated animal fats have highly significant statistical correlations with cardiac infarction. A diet rich in starch and sugar has a similar effect.

Platelet aggregation If this occurs on undamaged endothelium, the release of lysosomal enzymes from the platelets will destroy the integrity of the endothelium and allow lipoproteins to enter the intima. Many of the factors which cause a rise in LDL also induce platelets to aggregate, due perhaps to the high levels of circulating free fatty acids which are associated with elevated concentrations of LDL in the blood. In addition, disturbances which strain the endothelial lining of vessel walls, e.g. adrenaline secretion or cigarette smoking, may also make platelets more liable to clump.

Hypertension This may directly produce injury via mechanical stress on endothelial cells; it may also alter endothelial permeability and increase lysosomal enzyme activity.

Diabetes mellitus It is thought that diabetes directly results in a decreased life span of individual cells. This accelerates atherosclerosis.

Cigarette smoking This may result in repetitive toxic injury to endothelial cells. Further damage may also be caused by high levels of carboxyhaemoglobulin and low oxygen delivery.

Genetics Certain families exhibit a strong predisposition to premature ischaemic heart disease. At the age of 45 years heart attacks are seven times more common in men than in women. Genetic factors may affect arterial wall cell structure and metabolism and may influence hypertension, hyperlipidaemia, diabetes and obesity.

Occupation Occupation appears to be related to cardiac infarction since those in sedentary jobs appear to be more at risk than those obliged to exercise.

Stress Psychological stress is also a risk factor although it is not easy to assess.

Social class Low social class is an independent risk factor, even after accounting for these factors.

Ageing This may affect arterial wall metabolism and may be associated with other metabolic factors. Almost all middle-aged or elderly people dying of other causes or diseases show atheroma, certainly of the aorta, and probably of the coronary, femoral and cerebral arteries. In such cases there is often no evidence that atheroma caused any symptoms or contributed to death. Of all individuals dying, however, almost half do so as a result of the complications of atheroma.

Pathogenesis of atherosclerosis

There are a number of theories, listed below.

Reaction to injury hypothesis

It is thought that endothelial cells lining the intima are exposed to repeated or continuing injury. This results in loss of their normal function and they no longer act as a permeability barrier. Examples of the injury that may occur are chronic hypercholesterolaemia, hypertension resulting in increased mechanical stress and inflammation secondary to rejection after organ transplantation.

Once subendothelial tissue is exposed to plasma constituents, monocytes may travel into the intima and platelets may adhere, aggregating and forming microthrombi. Once this occurs, various platelet and macrophage secretory products may be released (e.g. platelet derived growth factor, interleukin-1, coronary stimulating factors), together with plasma constituents, including lipoproteins. The proliferation of intimal smooth muscle may be stimulated. A connective tissue matrix may be deposited by proliferating smooth muscle cells and this would accumulate lipid.

Monoclonal hypothesis

This theory suggests that there is multiplication of individual muscle cells due to the stimulation of single cells by mitogens.

Focal clonal senescence

Feedback control mechanisms may normally prevent intimal smooth muscle cells from proliferating. This system may fail with age when controlling cells die and are not replaced.

The lysosomal theory

Lysosomal function may contribute to atherosclerosis. It is thought that the deposition of cholesterol esters arises from a deficiency in the activity of lysosomal cholesterol ester hydrolase. These lysosomal enzymes may then cause degradation of cellular components.

PLASMA LIPIDS AND LIPOPROTEIN DISORDERS

Plasma lipid disorders are important because they are associated with an increased risk of atherosclerosis related disease, particularly *coronary heart disease*. More rarely, plasma lipid disorders can be associated with an increased risk of *pancreatitis*.

Lipid and lipoprotein metabolism

The major plasma lipids are cholesterol and triglyceride. They are relatively insoluble in water and are transported in the plasma as multimolecular micelle-like particles known as lipoproteins (Fig. 19.2). The insoluble cholesterol ester and triglyceride forms a lipid

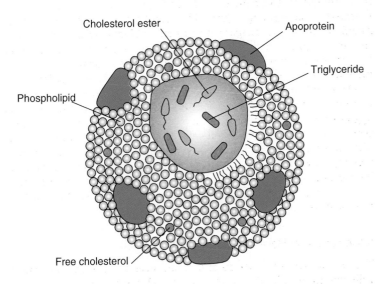

Fig. 19.2 Structure of lipoprotein.

droplet at the centre of these particles while more polar substances such as free cholesterol, phospholipid and apoproteins are found at the interface with the plasma.

The nomenclature of the plasma lipoproteins is based on their separation by density gradient ultracentrifugation (Table 19.2). The lipoproteins differ in size, lipid content and content of apoproteins. The apoproteins not only have a structural role, but also have important effects on lipid and lipoprotein metabolism (Table 19.3).

Dyslipoproteinaemia and the cause of atheroma

Dyslipoproteinaemias

Lipid disorders are classified as either primary or secondary (Tables 19.4 and 19.5). The nomenclature of the primary lipid disorders is based where possible on the underlying metabolic and/or genetic abnormality.

Familial hypercholesterolaemia

Familial hypercholesterolaemia is the most severe of the familial disorders of lipid metabolism in terms of its associated risk of premature heart disease. It affects approximately 1 in 500 of the population. The homozygous form is rare and affects approximately one in a million of the population. The average age of onset of coronary heart disease is the early 40s in men and early 50s in women. The condition is inherited as an autosomal dominant trait and is more common (approximately 1:100) in some population groups, notably South African Boers and Lebanese.

The genetic defect is at the LDL receptor: LDL is not removed efficiently from the circulation by the liver and its half-life is prolonged.

Familial combined (mixed) hyperlipidaemia

The incidence of this autosomal dominant inherited condition is approximately 1 in 200–300. The genetic defect of familial combined hyperlipidaemia remains to be determined, but the underlying metabolic abnormality appears to be an overproduction by the liver of lipoproteins containing apoprotein B. Affected members from the same family show varying abnormalities of their plasma lipids. They may have a raised cholesterol, a raised triglyceride, or both. The plasma lipid abnormality may also vary within the same individual depending on diet and weight.

Table 19.2 Classification of lipoproteins

| Class | Diameter (Å) | Density (g/ml) | Electrophoretic mobility | Chemical composition (% of dry mass) | | | | | |
				Triglycerides	Cholesterol esters	Cholesterol	Phospholipids	Proteins
Chylomicrons	800–5000	0.93	α_2	86	3	2	7	2
VLDL	300–800	0.96–1.006	Pre-β	55	12	7	18	8
IDL	250–350	1.006–1.019	Slow pre-β	23	29	9	19	19
LDL	216	1.019–1.063	β	6	42	8	22	22
HDL$_2$	100	1.063–1.125	α_1	5	17	5	33	40
HDL$_3$	75	1.125–1.210	α_1	3	13	4	25	55

IDL, intermediate density lipoprotein;
LDL, low density lipoprotein;
HDL, high density lipoprotein;
VHDL, very high density lipoprotein

Table 19.3   Classification and function of apoproteins

Type	Number of amino acids	Molecular weight (~)	Origin	Lipoprotein distribution	Principal function
A-I	243	28 000	Liver, intestine	HDL, chylomicrons	LCAT activator
A-II	154	17 000	Liver, intestine	HDL, chylomicrons	Structural protein in HDL
A-IV	391	40 000	Liver, intestine	HDL, chylomicrons	Non-specific LCAT cofactor
B_{48}	2152	246 000	Intestine	Chylomicrons chylomicron remnants	Mediates chylomicron formation and secretion by enterocytes
B100	4536	513 000	Liver	VLDL, LDL	Mediates hepatic VLDL formation Ligand for LDL receptor
C-I	57	7000	Liver	Chylomicrons, VLDL, HDL	Inhibitor of chylomicron uptake
C-II	78	9000	Liver	Chylomicrons, VLDL, HDL	LPL activator
C-III	79	9000	Liver	Chylomicrons, VLDL, HDL	Inhibitor of chylomicron? Inhibitor of LPL
D	?	2000	Liver	HDL	?Involved in cholestrol ester transfer
E	299	3400	Liver	Chylomicrons, VLDL, HDL	Ligand for chylomicron receptor and LDL receptor

Table 19.4 Classification of primary hyperlipidaemias

Type	WHO phenotype	Cholesterol	Triglycerides	Lipoproteins	Clinical signs
		Typical lipid levels (mmol/l)			
Polygenic hypercholesterolaemia	IIa	6.5–9.0	< 2.3	LDL ↑	Xanthelasma, corneal arcus
Familial hypercholesterolaemia	IIa	7.5–16.0	< 2.3	LDL ↑	Tendon xanthoma, arcus, xanthelasma
Familial defective apoprotein B-100	IIa	7.5–16.0	2.3	LDL ↑	Tendon xanthoma, arcus, xanthelasma
Familial combined hyperlipidaemia	IIa, IIb, IV or V	6.5–10.0	2.3–12.0	LDL ↑, VLDL ↑, VLDL ↓	Arcus, xanthelasma
Remnant particle disease	III	9.0–14.0	9.0–14.0	IDL ↑	Palmar striae, tuberoeruptive xanthomata
Familial hypertriglyceridaemia	IV, V	6.5–12.0	10.0–30.0	VLDL ↑	Eruptive xanthomata, lipaemia, retinalis, hepatosplenomegaly
Lipoprotein lipase deficiency	I	< 6.5	10.0–30.0	Chylomicrons ↑	Eruptive xanthomata, lipaemia, retinalis, hepatosplenomegaly
Primary HDL abnormalities					
Hyperalphalipoproteinaemia	—	HDL >2.0	—	HDL ↑	—
Hypoalphalipoproteinaemia	—	HDL >0.9	—	HDL ↓	—

Table 19.5   Classification of secondary hyperlipidaemias

Hormonal factors
Pregnancy
Diabetes mellitus
Hypothyroidism

Nutritional factors
Obesity
Anorexia nervosa
Alcohol abuse

Renal dysfunction
Nephrotic syndrome
Chronic renal failure

Liver disease
Primary biliary cirrhosis
Extrahepatic biliary obstruction

Iatrogenic
High-dose thiazide diuretics
Beta-adrenergic receptor antagonists which lack alpha-blocking effects, intrinsic sympathetic activity or vasodilator properties
Corticosteroids
Exogenous sex hormones
Retinoids

Remnant particle disease

This rare disease affects 1 in 3000–5000 individuals. The majority of patients with remnant particle disease are homozygous for apoprotein E_2, which occurs with a frequency of approximately 1:100 of the population. An additional metabolic defect is required for full expression of the disease: this is either another familial form of hyperlipidaemia or a secondary hyperlipidaemia such as diabetes mellitus, hypothyroidism or renal disease.

Apoprotein E_2 is a less effective ligand than apoprotein E_3 for removing remnant particles. Remnant particle disease is characterised by a marked elevation in cholesterol and triglyceride because of an accumulation of the cholesterol-rich remnant particles. These show up as a characteristic broad beta brand on lipoprotein electrophoresis, but definitive diagnosis requires isolation of very low density lipoprotein (VLDL) by ultracentrifugation, which shows a molar ratio of cholesterol to triglyceride greater than 0.6.

Polygenic hypercholesterolaemia

This is the most common form of hypercholesterolaemia. It is polygenic and comprises a heterogeneous group of disorders with multiple genes interacting with environmental factors such as diet. The genetic factors responsible remain to be fully documented.

Chylomicronaemia syndrome

Chylomicronaemia syndrome is characterised by the persistence of chylomicrons in the fasting state. Triglyceride levels are very high, but cholesterol levels may be normal or moderately raised. Usually the syndrome is secondary to other causes such as diabetes mellitus or alcohol excess. Rarely it is the result of inborn errors of lipid metabolism.

Lipoprotein lipase deficiency

The condition affects about one in a million individuals and is autosomal recessive. Lipoprotein lipase deficiency is characterised by an absence or limited activity of the lipoprotein lipase. An additional cause of absent lipoprotein lipase activity is a deficiency of apoprotein C_2, which is the major activator of this enzyme.

The interrelationship of blood lipid, arterial damage and platelet aggregation in the causation of atheroma is shown in Figure 19.3.

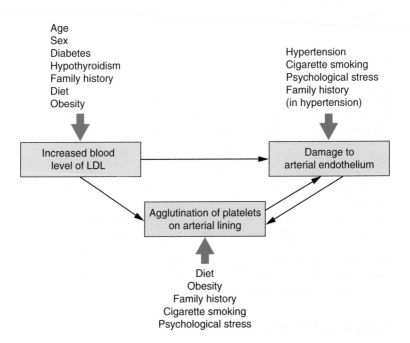

Fig. 19.3 Interrelationship of blood lipid, arterial damage and platelet aggregation in the causation of atheroma.

Hyperlipidaemia, arterial damage and platelet aggregation may act alone or in deadly cooperation. In other words, the characteristic lesions of atheroma result from increased entry of LDL into the vessel wall due to high levels of circulating LDL alone or in combination with local aggregation of platelets, or with increased permeability of the endothelial barrier which separates the intima from the blood. High blood pressure could increase filtration of LDL into the artery and also damage the endothelium and make it allow the entry of LDL in abnormal amounts. The high incidence of atheroma and ischaemic heart disease in youngish black women in the USA appears to be due almost entirely to hypertension.

There is no doubt that interference with the integrity of the lining endothelium allows atheromatous plaques to form in the intima (Figs 19.4, 19.5). There is also no doubt that these plaques contain LDL identical with that found in plasma. They also contain fibrinogen but other plasma proteins are generally not demonstrable. The retention of LDL and fibrinogen is due partly to their high molecular weight and partly to selective precipitation with charged calcium-rich sulphated glucosaminoglycans which are also present in the plaques. Since fibrinogen is an important constituent of atheromatous lesions, it is of interest that the erythrocyte sedimentation rate (p. 132), which largely depends on blood fibrinogen concentration, has a linear correlation with overall mortality in men over 55 years old.

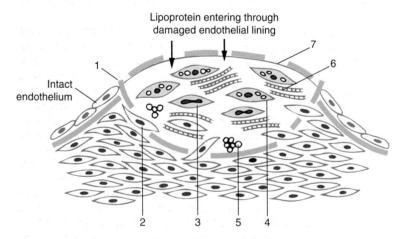

Fig. 19.4 Atheromatous plaque. 1. Fragmented internal elastic lumen. 2. Smooth muscle cells migrating into intima. 3. Dividing smooth muscle cells. 4. Lipid in smooth muscle cells. 5. Extracellular lipid. 6. Newly synthesised collagen. 7. Naked subendothelial surface.

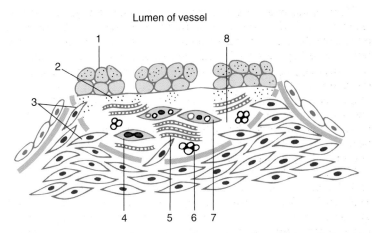

Fig. 19.5 Atheromatous plaque. 1. Adherent platelets. 2. Lysosomes discharged from platelets. 3. Migrating smooth muscle cells. 4. Dividing smooth muscle cell. 5. Newly synthesised collagen. 6. Extracellular lipid. 7. Lipid-laden smooth muscle cell. 8. Lipoprotein entering from plasma.

Smooth muscle proliferation into the intima is an early manifestation of atherosclerosis. *Platelet derived growth factor* (PDGF) as well as 12-lipoxygenase products stimulate proliferation and migration of smooth muscle cells. The fibrosis in atheroma is caused by the smooth muscle cells in the aortic intima that can synthesise collagen and glucosaminoglycans.

Platelets contain several growth factors; of these PDGF is the best characterised. It is a glycoprotein of about 30 000 daltons consisting of two peptide subunits joined by disulphide bonds. PDGF probably plays an important role in inflammation and repair. Its release from platelets mediates the chemotactic response of monocytes and neutrophils to platelet aggregation. After endothelial injury, it stimulates the migration and replication of smooth muscle cells and fibroblasts. Furthermore, PDGF modulates the binding of low density lipoprotein to its receptor. It is this wide range of actions which has led to suggestions that its release from platelets adhering to injured endothelium plays a role in the pathogenesis of atherosclerosis.

Other potential actions of platelets in the production of atheroma have attracted attention. In particular, *prostacyclin,* a potent vasodilator and inhibitor of platelet aggregation, is produced in consistently lower quantities by smooth muscle cells obtained from atherosclerotic lesions than by normal smooth muscle cells in vitro. The increased generation by atherosclerotic vessels of lipoxygenase products which are selective inhibitors of prostacyclin formation may be responsible for this.

Prostacyclin has a regulatory role in aortic cholesterol metabolism. Its defective production may predispose to atheroma. Thus, as atheromatous lesions develop, cholesterol and cholesterol esters are deposited in the extracellular matrix of the aortic smooth muscle cells as well as in lysosomal and cytosolic compartments of these cells. Prostacyclin stimulates the hydrolysis of the cholesterol esters via an increase in adenylate cyclase activity. Further, in smooth muscle cells derived from human atherosclerotic lesions in culture, cholesterol ester metabolism is enhanced by two stable prostacyclin analogues, so that the triglyceride and cholesterol levels in these cells are substantially reduced. Prostacyclin also inhibits the mobilisation of fibrinogen binding sites on human platelets in vivo, which may limit the extent of fibrinogen–platelet interactions.

To make all these observations fit a simple scheme of pathogenesis it is necessary to visualise a pathway which starts with initial damage to endothelium due to age, hypertension or increased lipid entry due to high LDL (Fig. 19.6). This could lead to platelet aggregation which, in turn, would cause smooth muscle cell hyperplasia and connective tissue overgrowth. With disorganisation of the intima there would be further entry and binding of lipoproteins, naturally accelerated if there are high levels of circulating LDL.

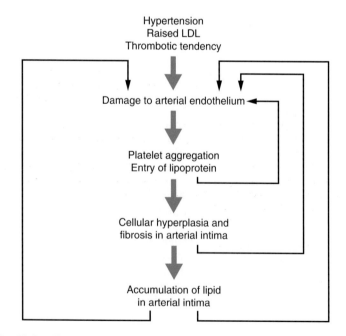

Fig. 19.6   The self-perpetuating factors in the development of atheroma.

COMPLICATIONS OF ATHEROMA

Thrombosis is not the only serious complication. Atheroma also causes *aneurysms of the aorta* due to local dilatation, as a result of destruction of normal constituents, especially elastic fibres. Aneurysms may rupture and cause death but if diagnosed earlier the affected aortic segment can be excised and replaced by a tube of woven synthetic fibres. A form of aneurysm not due to atheroma but also prevalent in middle-aged or elderly males is *dissecting aneurysm of the aorta*. This is due to degeneration of the media, often associated with hypertension. Blood appears in the medial coat either by a crack in the intima or from a ruptured vasa vasorum. The blood finds its way between the middle and outer thirds of the media and dissects them.

Another risk in atheroma is that a portion of fatty necrotic tissue may become sufficiently soft to detach and be swept to another part of the arterial tree where it may block a vessel and cause an *infarct*. A similar effect may arise from the dislodgement of an adherent thrombus. The process of detachment, circulation and lodgement is known as *embolus formation* and is an important pathological mechanism.

Atheroma may also affect the valves of the heart, causing interference with the opening and closing of the valves and leading to heart failure.

KEY POINTS

- The complications of atheroma kill more people in the western world than any other disease, being the major cause of heart attacks and strokes.
- The aorta, cerebral, coronary, mesenteric and femoral arteries are most severely affected.
- The essential pathological change is the accumulation in the intima of collagen and lipid material which consists mainly of cholesterol and triglycerides.
- Atheromatous plaques form in stages and the first lesions may be seen in childhood. Various mechanisms have been proposed for their pathogenesis.
- Plasma lipid disorders are associated with an increased risk of atherosclerosis related disease.
- The complications of atheroma include:
  — thrombosis
  — aneurysm of the aorta
  — embolus formation
  — infarct.

20 Thrombosis, embolism, infarction and clotting

THROMBOSIS

Thrombosis is the formation of a solid mass (*thrombus*) within the vascular system from the components of the blood in which activation of the coagulation pathways plays an integral part. By distinction, a blood clot is the result of activation of the coagulation system in isolation and may occur either outside the vascular system (haematoma) or in the test tube. Thrombosis is a well-ordered event, set along well-ordered lines, that has the purpose of arresting haemorrhage. The pathological nature of thrombosis arises from the initiating event, and the complications of having thrombus within the vascular system.

Thrombosis in its many and varied clinical manifestations is a major health problem. The disorders in which thromboembolic mechanisms occur include:

- myocardial infarction
- cerebral infarction
- pulmonary embolism.

All organs may be affected, however some tissues, e.g. brain and myocardium, are more vulnerable than others.

In the nineteenth century Virchow described the initiation of thrombosis, postulating that one or more aspects of a triad must exist for thrombus to form. *Virchow's triad* consists of:

- changes in the intimal surface of the vessel
- changes in the pattern of blood flow
- changes in the blood constituents.

THE MECHANISMS OF THROMBOSIS AND EMBOLISM

In thrombosis the first essential event is *activation of platelets* which stick to the vessel wall (adherence) and to each other (aggregation) (Fig. 20.1). Following this the blood coagulation system is activated, terminating in the formation of stable fibrin. The fibrin filaments enmesh red blood cells and upon this dark red mass more platelets alight. The only balancing force at this point is the body's fibrinolytic system which prevents the process of thrombosis continuing.

Seen with the naked eye a thrombus often takes the shape of the vessel in which it has formed (Fig. 20.2). The solid lines of platelets are visible within a thrombus as lighter bands in the dark red

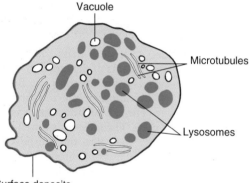
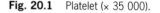

Fig. 20.1 Platelet (× 35 000).

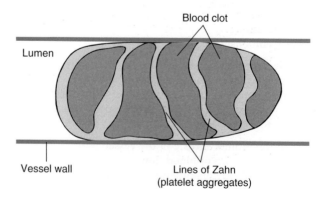
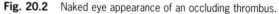

Fig. 20.2 Naked eye appearance of an occluding thrombus.

background of red blood cells and fibrin (Fig. 20.3). These platelet lines are called the lines of Zahn. This basic appearance may be slightly altered by the circumstances of the thrombosis. The thrombus grows in the direction of blood flow, a process called *propagation*. If flow is sufficiently sluggish to allow rapid obliteration of the vessel in which the thrombus forms, and back flow is not too strong, then downstream of the initial plug there will be complete stasis of blood, and coagulation will occur.

Most venous thrombi begin at valves as this is where there is maximum turbulence. Reduced blood flow may result from reduced blood pressure during surgery or immobilisation of the elderly and increase the predisposition to thrombosis. This is best seen in the deep veins of the leg (deep vein thrombosis or DVT), where long stringy thrombus forms and completely occludes the venous system (Fig. 20.4).

Venous thrombosis may result in inflammation, termed *thrombophlebitis*. The reverse may occur and inflammation result in thrombosis; this condition is called *phlebothrombosis*. Within the arterial system the thrombus usually remains smaller and firmer, though complete occlusion of vessels may occur as in the coronary circulation.

Disruption of the blood supply to an organ by a thrombus has two effects: ischaemia and/or infarction. *Ischaemia* is the term used to describe the deprivation of a tissue of oxygenated blood, causing a disruption or loss of function within that organ. *Infarction* describes the death of that tissue following acute ischaemia when irreparable

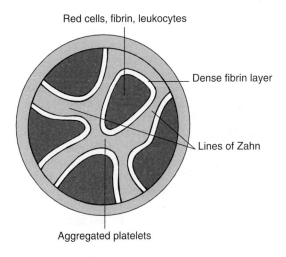

Fig. 20.3 Cross-section of thrombus.

1. Initial thrombus in vein pocket

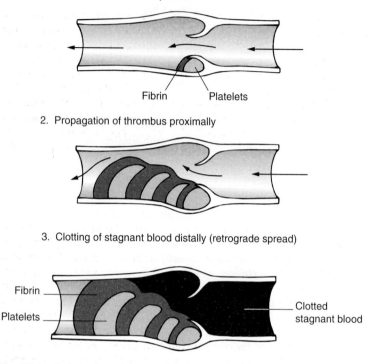

2. Propagation of thrombus proximally

3. Clotting of stagnant blood distally (retrograde spread)

Fig. 20.4   The stages of venous thrombosis.

damage has occurred. The time from ischaemia to infarction varies from organ to organ: it is very short in the brain (a few minutes), slightly longer in the heart (2–4 hours) and may be very much longer in the limbs. This has important consequences in the presentation of the clinical condition, being sudden and catastrophic in the case of cerebral infarct (stroke), and the potential for therapy.

A special case of infarction is *gangrene,* in which death of whole areas of the body, e.g. a limb or region of the gut, occurs because the arterial supply is cut off. Gangrene may become infected by putrefactive microorganisms. This is most likely to happen to the parts of the body most exposed to environmental organisms (i.e. toes, bowel).

Disruption of the blood supply to an organ can occur as a consequence of blockage at a fixed site, as in the case of thrombus formation. This usually arises on an atheromatous plaque and accounts for most myocardial infarctions.

EMBOLISM

Thrombus from a central source, such as the left atrium in atrial fibrillation, or dislodgement from a non-occlusive thrombus more proximally in the vessel, may cause obstruction. This process of matter being transported through large vessels and finally impacting in smaller distal vessels is called embolism. Usually embolism results from thrombus, but the term is also used for the passage of other material within the cardiovascular system. The inflammatory vegetation that sits on infected heart valves commonly embolises and may be seen as tiny blockages within the retina, or it may carry the infection (septic embolus) to the skin, where it can grow and infect the vessel in which it lodges causing a *mycotic aneurysm.*

Pulmonary embolism

Venous embolism occurs in leg veins, pelvic veins and intracranial venous sinuses; emboli may break off and travel to the pulmonary circulation causing pulmonary embolism. After a surgical operation, the immobile patient suffers from severe stasis of blood in the leg veins where it may clot and cause venous thrombosis. As this thrombosis is slowly dealt with by the fibrinolytic system, pieces of the thrombus may dislodge and float off into the inferior vena cava, pass on through the right heart and embolise to the lungs. Small emboli may be lysed within the lung or become organised and cause permanent damage, which may result in progressive respiratory deficiency. Large emboli may cause acute respiratory and cardiac problems. Very large pulmonary emboli will result in sudden death. If such an embolus impacts across the bifurcation of one of the major pulmonary arteries it is referred to as a *saddle embolus.*

The lung receives its own supply of oxygenated blood from the bronchial circulation. It seems likely that the bronchial microcirculation becomes blocked by the oedema and inflammation associated with embolus and hence infarction takes place. Pulmonary embolism that does not cause immediate death but results in some degree of circulatory impairment is eminently treatable with thrombolytic therapy.

Systemic embolism

In this case thrombus arises from the arterial system and its effects are relative to its size.

Thrombi commonly form on dead cardiac muscle as a result of *myocardial infarction.* These areas have lost their endothelial lining, exposing underlying collagen to circulating platelets. There is also disruption of normal blood flow as the myocardium is adynamic. This creates turbulence and predisposes to thrombus formation at that site. Emboli from the heart are usually left sided and travel to the brain causing cerebrovascular incidents such as transient ischaemic attacks or strokes. They also travel to organs or the limbs. A large embolus may lodge at the bifurcation of the aorta as a saddle embolus which cuts off the blood supply to the lower limbs.

Another material that can enter the blood from the body is *amniotic fluid* at the time of a complicated labour. This is very serious, because not only is the amniotic fluid infected, but it can also activate the components of the coagulation system and cause a severe intravascular coagulopathy.

Fat may embolise from the marrow of large bones at the time of fracture; small fat particles lodge in the lung and cause a severe disruption in gas transfer rather than infarction of the lung, as this organ receives its blood supply separately from the bronchial circulation.

Air embolism is usually the result of medical intervention. Usually air passes into the lungs where it is breathed off. However, larger amounts of air (about 50 ml) will cause circulatory arrest and death. This is because the heart, as a pump, relies upon fluid being relatively incompressible. Air, however, is not, and when the right heart fills with air the beating of the ventricle causes compression and expansion of the gas, resulting in nothing more than foaming of the surrounding blood which gives rise to the characteristic *mill wheel murmur*.

Parts of an *atherosclerotic plaque* (usually in the form of platelet clumps sitting on the surface of the diseased area) may embolise. This condition is important only when embolisation occurs to those parts which are sensitive to ischaemia. Platelet emboli usually disperse, even in the microvasculature, so the period of circulatory interruption is small. Their presence therefore only comes to light when they transiently lodge in the cerebral circulation. This causes a sudden but brief loss of function—a hemiplegia, a loss of speech, etc., depending on the site—termed a *transient ischaemic attack (TIA)*. The importance of this is that it may herald a more major event, and it is clear that the anti-platelet drug, aspirin, does seem to prevent recurrences of the condition.

Sources of emboli

These include:

- Atheroma.
- Infection, e.g. vegetations on rheumatic heart valves.
- Fat. Usually follows severe trauma with fracture to long bones.

- Gas, e.g. Caisson disease. This is experienced by divers when they undergo rapid decompression resulting in gas bubbles coming out of the blood.
- Amniotic fluid. During delivery amniotic fluid may be forced into the maternal uterine veins. From there the amniotic fluid emboli can travel in the circulation and lodge in the lungs causing respiratory distress.
- Tumour: uncommon.
- Iatrogenic: from intravenous fluid or through drug abuse, e.g. talc.

INFARCTION

Infarction is defined as death of tissue due to restricted blood supply. Infarction means 'stuffed full' and the term originated from the oxidation of organs following venous infarction in which arterial supply continues to pump blood into the organ.

Infarction, when it occurs, is treated like any other wound by the body's immune and repair system. Like all wounds, it consists initially of dead tissue. If the patient survives the consequences of the infarct, the wound will heal, i.e. become organised into connective tissue with or without regeneration of specialised structures and cells. In practice, regeneration is rare. Organisation (conversion to fibrous or scar tissue) is, however, predominant and is inevitably preceded by inflammation and phagocytosis of the dead debris by macrophages. The usual end result of an infarct is, therefore, a fibrous scar.

Under the microscope there are features of cell necrosis, i.e. shrinkage (pyknosis) or disintegration (karyorrhexis) of the nuclei. The cellular outlines may be faintly visible or may disappear, depending on the degree of *autolysis* (autodigestion of the cell). The area of dead tissue is surrounded by a zone of congested blood vessels in the surviving peripheral parenchyma. It is from there that new blood vessels will grow (*angiogenesis*) and fibroblasts will migrate to *organise* the infarct.

Chemicals may be released by dead cells into the circulation and are used to diagnose these events. In the case of myocardial infarction the activity of various heart muscle enzymes may be measured in the plasma. Inflammatory mediators and free radicals, polyamines, etc., may all have a deleterious effect on the juxtaposed but surviving tissue. This is best seen in the large area of cerebral oedema that surrounds a cerebral infarct, causing serious loss of function over and above that attributable to the infarct itself. Further, at the periphery of an infarct there may be an ischaemic zone. Here the tissue is not working and is relatively deprived of blood. The presence or absence of this zone is generally related to how well the tissue is supplied by blood from other vessels (collaterals). If there are almost no collaterals the ischaemia will be small around the infarct (e.g. a segmental infarct in the kidney). However, where collaterals are profuse, the area of ischaemia may be much larger than the area of infarction (e.g. the lower limb).

Susceptibility to ischaemia may occur in the following situations:

- absence of additional arterial supply, e.g. the retinal artery
- watershed areas:
  — the subendocardial zone in the heart which relies upon the coronary supply from outside and diffusion from blood within heart chambers
  — the splenic flexure of the colon, between the territories of the superior and inferior mesenteric arteries
  — regions of the cerebral hemispheres, between the territories of the major cerebral arteries.

Ischaemia may develop in patients who are severely shocked and *hypotensive*. This type of injury may occur in the portal vasculature, which is a vascular supply leading from a set of capillaries; a drop in intravascular pressure across the first set means that the tissue perfused by the second set of capillaries may be vulnerable to ischaemic injury.

Other possible examples include:

- the anterior pituitary, perfused by blood from the median eminence of the hypothalamus; ischaemia results in pituitary infarction
- the renal tubular epithelium, perfused by blood from glomerular capillaries; ischaemia results in renal tubular necrosis;
- the exocrine pancreas, perfused by blood already perfused by islets of Langerhans; ischaemia results in acute pancreatitis.

Atheromatous narrowing or stenosis of arteries may not cause infarction when the patient is normotensive but may result in ischaemia if the blood pressure drops.

The consequences of infarction reside in the site in which it occurs and some of the more important will now be considered in particular detail.

Myocardial infarction

Coronary thrombosis and resultant myocardial infarction is the major cause of death in the western world. In the vast majority of cases of myocardial infarction, there is an associated and causative thrombus.

When a coronary vessel becomes occluded by a thrombus, the area of heart supplied by that vessel becomes ischaemic and this causes an immediate alteration in function (seen as a change in the ECG), perhaps even before the chest pain. The area at risk will depend on the

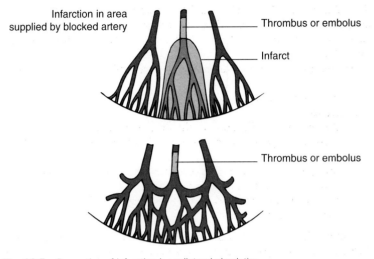

Fig. 20.5   Prevention of infarction by collateral circulation.

collateral supply to the heart. In a dog, when the coronary artery is tied off, there is almost no blood supply to the heart, but in humans with longstanding coronary artery disease there may be considerable collateral development and consequently less infarction (Fig. 20.5).

Ischaemia of heart muscle makes its presence felt as *pain,* and its consequences are often *heart failure* or *rhythm disturbance.* The latter may be any of the rhythm abnormalities, but *ventricular fibrillation* is a common consequence of coronary thrombosis; organised contraction of the ventricle is lost and the heart cannot expel a useful stroke volume. The ischaemia therefore worsens and, left untreated, can only lead to death. This accounts for the vast majority of 'sudden deaths' as they are described. If, by good fortune, the heart does not fibrillate, pump failure becomes more of a feature and *left ventricular failure* occurs. Other possible sequelae are *rupture* and *aneurysm* (Fig. 20.6).

The recognition that myocardial infarction is caused by thrombosis and that in the early hours of the event the heart muscle may recover if reperfused has led to great interest in treatment that dissolves the thrombus (thrombolytic therapy). There is good evidence that with such therapy not only is the size of the infarct reduced but the chances of survival are also improved. If the thrombus remains, the heart muscle will die. This has several consequences as outlined in Figure 20.6.

Cerebral infarction

A *stroke* is caused by death of cerebral tissue. This may result from either a *cerebral infarct* or a blood vessel bursting into the brain

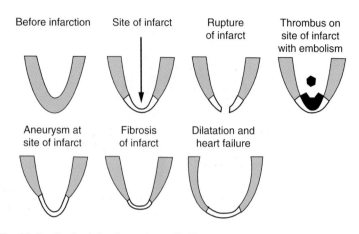

Fig. 20.6   Cardiac infarction and complications.

(*cerebral haemorrhage*). It is difficult to assess which event is the cause in a particular patient. The subject is further complicated by the knowledge that a major risk factor for stroke—high blood pressure—is associated with both atheroma in the cerebral vessels and weaknesses in the little arterioles in the substance of the brain, known as Charcot–Bouchard aneurysms. When the blood pressure rises, these aneurysms may burst into the brain causing haemorrhage and infarction.

It is important to distinguish Charcot–Bouchard aneurysms from berry aneurysms; the latter are probably an inherited weakness of the vessels that supply the brain but they occur outside the substance of that organ and if they rupture cause subarachnoid haemorrhage because of their site. Cerebral infarction may follow upon subarachnoid haemorrhage but usually occurs at a later date when the blood in the cerebrospinal fluid causes cerebral vasospasm which may be intense enough to cause infarction. These differences in mechanism are outlined in Figure 20.7.

Aspirin therapy

Aspirin inhibits thromboxane synthesis in situations where platelet activation is deleterious, e.g. transient cerebral ischaemia. Aspirin is an irreversible inhibitor of cyclo-oxygenase: after one dose all the platelets in the circulation are inhibited for the rest of their lives. There is, however, only transient inhibition of endothelial cyclo-oxygenase, due to the presence of nuclei within the cells which can synthesise more enzyme. Indeed, prostacyclin release returns to normal 90 minutes after a dose of aspirin. In this way the favourable

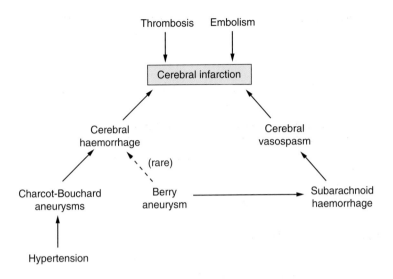

Fig. 20.7   Mechanisms involved in cerebral infarction.

situation whereby prostacycline production remains unchecked while thromboxane synthesis is inhibited is achieved.

THE VESSEL WALL, PLATELETS AND CLOTTING

One of the fundamental properties of the circulatory system is its ability to prevent or arrest the flow of blood from an injured vessel. The efficiency of this depends on a complex interaction between the vessel wall, platelets and the coagulation and the fibrinolytic systems. Failure of any one of these components can result in either a *haemorrhage* or a *thrombotic tendency*. For simplicity each component will be considered independently although in life their functions are interactive.

Vessel wall

The role of the vessel wall endothelial cell in coagulation has only recently been appreciated. It is not merely a passive structural element separating platelets from subendothelial connective tissues, but possesses both procoagulant and anticoagulant properties.

When this rather dull-looking cell is put under the electron microscope, a dense glycocalyx and a pitted cell surface are revealed. It now appears to play an integral part in the control of thrombosis, vascular tone and components of the immune system. Within the control of thrombosis, this cell also has the ability to both promote and prevent coagulation.

Endothelial cell anticoagulant activity

The three main mechanisms of endothelial cell anticoagulant activity are prostacyclin production, protein C activation and fibrinolysis as follows:

1. *Prostacyclin* is synthesised and secreted by endothelial cells and is a powerful inhibitor of platelet aggregation by stimulating adenylate cyclase and thereby increasing platelet cyclic AMP levels.
2. *Protein C* is a vitamin K dependent coagulation factor that inhibits coagulation following activation by the binding of thrombin to the endothelial cell surface protein thrombomodulin.
3. *Fibrinolysis.* Tissue plasminogen activator (tPA) and its inhibitor (tPAI) regulate the fibrinolytic system. They are synthesised and released by endothelial cells.

Disruption of the endothelium is probably one of the most important causes of thrombosis within the arterial system. *Atheroma* is the most usual cause of endothelial disruption, causing abnormalities within the cells and their eventual loss at very early stages of the atherosclerotic process. It is thrombosis forming upon the atheroma found within the coronary circulation that causes myocardial ischaemia and infarction. *Homocysteine*, which accumulates in the inherited disease homocysteinuria, also causes endothelial damage and the condition is associated with a high risk of venous and arterial thrombosis.

Absence of the endothelium exposes a subendothelial space which leads to thrombus formation by initiating both platelet adhesion and the activation of clotting (Fig. 20.8). In addition, the lack of endothelium removes protective antithrombotic systems such as prostacyclin production or anti-aggregatory adenosine. Table 20.1 lists the products of endothelium and how they are involved with the control of thrombosis.

The effect of the *flow component* of Virchow's triad is crucial and even slight disruption in flow may cause thrombosis.

When atheromatous plaque protrudes into the vessel lumen turbulent blood flow results. Loss of intimal cells results in presentation of denuded plaque surface to blood cells; turbulence results in fibrin deposition and platelet clumping and exposure of collagen which results in platelet adhesion. There will be greater predisposition if the individual has high cholesterol and high levels of LDL. The process is self-perpetuating.

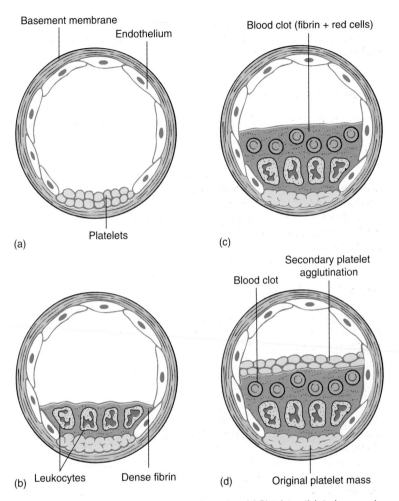

Fig. 20.8   The four stages of thrombus formation. (a) Platelets stick to basement membrane. (b) A dense layer of fibrin and leukocytes adheres to the surface of the platelets. (c) Blood clot forms on the surface of the leukocyte/platelet layer. (d) Fresh platelets agglutinate on the surface of the blood clot.

Platelets

Circulating platelet mass (i.e. platelet count, mean platelet volume) is maintained at a fairly constant level by a humoral factor called *thrombopoietin*. Platelets circulate for 8–14 days before sequestration by the reticuloendothelial system. The splenic pool contains about 30% of blood platelets and is in dynamic equilibrium with the general circulation.

Table 20.1   The endothelium and its role in haemostasis

Prothrombotic	Antithrombotic
Modulation of platelet function	
Synthesis of basement membrane collagen	Generates prostacyclin
Synthesis of von Willebrand factor	Inactivates thrombin
	Adenosine
	Endothelium derived relaxing factor (EDRF)
Modulation of coagulation	
Synthesis of basement membrane collagen	Synthesis of antithrombin III
Synthesis of factor V	Synthesis of protein S
Synthesis and expression of tissue factor	Synthesis of plasminogen activator
Binding site for thrombin	Binding site for plasmin
	Activation of protein C

Platelets (Fig. 20.1) are fragments of cytoplasm derived from megakaryocytes, mainly within the bone marrow. Resting and unstimulated, they are flattened disc-shaped structures with a diameter of 2–4 μm. They have a trilamellar surface membrane that invaginates into the cytoplasm to form an open canalicular system. This greatly increases the surface area of membrane phospholipid, termed platelet factor 3, onto which clotting factors attach.

Platelet cytoplasm contains a number of organelles, including alpha granules containing growth factors, von Willebrand factor and fibrinogen, and dense bodies storing calcium and adenosine nucleotides. When platelets adhere to exposed subendothelial structures:

1. the granular contents are released, activating and aggregating neighbouring platelets
2. arachidonic acid is liberated from membrane phospholipids and converted by cyclo-oxygenase to cyclic endoperoxides and the powerful platelet aggregating agent thromboxane A_2.

Platelet activation

The platelet is a key initiating cell in thrombosis. To achieve this the platelet becomes 'activated', and this process is usually divided into:

- adhesion
- release
- aggregation
- participation in the clotting system
- clot retraction.

Whilst these stages are theoretically distinct, they all follow sequentially and inevitably one upon the other, following the release of the contents of the platelet granules (Fig. 20.9).

Platelet adherence Upon exposure of the subendothelial surface, platelets adhere. This is not a haphazard event but requires the presence of specific platelet glycoproteins which interact with von Willebrand factor in the subendothelial matrix. Disruption of either causes abnormal haemostasis as seen in von Willebrand's disease or the qualitative platelet disorders of Bernard–Soulier disease and Glanzmann's syndrome, in which the surface glycoproteins are abnormal.

Release Following this there is release of the contents of the dense granules of the platelets. The contents of the granules are numerous, and the role of many of the compounds identified is still being elucidated. Notable, however, are ADP, 5HT and platelet derived growth factor (PDGF).

Platelet aggregation *ADP* is the compound that perpetuates the whole activation process since it causes the next stage, aggregation of that individual platelet, and also activates additional platelets, recruiting more cells to the site of injury. *5HT* is a vasoconstrictor and

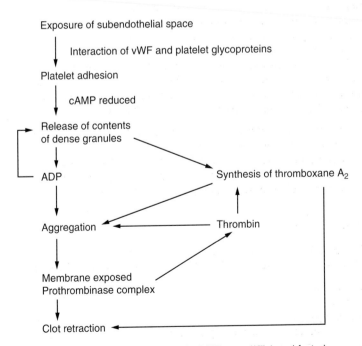

Fig. 20.9 Platelet activation in fibrinolysis. (vWF = von Willebrand factor)

causes vasospasm of the local microcirculation. *PDGF* is probably important in the process of platelet activation, but is of additional interest for its capacity to cause smooth cell division. It has been implicated as the link between platelet adherence and smooth muscle hypertrophy in atheroma.

Aggregation occurs because of conformational changes within the platelet which cause the surface to become more sticky. It seems that an energy-dependent mechanism activates a change in the cell shape via the platelet's complex cytoskeleton, bringing about exposure of the membrane glycoprotein and allowing adhesion of adjacent platelets. They thus form a mass that covers the vessel wall defect until endothelial cells have regenerated and permanently repaired the vessel. A thrombus results if this process is activated within an intact vessel.

Platelet binding properties depend on the presence of two bridging proteins, vWF:Ag and fibrinogen. vWF:Ag is an endothelial cell-derived protein which polymerises in plasma into a high molecular weight species capable of bridging the gap between platelet membrane glycoprotein Ib and subendothelial collagen (Fig. 20.10). The

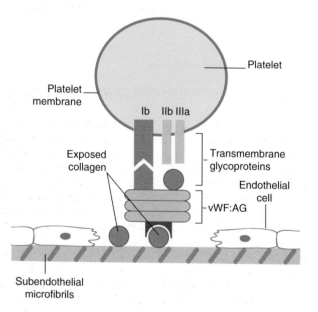

Fig. 20.10 Platelet adhesion to damaged endothelium. The adhesion of platelets to damaged vascular endothelium is mediated by multimeric von Willebrand factor (vWF:Ag). It binds to glycoprotein Ib on the platelet membrane as well as to subendothelial collagen. Deficiencies of glycoprotein Ib (i.e. Bernard–Soulier syndrome), IIb/IIIa (i.e. Glanzmann's thrombasthenia), and vWF:Ag (i.e. von Willebrand's disease) all result in haemorrhagic disorders.

glycoprotein complex IIb/IIIa is the receptor for fibrinogen, and binding with fibrinogen enables interplatelet aggregation. Platelet activation causes a conformational change in IIb/IIIb enabling it to bind fibrinogen. ADP, however, is not the only agonist that causes aggregation; others include thrombin, thromboxane A_2, and platelet activating factor (PAF).

The platelets are now joined together at the site of injury but there remains more work to be done. The platelet membrane contains enzymes of the coagulation pathway (e.g. prothrombinase complex) and this focuses the activation of coagulation to the site of damage. This ingenious mechanism will then generate more thrombin which in turn activates more platelets and the system continues.

Platelet disorders

Platelet defects may be qualitative, in which platelet function may be abnormal despite normal counts, or quantitative from either impaired production or increased consumption. Haemostasis usually remains intact unless the platelet count falls below $40 \times 10^9/l$ (the normal range being 120 to 160). This is discussed in more detail later (p. 252).

THE COAGULATION AND FIBRINOLYSIS SYSTEM

Our understanding of the control of blood coagulation (Fig. 20.11) is growing ever more complicated. The main aim of coagulation is the conversion of soluble fibrinogen into an insoluble cross-linked fibrin clot (Fig. 20.12), and this is achieved by activation of two cascade systems made up of coagulation factors which are either enzymes or their co-factors. The two pathways are called the *intrinsic* and *extrinsic pathways*. When blood is put in a glass tube it takes about 10 minutes to clot. This occurs as a result of activation of the intrinsic pathway by the presence of a negatively charged surface. In life the negatively charged surface is provided by the subendothelium, and this activates kallikrein and attaches factor XII. The extrinsic pathway, however, can only be activated in the test tube by addition of a tissue factor (the usual source being brain) which activates factor VII. This is much faster and causes clotting within 15 seconds. In life (i.e. tissue) factors released from damaged cells activate factor VII, which in turn activates factor X (the extrinsic pathway). It now appears that a very important part of the coagulation pathway is direct activation of factor IX by the activated factor VII–tissue factor complex. The clotting pathways meet at factor X, which in its activated form is bound into the prothrombinase complex in the platelet membrane. This clearly helps to localise clotting to the site of platelet accumulation. In

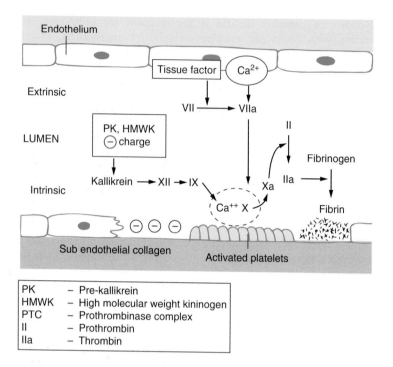

Fig. 20.11 The pathways involved in blood coagulation.

addition contact with damaged surfaces activates factor XII, which, via factors XI, IX and VIII, leads to factor X activation (the intrinsic pathway). From this point factor X converts prothrombin to thrombin. Thrombin then acts on fibrinogen to form fibrin.

- Fibrin polymerises and is stabilised by cross-linking in the presence of factor XIII.
- Clot formation is controlled (localised to the site of damage) by naturally occurring coagulation inhibitors (antithrombin III, protein C, protein S).

Predisposition to thrombosis

Fibrin forms the structural framework of the thrombus, and the conversion of fibrinogen to fibrin is initiated by the enzyme thrombin. Two regulatory mechanisms modulate thrombus formation in vivo:

1. an anticoagulant system that inactivates serum proteases including thrombin
2. a fibrinolytic system that proteolytically degrades fibrin.

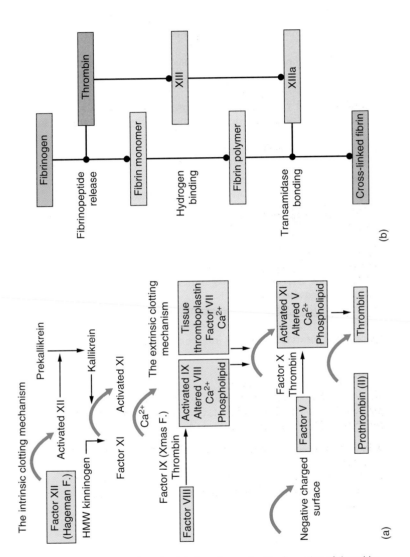

Fig. 20.12 (a) The intrinsic and extrinsic pathways for the formation of thrombin. HMW = high molecular weight. (b) Conversion of soluble fibrinogen into a cross-linked fibrin clot. Thrombin specifically cleaves small peptides from A· and B chains of fibrinogen. The resultant fibrin is stabilised by activated factor XIII (XIIIa).

Inherited deficiencies of protein C, protein S, antithrombin III and tissue plasminogen activator predispose to thrombosis. Such inherited 'thrombophilias' have a prevalence of 1:7500 and are more common in the general population than inherited bleeding disorders, which affect 1:20 000.

People with inherited abnormalities of either of these regulatory mechanisms have an increased risk of developing venous and, more rarely, arterial thromboembolism.

Protein C is a vitamin K dependent protein that in the presence of a co-factor (protein S) destroys the activity of factor V in the prothrombinase complex. It also has anti-factor VIII activity. Families with protein C deficiency are now recognised and often present with venous thrombosis. Protein C, being a vitamin K dependent compound, will be reduced still further by warfarin treatment and this often leads to thrombosis in the microcirculation of the skin.

Antithrombin III is a protein capable of binding to thrombin and factors XIIa, XIa, IX, VIIa and Xa, rendering them inactive. Deficiency of antithrombin III is quite common and is familial. Patients suffering from this condition are at risk of thrombosis. An important feature of this condition is that heparin acts via antithrombin III, and anticoagulation in these people will not be achieved using this compound.

Increased levels of clotting factors may promote thrombosis. Elevated factor VII levels are found to be associated with increased risk of myocardial infarction and, by inference, with coronary thrombosis.

Acquired risk factors include:

- immobility
- obesity
- pregnancy
- the puerperium
- the contraceptive pill
- surgery (especially abdominal or hip surgery)
- smoking
- burns
- dehydration
- autoimmune disorders
- the presence of lupus anticoagulant.

Vascular bleeding disorders

These may result in subcutaneous bleeding (purpura). Such conditions may be either hereditary or acquired and may result from:

- hereditary vascular disorders (hereditary haemorrhagic telangiectasia)

- hereditary connective tissue defects (Ehlers–Danlos syndrome, Marfan's syndrome, osteogenesis imperfecta)
- acquired allergic diseases (e.g. Henoch–Schönlein syndrome, drug reactions)
- acquired atrophic conditions (e.g. senile purpura, scurvy, corticosteroid therapy, Cushing's syndrome)
- acquired infection, which may be bacterial (e.g. meningococcal), viral (e.g. haemorrhagic fever), rickettsial or purpura fulminans
- acquired miscellaneous causes such as easy bruising syndrome.

Hereditary haemorrhagic telangiectasia (Osler–Rendu–Weber syndrome)

This condition is rare and may present at any age. There is autosomal dominant inheritance. Hereditary haemorrhagic telangiectasia is characterised by small vascular malformations, particularly in the nose, mouth and gastrointestinal tract.

Epistaxis and chronic severe iron deficiency are common symptoms and may not develop until adulthood.

Hereditary connective tissue defects

A number of genetic defects are characterised by defects in capillary support including Marfan's syndrome, osteogenesis imperfecta and pseudoxanthoma elasticum. The purpura of patients with Ehlers–Danlos syndrome is due to defective platelet aggregation due to abnormal skin collagen.

Acquired atrophic vascular bleeding disorders

Acquired atrophic vascular bleeding disorders include senile purpura, which results in characteristic lesions (ecchymoses) in the elderly due to the progressive loss of supporting collagen. The lesions usually occur on the backs of the hands, wrists and forearms. Patients on long-term corticosteroid therapy and with Cushing's syndrome may also have thin skin and associated purpura.

Acquired infection-associated vascular bleeding disorders

Purpura may be associated with infections that produce endothelial damage directly or via immune complex-type hypersensitivity.

Hereditary blood coagulation disorders

Disorders of blood coagulation are uncommon and include haemophilia A, haemophilia B (Christmas disease) and von Willebrand's disease.

Haemophilia A

The prevalence of this condition is 1:10 000; spontaneous haemarthrosis and soft tissue haemorrhage may be present from birth. The disorder is X-linked recessive and males of all races are affected.

Haemophilia A results from an absence or a low level of plasma FVIII:C; this may arise from a number of different factor VIII gene deletions or single point mutations.

Factor VIII complex is composed of a large multimeric protein vWF:Ag (von Willebrand factor antigen) and the smaller coagulant protein FVIII:C (Fig. 20.13). In addition to involvement in platelet formation vWF:Ag is important in the binding and stabilisation of FVIII:C; von Willebrand's disease is therefore associated with low FVIII:C levels.

Haemophilia A has a spectrum of clinical severity that approximates with the assayed level of plasma FVIII:C. The most severely affected patients have FVIII:C of about 1% of normal levels. The disease is characterised by a prolonged kaolin cephalin clotting time (KCCT), and a normal prothrombin time (PT) and thrombin time (TT). Factor VIII:C is low, but vWF:Ag, platelet count and bleeding time are normal.

Haemophilia B (Christmas disease)

This is less common than haemophilia A, having an incidence of 1:100 000. It is characterised by a deficiency of factor IX and is an X-linked recessive condition.

The clinical presentation is identical to haemophilia A, and investigation shows:

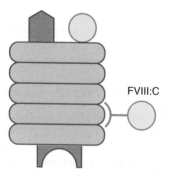

FVIII:C

Fig. 20.13   Diagram of the factor VIII complex. VWF:Ag is a multimer of up to 80 units, each of molecular weight 270 000. Factor VIII:C is bound to vWF:Ag via specific receptors.

- prolonged KCCT
- normal PT/TT
- reduced factor IX.

von Willebrand's disease

von Willebrand's disease (vWD) is an inherited bleeding disorder affecting 1% of the population. It can occur at any age depending on the type. There is no sexual predisposition and the majority show autosomal dominant inheritance.

Patients have either reduced vWF:Ag (classical, Type I vWD) or an abnormal vWF:Ag molecule (Type II vWD).

A diagnosis of vWD is established by demonstrating a prolonged bleeding time, reduced or abnormal vWF:Ag, low FVIII:C and impaired ristocetin-induced platelet aggregation. (Ristocetin aggregates platelets only in the presence of normal vWF:Ag.)

Acquired blood coagulation disorders

Unlike the inherited diseases, acquired blood coagulation disorders usually involve multiple clotting factor deficiencies. They may be associated with:

- vitamin K deficiency (haemorrhagic disease of the newborn)
- biliary obstruction
- malabsorption syndrome
- drugs
- liver disease
- uraemia
- disseminated intravascular coagulation (DIC).

Disseminated intravascular coagulation (DIC)

The causes of disseminated intravascular coagulation are listed in Table 20.2. Disseminated intravascular coagulation results from activation of the coagulation system in response to both direct and indirect triggers. Thrombin production is the postulated common mechanism, causing fibrin and platelet deposition and secondary fibrinolysis. Consumption of clotting factors may be acute and lead to total defibrination. Acute DIC is typically seen in specific obstetric situations (intrauterine death, amniotic fluid embolism) and after acute Gram-negative infection. The initiating events are systemic release of placental thromboplastin and endotoxin, and the resulting coagulopathy may be life-threatening.

A reduced PT, KCCT, TT, plasma fibrinogen and platelet count, together with raised fibrin degradation products (FDPs) confirm the diagnosis.

Table 20.2   Causes of disseminated intravascular coagulation

Infections
Gram-negative, meningococcal, clostridial or viral

Malignancy
Solid tumours, leukaemia

Obstetric
Amniotic fluid embolus, antepartum
haemorrhage, intrauterine death, eclampsia or retained placenta

Immunological
Incompatible blood transfusion, anaphylaxis

Liver disease
Acute liver failure, cirrhosis, Reye's syndrome

Snake bite
Rattlesnakes, other vipers

Fibrinolytic system

Fate of thrombi

Thrombus has a number of possible fates:

- Degradation and dissolution: this probably happens to the majority.
- Organisation: macrophages will invade and clear away the thrombus but fibroblasts replace it with collagen and may leave a stricture.
- Recanalisation: small capillaries may grow into the thrombus and regain patency of the vessel.
- Embolisation: small fragments of the thrombus may break off into the circulation.

The process of thrombus resolution

Once a thrombus is formed the body has to consider its resolution. The process of organisation of the clot is to some extent similar to the organisation and healing found in other systems. The main aim of any such process is the restoration of function; in the case of blood vessels this is recanalisation and the re-establishment of flow. This may occur in both venous and arterial thrombi. This process requires a system to digest the stable fibrin (fibrinolysis), with the formation of new capillary channels.

Histologically, a resolving thrombus becomes invaded by fibroblasts and macrophages. Adjacent endothelium grows into the crevices on the surface of the thrombus that result from fibrinolysis.

The dead cells within are removed by macrophages, and the endothelial pouches descend deeper into the thrombus; some of them, like tunnellers, meet in the middle and recanalisation is achieved.

Degradation of fibrin

Fibrinolysis is the enzymatic degradation of fibrin into soluble fibrin degradation products (FDPs). It maintains vascular patency by preventing excess fibrin deposition on blood vessel walls.

The process of fibrinolysis is complex. The stable fibrin protein is digested by an enzyme called *plasmin*. As is so often the case plasmin circulates as its inactive form *plasminogen*. There are groups of compounds that cause the conversion of plasminogen to plasmin, and these are called *plasminogen activators* (Figs 20.14, 20.15). The body has its own natural activator called *tissue plasminogen activator (tPA)*. tPA is made by endothelium, and by itself does not activate much

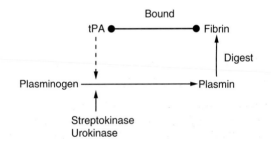

Fig. 20.14 Fibrinolysis.

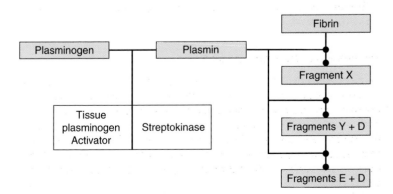

Fig. 20.15 Fibrin digestion. Plasma cleaves fibrin into a number of soluble fragments called fibrin degradation products (FDPs).

plasminogen, but upon binding to fibrin tPA undergoes a conformation change that allows exposure of its active site. Plasminogen is thus only activated to plasmin at sites where fibrin is bound.

Various exogenous activators of plasminogen exist and these are used therapeutically. A protein found in the urine called *urokinase* activates plasminogen, as does the streptococcal product *streptokinase*. These two agents are widely used for the treatment of thrombotic conditions (e.g. acute myocardial infarction and pulmonary embolism) with considerable success when introduced early enough. Recombinant DNA technology has allowed the production of large amounts of tPA, and this too is being used in the treatment of these conditions.

KEY POINTS

- Thrombosis has the vital purpose of arresting haemorrhage. Platelets are activated, sticking to the vessel wall and to each other. The blood coagulation system is then activated, resulting in the formation of stable fibrin. The fibrin filaments enmesh red blood cells, and more platelets alight on the mass.
- Embolism is the process of matter being transported through large vessels and finally impacting in smaller distal vessels. Embolism usually results from thrombus, but may also be caused by air, fat, amniotic fluid, atheroma, tumour or infection.
- Infarction is the death of tissue due to restricted blood supply.
- Coronary thrombosis and resultant myocardial infarction is the major cause of death in the western world.
- A stroke is caused by ischaemia and death of cerebral tissue. This may result from either a cerebral infarct or a cerebral haemorrhage.
- The efficiency of blood clotting depends on a complex interaction between the vessel wall, platelets and the coagulation and the fibrinolytic systems. Failure of any of these can result either in haemorrhage or in a thrombotic tendency.

21 | Failure of body systems

HEART FAILURE

The term 'heart failure' is a pathophysiological description rather than a purely pathological entity. It describes the situation where the cardiac output is not sufficient for the body's demands. Heart failure can be classified on the severity of the symptoms and ranges from mild to severe. Many of the mechanisms present in the severe form of the condition are also present in mild failure, although they are of a transient nature in the latter.

Heart failure can be divided into left or right heart failure or a combination of both, and may be further subdivided into acute and chronic. The term 'congestive cardiac failure' refers to the situation where chronic left and right heart failure coexist. The feature common to all the above is that there is insufficient cardiac output, the consequences of which tend to make matters worse. As cardiac output falls there is increased sympathetic activity. This results in peripheral vasoconstriction (patients are often pale, cool to the touch, sweaty and in fear for their lives).

This peripheral vasoconstriction is teleologically thought of as the redirection of blood from parts that do not require 'luxury perfusion' to other parts that do (heart and brain). This simplistic view may act as an *aide memoire* but is incorrect. Firstly, the whole sympathetic discharge is usually overdone and increases the peripheral vascular resistance to such a degree that the work the heart has to do is increased (*afterload*). The realisation of this fact is responsible for the increasing use of vasodilators in heart failure. Secondly, the kidney also undergoes vasoconstriction in this process. This is detrimental and leads to a number of events. The best understood is activation of the *renin angiotensin system*, which causes more peripheral vasoconstriction (via angiotensin II) and stimulation of aldosterone production (Fig. 21.1).

Renin is a proteolytic enzyme that is made by the kidney. When in the plasma it converts *angiotensinogen* to *angiotensin I,* an inactive amino acid nonapeptide. Angiotensin I is then converted to the heptapeptide *angiotensin II* (the active component of the pathway) by the action of *angiotensin converting enzyme (ACE).* The enzyme ACE is found on the surface of endothelial cells throughout the cardiovascular system. Angiotensin II has a direct pressor action and intensifies the vasoconstriction. It also facilitates adrenergic vasoconstriction, thereby worsening vasoconstriction caused by the sympathetic. Finally, it stimulates the zona glomerulosa cells of the adrenal to produce *aldosterone,* a steroid hormone that favours salt resorption by the distal nephron, thus increasing total body fluid. Salt handling by the kidney is also disrupted as a result of the reduction in glomerular perfusion pressure brought about by renal vasoconstriction. This leads to the disruption of tubulo-glomerular feedback and increased salt retention.

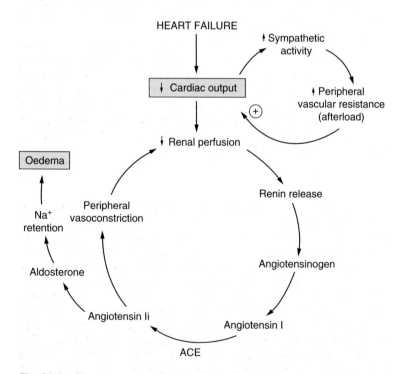

Fig. 21.1 The renin angiotensin system in heart failure.

These mechanisms all work to exacerbate heart failure, and this observation prompted the search for an endogenous natriuretic hormone which might redress the balance. One such substance is *atrial natriuretic peptide (ANP)*, a powerful natriuretic compound released by the atria following expansion of blood volume. Another possible hormone is *endogenous digitalis-like factor* which reduces sodium reabsorption and constricts blood vessels. The precise role of these endogenous factors remains unclear.

Left heart failure

The clinical picture of acute left heart failure is dramatic. There is massive vasoconstriction, producing a cold, sweaty, pale patient who is severely breathless due to pulmonary oedema, often with pink, frothy sputum (actually oedema fluid). Acute left heart failure results from a sudden event that does not allow the left heart time to dilate and compensate. This event is usually acute myocardial ischaemia at the time of a myocardial infarct (p. 216). Very severe infections of heart muscle, such as certain viruses (myocarditis) or depression of function by the toxin of diphtheria, may also cause this picture. Alternatively the left ventricle may fail because of acute overload, often as a result of valvular leakage.

From the moment of the insult the pressure in the left atrium rises, usually reflecting the raised left ventricular end diastolic pressure in LVF. The formation of pulmonary oedema in these circumstances can largely be related to the left atrial pressure, and is the reason for its measurement in assessing treatment. Pulmonary oedema does not usually occur until the left atrial pressure rises above 30 mmHg; a massive transudate then occurs, filling the alveoli and causing hypoxia, breathlessness and sometimes cough.

Congestive cardiac failure

This is usually a chronic problem with failure of both ventricles on both sides of the heart. A persistent left heart problem leads to chronic pulmonary venous congestion with resultant pulmonary hypertension. Faced with a hypertensive pulmonary circulation the right ventricle will hypertrophy and eventually dilate. The Starling curves relating force of contraction to ventricular volume are much flatter for the right ventricle and right ventricular failure occurs at an earlier stage, often associated with a functional leakage of the tricuspid valve (*tricuspid regurgitation*). This leads to marked *venous congestion* and oedema in the dependent part of the body (usually the ankles). The venous congestion often affects the liver, initially causing enlargement. Red blood cells and their pigments may collect within the liver, and cells in this area may become smaller and atrophic.

Surrounding this area the normal liver tissue appears lighter and the resulting appearance resembles a half-ground nutmeg. If the venous congestion is longstanding, fibrosis of the liver lobules may occur, a state known as *cardiac cirrhosis*, with resultant abnormalities of hepatic function. The bowel may also become distended with oedema, interfering with drug absorption.

Acute right heart failure

This occurs in two situations:

1. massive pulmonary embolus
2. right ventricular infarction.

The patient is usually breathless, mainly as a result of *hypoxia*. The importance of making an accurate diagnosis cannot be overemphasised. When the right ventricle fails in isolation, the patient will die of low cardiac output rather than of congestion. The cardiac output is only improved by increasing the filling pressure of the right ventricle (i.e. with fluids) rather than by reducing it with diuretics which aggravate the situation.

Cor pulmonale

Cor pulmonale is right heart failure secondary to a pulmonary lesion. A pulmonary lesion that affects gas transfer (emphysema, fibrosing alveolitis) leads to hypoxia and resulting pulmonary vasoconstriction. *Pulmonary hypertension* ensues, which in turn leads to right ventricular hypertrophy and failure. Pulmonary hypertension may also occur as a result of reduction of vascular territory by chronic pulmonary thromboembolism. The features of cor pulmonale, apart from oedema, are somewhat different from those of congestive cardiac failure. The patient is often warm because of hypercapnia (CO_2 retention), and the cardiac output is not usually low. Salt and water retention probably occurs more as a result of the electrolyte and acid–base disturbances.

RENAL FAILURE

The role of the kidney in homeostasis is so vital that any disturbance in its function is soon reflected in the body fluid and any major impairment is often incompatible with life.

In the kidney the glomerulus filters plasma in such a way as to clear it of waste products, leaving high molecular weight protein unfiltered. The kidney tubules then modify the filtrate in such a way as to form a urine of the concentration appropriate to the body's current fluid status and acid–base balance. An insult to the kidney will, therefore, cause different clinical problems according to which structure is damaged. The term 'renal failure' is reserved for conditions where the kidney is damaged to such an extent that urea and creatinine collect in the plasma. However, other stresses on the kidney leave this aspect of function unaltered, but may allow the passage of large amounts of protein or blood in the filtrate. Whilst these states are technically not called renal failure, it is clear that major renal damage is present.

Glomerulonephritis

Glomerulonephritis is damage, usually by an immune process, to the glomerulus. The pathology is classically divided into different types on the basis of histology. The clinical result of glomerulonephritis is divided into a group of conditions characterised by the symptoms and signs seen in the patients. Whilst there are sometimes correlates between the clinical and pathological picture (e.g. minimal change type glomerulonephritis and nephrotic syndrome), this is not always the case.

The nephrotic syndrome

The nephrotic syndrome is the combination of proteinuria, hypoalbuminaemia and oedema. The cause is damage to the glomerulus from any cause (drugs, poisons, etc.) but immune glomerulonephritis is the most common. For hypoalbuminaemia to exist the proteinuria has to be greater than 3 g/day to exceed the amount synthesised by the liver. Hypoalbuminaemia is a prerequisite for oedema formation by reducing the oncotic pressure (p. 242). Hypoalbuminaemia also causes a reduced circulating volume; as always, this stimulates salt and water retention.

Nephritis

Glomerulonephritis may also present with a nephritic illness, most commonly seen following a group A streptococcal infection or in SLE (p. 71). Here the glomerular injury results in hypertension, impaired glomerular filtration rate (GFR) and mild proteinuria. Confusingly, mild oedema, usually of the face, is also a feature of nephritis, despite the lack of hypoalbuminaemia. Oedema probably occurs due to the low GFR of the damaged kidney causing significant sodium retention. Progression from nephritis to acute renal failure is seen, but usually only occurs with the acute vasculitides (polyarteritis nodosa, Goodpasture's syndrome) and is extremely uncommon in poststreptococcal glomerulonephritis.

Acute renal failure (ARF)

Acute renal failure is a clinical entity and glomerular damage is but one of its many causes. It is characterised by a falling GFR which causes a rise in urea and creatinine. Clinically the causes are classified into:

- prerenal (renal hypoperfusion)
- renal (renal damage)
- post-renal (obstruction to outflow).

These groups do have their pathological correlates, but they are sometimes confusing. When the blood supply to the kidney is reduced for whatever reason (haemorrhage, heart failure), intense vasoconstriction occurs which usually shunts blood away from the renal cortex. There is a critical period when, if the perfusion pressure can be normalised, the GFR starts rising and the kidney recovers. However, if renal ischaemia persists, a cycle of events occurs where the renal tubules become swollen and do not function even when the perfusion pressure returns to normal. This situation is called *acute tubular necrosis* and is the renal lesion secondary to hypoperfusion that causes sustained renal failure. Some confusion arises as acute tubular necrosis can also be caused directly by nephrotoxic agents and drugs, especially aminoglycosides.

Acute renal failure is characterised by the production of small amounts of poorly concentrated urine. The fluid retention results in systemic and pulmonary oedema. Hyperkalaemia occurs because of the body's inability to excrete potassium, and may lead to disturbances of cardiac rhythm. The failure to clear urea and other waste products makes the patient feel sick. Disturbance of the kidney's role in acid–base balance renders the patient acidotic, causing hyperventilation. Obviously acute renal failure is a medical emergency.

Chronic renal failure (CRF)

Chronic renal failure is often revealed by the history which includes polyuria, nocturia and a story of chronic ill-health with clinical evidence of a longstanding problem, i.e. anaemia due to low erythropoietin (p. 250), or bone disease (osteomalacia) due to reduced vitamin D hydroxylation. The kidneys are usually small and shrunken and the blood urea is elevated. Some of the most common causes of CRF (as opposed to ARF) are diabetes mellitus and hypertension, as well as polycystic disease and occasionally recurrent urinary tract infection. However the condition can present as an acute episode of, say, vomiting and diarrhoea which puts an undue stress on an already damaged kidney deprived of nephrons.

LIVER FAILURE

The liver, with its multiple functions, when failing presents with protean features. Failure, as in any organ system, may be acute or chronic, or indeed acute on chronic.

Acute liver failure

In acute liver failure, which in this country usually results from either *viral hepatitis* or *paracetamol* poisoning, the detoxification process normally performed by the liver of removing ammonia and amino acids from the bowel is abolished at an early stage. This probably accounts for the encephalopathy that is seen. Bilirubin is not cleared from the blood and the patient becomes jaundiced. The absence of gluconeogenesis results in hypoglycaemia and the disruption of protein synthesis causes reduced levels of albumin and clotting factors. The condition has a high mortality rate but complete recovery, ultimately with a normal hepatic architecture, is possible.

Chronic liver failure

Chronic hepatic failure results usually from either *chronic active hepatitis* or *cirrhosis*. In this condition the structure of the liver is distorted such that a rise in portal perfusion pressure occurs. This causes increased formation of hepatic lymph. The hepatic sinusoids are permeable to protein, so the restraining oncotic influence is unchecked and small rises in pressure lead to large rises in lymph formation. When this exceeds the capacity of the lymphatics, free fluid, known as *ascites*, collects in the abdomen. The formation of ascites is also contributed to by leakage from the mesenteric capillaries. Similarly, in chronic hepatic failure salt retention occurs from renal hypoperfusion and secondary hyperaldosteronism, further promoting ascites.

RESPIRATORY FAILURE

Although deteriorating lung function can cause increasing breathlessness, a reduction in exercise and cough, the ultimate, often fatal, outcome is an inability to maintain gas exchange at normal levels. This is known as respiratory failure and is usually defined as being present when the P_{O_2} is less than 8 kPa and the P_{CO_2} is greater than 6.5 kPa. The functional capacity of the lungs is such that, using compensatory mechanisms, considerable reduction is possible before gas exchange is impaired. These mechanisms include an increased ventilation rate and local alterations in vascular and airway resistance.

Once the system can no longer compensate, however, rapid deterioration ensues.

Although blood gas abnormalities occur in combination, a disturbance in oxygenation (perfusion) can occur in isolation and is classified as *Type I respiratory failure*. This commonly occurs against a background of chronic lung disease, such as pulmonary fibrosis or chronic obstructive lung disease, or following pulmonary congestion or pulmonary embolus.

Ventilatory failure or *Type II respiratory failure* occurs when the normally powerful compensatory mechanisms controlling P_{CO_2} levels fail and the levels rise. This is usually the result of an inability to blow off CO_2 from the lungs, and leads to *acidosis*. Ventilatory failure can occur in severe asthmatic attacks or in chronic bronchitis.

Often Type I and Type II failure can coexist in the same patient; as with other systems the failure can be acute or chronic or a combination of both.

OEDEMA

Oedema is an abnormal amount of fluid in an extracellular compartment. We have seen how it commonly results from the dysfunction of the heart or kidneys. It can occur in any organ but is clearly and commonly seen in the swollen ankles of elderly women with mild congestive heart failure. Its formation is due to the disruption of the homeostatic mechanism described by Starling's hypothesis, namely the balance between hydrostatic and oncotic pressures. Wherever perfusion of a capillary bed occurs, because of the thinness of the blood vessel walls there is a tendency for the perfusion pressure to cause the formation of a filtrate out of the vessel. This hydrostatic pressure is in balance between the intracapillary pressure and the extracellular pressure, i.e. it is a transmural pressure. In general the *extracellular pressure* does not alter within an organ but does vary between different organs, explaining why oedema tends to occur preferentially in certain sites. The *intracapillary pressure* may, however, vary considerably, either from increased perfusion or increased venous pressure resulting in back pressure on the capillary bed. Such variation may cause a greater filtration or tendency towards the formation of a filtrate.

The restraining influence is the presence of protein within the circulation, resulting in an *oncotic pressure* that favours resorption of fluid from the extracellular spaces to the vessel. Oedema formation may result, therefore, if the plasma proteins fall below the minimum level necessary to restrain the hydrostatic tendency to form a filtrate.

The only other possible variables in this model arise if the *permeability of the vessels* is altered. This can occur as a result of a number of insults, all of which disrupt the functional integrity of the microvascular endothelium. This occurs within life as part of the homeostatic mechanism of inflammation. Vasoactive kinins, complement fragments and even neuropeptides can alter vascular permeability, usually as part of the well-ordered sequence of events in the formation of inflammatory exudate. Rarely, excessive amounts of complement products collect within the circulation due to the congenital absence of an inhibitor of the pathway (C1 esterase inhibitor) and this gives rise to the rare condition hereditary angio-oedema.

It is clear therefore that two mechanisms for oedema formation exist:

- hydrostatic/oncotic changes
- changes in permeability.

The resultant oedema formed under the two circumstances varies accordingly. The former gives rise to *transudates* and the latter to *exudates*. The major differences between the two are outlined in Table 21.1 and can easily be predicted from the understanding that an increase in permeability in the vessel wall not only results in increased amounts of fluid but also in an increase in the molecular weight of the contents of the filtrate. Although in individual situations oedema may occur as a result of multiple mechanisms, oedema seldom results if the above systems remain intact; for example, oedema is not seen in primary hyperaldosteronism (Conn's syndrome) despite considerable salt retention with hypertension.

A small amount of extracellular fluid is constantly being formed, and is in exchange with the cells of the body. This fluid is drained by the lymphatic system. Two changes may occur in the lymphatics that concern the extracellular fluid: they may be blocked or they may increase in capacity. *Blockage of the lymphatic system* may be congenital (congenital lymphoedema) or acquired. In this country the latter is nearly always the result of invasion by malignancy. Carcinoma of the breast often spreads to the axillary nodes and this may result in

Table 21.1 The characteristics of transudates and exudates

Characteristic	Transudate	Exudate
Protein content	Low < 30 g/l	High > 30 g/l
Protein pattern	Albumin only	As in plasma
LDH enzyme level	Low < 200 iu	High > 200 iu
Fibrinogen	Absent	Present (clots)
Specific gravity	1.012	1.020
Cells	Few mesothelial	Present

lymphoedema of the arm on that side. Worldwide, however, blockage of the lymphatics by the nematode *Wuchereria bancrofti* (filiariasis) is probably the most common cause. *Increase in lymphatic capacity* results when there has been a slow increase in the amount of extracellular fluid formed over the years and the lymphatics have grown accordingly. This probably explains why patients with raised left atrial pressure in mitral stenosis are not in pulmonary oedema at rest.

Pulmonary oedema

Pulmonary oedema is commonly seen in *acute left heart failure* when the left atrial pressure rises causing back pressure on the pulmonary capillary bed and thence filtration into the alveolar space.

Permeability changes do occur in the pulmonary circulation and, when they are severe, massive pulmonary oedema will occur even with the lowest of left atrial pressures. The usual situation in which this occurs is massive *sepsis*. Following Gram-negative septicaemia the lungs become more permeable to fluid, which fills up the alveolar spaces and causes hypoxia.

Interestingly, changes in permeability can occur without direct insult, as pulmonary oedema can occasionally be seen following a head injury or neurosurgery. The cause of this neurogenic pulmonary oedema is not clear.

FAILURE OF THE RED BLOOD CELL SYSTEM

The important pathology of red cells is *anaemia*—a deficiency of red cells defined as a concentration of haemoglobin of less than 13 g/dl in men and 11.5 g/dl in women.

Erythrocytes, or red blood corpuscles, are by far the most numerous of the cells of the blood. Each mm^3 (microlitre) of blood should contain about 4.5 to 6.2 million red cells. Their importance is that they contain the body's supply of haemoglobin which is required for the transport of oxygen to the tissues, the red cell haemoglobin having become oxygenated in the lungs.

There are several different varieties of anaemia, each of which in turn depends on a disturbance of some facet of red cell production or metabolism. In addition, each of the main subgroups usually needs to be further divided to make a comprehensive classification. As in the case of malignant disease, the taxonomy of anaemia is not an exercise in memory but an essential prelude to understanding. Table 21.2 outlines the classification of anaemias, which basically arise either from a failure of production or from an increase in red cell loss.

Table 21.2 A classification of anaemia

Anaemia	MCV	Platelets	White cell count	Diagnosis
Microcytic	< 80 fl			Iron deficiency
				Thalassaemia
Normocytic	80–96 fl	Normal	Normal	Anaemia of chronic disorder, rheumatoid arthritis
		Low/normal	Abnormal	Marrow invasion by cancer (leukoerythroblastic anaemia)
				Haematological malignancy
		Normal	Increased	Chronic haematological malignancy
Macrocytic	> 96 fl	Normal	Normal	Vitamin B_{12} or folate deficiency, liver disease, haemolysis
		Low	Normal/low	Vitamin B_{12} or folate deficiency, acute haematological malignancy
		Normal/low	Abnormal	Myelodysplastic syndrome

Haemolytic anaemias

In this group, anaemia occurs because there is an *excessive destruction* of red cells. The normal life span of the red corpuscle is about 120 days. When the cells are old and effete they are destroyed (haemolysed) in the circulation and spleen and liver. It is this process which is exaggerated and accelerated in a haemolytic anaemia.

Haemolytic anaemias due to abnormalities of the red cell

The most important group numerically in this category is that of diseases due to *abnormalities of haemoglobin*. This substance, which carries the blood oxygen, consists of four haem molecules, each bound to a globin polypeptide chain. Most abnormalities of haemoglobin arise in the globin moiety.

In *sickle cell anaemia* (p. 189) the patients, usually of African origin, inherit a structural abnormality of the beta chain of the globin in which a glutamic acid molecule is replaced by a valine. This alters the physicochemical nature of the haemoglobin and reduces its solubility. As a result the red cells assume a sickle shape, are rendered fragile and are rapidly destroyed in the circulation.

In *thalassaemia*, an inherited disease of Mediterranean peoples, there is defective synthesis of either beta chains or, less commonly, alpha chains of haemoglobin. The defective chains are replaced by other chains of different structure but once again the red cells are abnormally fragile and rapidly destroyed, leading to anaemia.

Another group of corpuscular defects is due to genetically determined deficiency of intracellular glucose-6-phosphate dehydrogenase (G6PD). This results in impaired activity of the hexose monophosphate shunt pathway, leading in turn to failure to generate sufficient energy to maintain glutathione in a reduced state (GSH). GSH itself is needed to maintain the many SH groups of the red cell in a reduced state. Failure to do so makes the cell abnormally permeable. In these groups of disorders, haemolytic anaemia does not usually occur unless precipitated by exposure to an *oxidising agent* in a drug or foodstuff, e.g. primaquine, sulphonamides, aspirin or the fava bean. The genetics of these disorders are complex, some being sex-linked (p. 178) and occurring in both Mediterranean and African peoples.

The final group of corpuscular haemolytic anaemias arises from *abnormal permeability* of the red cell membrane. In this category is hereditary spherocytosis where the cells cannot resist the entry of water and sodium chloride and thus become spherical and fragile. In this disease, removal of the spleen is often curative because the abnormal corpuscles are no longer destroyed there.

Haemolytic anaemias due to extracorpuscular factors

The most important cause of these anaemias is *antibodies*, which have been discussed previously (p. 38). Extrinsic antibodies (*allo-antibodies*) or autologous antibodies (*auto-antibodies*) can be responsible. In either instance the antibody has the capacity to agglutinate the red cells in vitro, either directly or after the addition of antihuman globulin (the Coombs test). In the latter instance the haemolytic antibodies are said to be incomplete. The lack of 'completeness' is, however, merely a useful laboratory artefact. In the body, the cells are coated with the 'incomplete' IgG which is sufficient to render them highly sensitive to destruction in the spleen and liver and hence to produce a haemolytic anaemia.

The most important haemolytic anaemia due to extrinsic antibodies is that which occurs in a newborn baby which has *Rhesus positive* red cells, its mother being Rh negative and having therefore been able to produce antibody to the baby's red cells during fetal life, especially during parturition. The first-born child is usually unaffected, but the risk increases with subsequent births as sensitisation increases. The antibody-coated red cells of the baby are rapidly haemolysed in the liver and spleen causing distension (hydrops fetalis); bile pigment from the broken down haemoglobin stains and damages the basal ganglia of the brain (kernicterus); and death or spasticity of the child may ensue. It is, however, possible to prevent this catastrophe by injecting a blocking anti-Rh antibody into the mother in the two days following delivery.

Haemolytic anaemia may follow *drug sensitisation*. Thus penicillin may sometimes act as a hapten (p. 37), binding with red cell protein and causing complement and antibody binding with resultant haemolysis.

Autoimmune haemolytic anaemia is by no means rare but in almost no case is its causation clear. It can occur without apparent cause (idiopathic) or as a feature of a wide range of diseases including malignancy such as Hodgkin's disease, other lymphomas or carcinoma or known autoimmune conditions such as systemic lupus erythematosus (p. 69). In most cases the antibodies are of the 'incomplete' variety and haemolysis is due to excessive destruction of the antibody-coated cells by the mononuclear phagocyte system.

Finally, haemolytic auto-antibodies exist which can be demonstrated in vitro only by an agglutination reaction performed in the cold, at about 0–2°C (*cold agglutinins*). They occur in various diseases, notably mycoplasma pneumonia (p. 8) and certain rare autoimmune disorders. Unlike all the other antibodies discussed in this section, cold agglutinins usually haemolyse red cells in the circulation by the action of bound activated complement instead of merely rendering them more susceptible to destruction in the spleen and liver.

Iron deficiency anaemia

This is the most common cause of anaemia worldwide. A major constituent of the haem portion of the haemoglobin molecule is iron. It is obvious therefore that a bodily shortage of iron will lead to an overall deficiency of haemoglobin, i.e. an iron deficiency anaemia. It is equally obvious that iron deficiency might result from:

1. inadequate dietary intake
2. inadequate absorption from the intestine
3. excessive chronic loss of blood.

When red cells are destroyed at the end of their life span, their organic constituents are broken down, metabolised and excreted. Their iron however is recycled, being taken up by the iron-binding protein *apoferritin* to form *ferritin*. As a result, the dietary requirement for iron is low and man has evolved an elaborate mechanism for limiting absorption of inorganic iron. This mechanism consists of the presence in the intestinal epithelium of the protein ferritin which binds ionic iron from the diet and retains it in the intestinal wall.

In situations of chronic blood loss, such as a bleeding peptic ulcer or excessive menstrual bleeding, it has to be assumed either that the diet does not contain sufficient iron to replace that which is being lost, or that the ferritin mechanism is too insensitive to the body's needs to release the iron that is needed. The loss of blood is sometimes massive and prolonged; in such cases iron deficiency anaemia is easily explicable and often readily remedied by dosage with ferrous salts.

In other cases blood loss is modest and the anaemia less explicable. There is certainly evidence that the ferritin mechanism for preventing iron overloading of the body can sometimes be too efficient, in that even when iron deficiency anaemia is present, dietary iron supplements are not absorbed.

The *diet* itself may provide another clue. Poor diets may not contain enough ionic iron, due for example to lack of fresh vegetables. There is, however, another pathway for iron absorption in which the metal is taken up by the intestinal epithelium as part of a relatively intact haem molecule, mainly from the myoglobin of animal protein. From the point of view of iron intake the worst diet would be one lacking both ionic iron and animal protein, the next worse one lacking only the protein, and the best a diet rich in both fresh vegetables and meat.

As well as malnutrition, iron deficiency anaemia can be due to *intestinal malabsorption*, e.g. following major bypass surgery in the intestinal tract, although the mechanisms are unclear. Iron needs are also increased in pregnancy and childhood and a mild iron deficiency anaemia is quite common during pregnancy.

Megaloblastic or macrocytic anaemias

Iron can be regarded as an essential nutrient for the production of haemoglobin. The carriage of haemoglobin, however, requires healthy red cells. The formation of healthy corpuscles depends on the usual supply of amino acids, etc., and in theory any severe lack of nutrition should cause red cell production to fall. In practice, iron deficiency supervenes before lack of other dietary constituents becomes effective.

Two substances exist, however, which are specifically required for the production of normal red cells: *folic acid* (pteroylglutamic acid) and *vitamin B_{12}* (cyanocobalamin). They are required for the synthesis of nucleic acids, working independently. As might be expected their lack is felt not only by the red cells but also by leukocytes and platelets, and indeed may be observed even in epithelial cells. Nevertheless it is the nucleated red cell precursors in the bone marrow which suffer most. When either or both substances are deficient these cells acquire abnormal nuclei and are called *megaloblasts*. They give rise to red corpuscles which are larger than normal (*macrocytes*) but greatly reduced in number so that although each cell carries more than its full complement of haemoglobin the patient is nevertheless severely anaemic. The anaemia is worsened by the undue fragility of the megaloblastic corpuscles which gives rise to an associated haemolytic anaemia.

The most important cause of megaloblastic anaemia is *pernicious anaemia* (p. 70), an autoimmune condition in which atrophy of the mucosa of the upper two-thirds of the stomach leads to absence of a substance called intrinsic factor, essential for the absorption of vitamin B_{12}.

Malabsorption from the small intestine is also a common cause of megaloblastic anaemia, often complicated by an associated iron deficiency. Both folic acid and B_{12} may be deficient in such states. Such malabsorption may be due to a defect in the intestinal mucosa as in gluten enteropathy (coeliac disease), or to mucosal destruction and inflammation as in Crohn's disease, or to growth of abnormal bacterial flora which compete for the dietary folic acid or B_{12} as may occur after major intestinal surgery.

Aplastic (hypoplastic) anaemia

In this condition anaemia develops because the red cell precursors in the bone marrow are absent, destroyed or fail to mature into red corpuscles, even of the abnormal variety. It is essentially depression or destruction of the haemopoietic tissue in the bone marrow and as might be expected is likely to affect not only red cells but also leukocytes and platelets, causing a so-called *pancytopenia*.

The commonest cause is *toxic depression of the marrow*, as occurs for example in chronic renal failure, where retained metabolites prevent normal marrow function. Lack of erythropoietin, the red cell stimulating factor formed in the kidney (p. 240), is likely to play a contributory role which is partially reversed by therapy with synthesised erythropoetin. Many drugs have the unfortunate side effect of causing aplastic anaemia, e.g. benzene and cytotoxic drugs used in cancer chemotherapy. Common drugs, e.g. chloramphenicol, gold salts and phenylbutazone, cause the disease in a few susceptible individuals.

Ionising radiation is of course an important cause of marrow aplasia (p. 299). Sometimes the bone marrow becomes so heavily infiltrated by *malignant cells* that the erythropoietic cells are destroyed and replaced and aplastic anaemia results. A similar result may follow fibrosis or bony replacement of the marrow spaces due to diseases of obscure nature, e.g. myelofibrosis.

FAILURE OF THE WHITE CELL SYSTEM

Leukocytes are the 'white' (i.e. non-haemoglobin containing) cells of the circulation. They consist of the *polymorphonuclear leukocytes* (comprising neutrophils, eosinophils and basophils, according to their staining characteristics and in descending order of importance), the *lymphocytes* and the *monocytes*. All types of leukocytes can rise or fall in number in the circulation as a result of disease. With the exception of malignant transformation (leukaemia), a *rise* in number is called a leukocytosis, monocytosis or lymphocytosis and a *fall* in number a leukopenia, etc.

Polymorphonuclear leukocytes are the highly important phagocytes discussed elsewhere (p. 26 and p. 93 for leukocytosis). Lymphocytosis is a less important phenomenon seen mainly in viral diseases such as infectious mononucleosis. Monocytosis is unimportant.

Leukopenia

Leukocytes, unlike red corpuscles, do not appear to fall in number because of excessive destruction or, with the exception of B_{12} and folate deficiency, because of nutritional factors. A leukopenia is almost always the result of toxic depression of polymorph precursors in the bone marrow. The causes of such a depression are the same as those already listed for precipitating anaemia. By far the most important is the use of the cytotoxic antimetabolites, such as cyclophosphamide or methotrexate, used in the chemotherapy of cancer or autoimmune disease, but there are also rare leukopenias of unknown aetiology.

There are normally about 4000 neutrophil polymorphs per microlitre of blood. This level needs to fall to about 400 to make serious infection a likely consequence and to about 200 before acute inflammatory reactions containing substantial numbers of the cells cease to be produced.

Lymphopenia and monocytopenia are unimportant except as complications of malignant disease.

Leukaemia

This is a neoplastic proliferation of leukocytes and their precursors in the bone marrow and can be regarded as the result of malignant transformation (p. 262) of these cells. It may affect the polymorphonuclear (myeloid), lymphocytic or monocytic populations, the last being relatively uncommon.

Leukaemia exists in two forms:

- acute (blastic)
- chronic (cytic).

Thus it is customary to refer to *myeloblastic, myelocytic, lymphoblastic, lymphocytic* leukaemia. The essential difference between acute and chronic leukaemias is the presence in the circulation in the acute variety of very primitive leukocyte precursors, i.e. myeloblasts or lymphoblasts. As might be expected from the terminology, in the absence of treatment acute leukaemia would normally lead to death more rapidly than the chronic variety. However, with treatment many cases of 'acute' lymphatic leukaemia now have a better prospect of survival than many cases of 'chronic' myeloid leukaemia.

The uncontrolled proliferation of leukaemic cells in the bone marrow often spills over into the circulation and causes very high leukocyte counts, sometimes exceeding 100 000 per microlitre of blood. There are often deposits of the neoplastic leukocytes in many organs and tissues. More importantly, the replacement of normal bone marrow leads to severe anaemia and deficiency of circulating platelets (see below). In addition, a mysterious haemolytic anaemia due to auto-antibodies (p. 247) may complicate the clinical situation.

Paradoxically, all leukaemic patients are very susceptible to infection because of lack of bactericidal capability (p. 17). In blastic leukaemias there may indeed be very few mature polymorph neutrophils in the circulation, but in chronic myeloid leukaemia it is likely that the enormous numbers of polymorphs in the blood do not possess the antimicrobial activity of their normal counterparts.

Leukaemia is known to be provoked by exposure to *ionising radiation* and possibly by some *oncogenic viruses* (p. 278).

Platelets

These cells play a major role in thrombosis and have been discussed elsewhere (p. 225) in that capacity. Their numbers in the circulation, apart from some cases of rare diseases such as polycythaemia rubra vera, usually increase only as a transient phenomenon, e.g. after injury.

There are, however, many pathological situations in which the number of circulating platelets falls. This is serious, because the cells are vital for the prevention of bleeding from capillaries. It seems likely that they are required continuously to form haemostatic plugs in these tiny vessels. When their numbers fall below about 20 000 per microlitre of blood (the normal range being 120 000 to 600 000) spontaneous haemorrhages (purpura) take place in brain, skin, mucous membranes, intestinal tract, lungs and elsewhere, and fatal haemorrhage is likely to occur.

The most common cause of platelet deficiency (*thrombocytopenia*) is damage to the multinucleate platelet precursor in the bone marrow, the megakaryocyte, by antimetabolic drugs used in cancer chemotherapy. Similar bone marrow effects are produced by the physical and chemical agents which cause aplastic anaemia, for example ionising radiation or benzene poisoning. Thrombocytopenia is also a major feature of *leukaemia*, caused mostly by replacement of megakaryocytes by neoplastic cells.

In addition to the destruction or replacement of megakaryocytes, thrombocytopenia is a well recognised consequence of hypersensitivity to certain drugs, notably sedormid or quinidine. The drug acts as a hapten in combining with platelets, and the cells are destroyed by complement activated by the adherent antibody provoked by the drug/platelet combination. This is a classic example of Type II hypersensitivity (p. 61).

Needless to say there are several diseases in which circulating platelets are few in number for no known cause. The most important of these is *idiopathic thrombocytopenic purpura*, believed to be due to circulating anti-platelet antibodies and often relieved by removal of the spleen or immunosuppressive drugs. Another important cause of purpura of obscure pathogenesis is *chronic renal failure*. The platelets are of normal numbers but there is evidence of abnormal function, i.e. small wounds take an unduly long time to stop bleeding (prolonged bleeding time). It is likely that retained toxic metabolites interfere with platelet interactions with subendothelium. Massive spontaneous haemorrhage, often from the bowel, is a common terminal event in those dying of kidney failure.

Abnormalities of platelet function can also occur due to defects of the surface glycoproteins which become coated with immunoglobulin in the malignant transformation of B cells called *myeloma*.

KEY POINTS

- Failure of the heart, lungs and kidneys are common end points of many diseases and can be due to many factors.
- Oedema is excess water in tissues. It is a common consequence of heart or kidney failure caused by excess leakage of fluid from vessels or impaired reabsorption of fluid from tissues.
- Anaemias are a deficiency of red blood cells due either to a failure of production or an increased rate of loss, the most common type of which is iron deficiency anaemia.
- Leukopenia is usually due to toxic suppression of the bone marrow; levels of white cells have to drop from 4000/µl to 400/µl before infection becomes likely.
- Thrombocytopenia is platelet deficiency. It causes bleeding problems when levels fall from normal levels of 120–600 000 to below 40 000 per µl blood. The most common cause is now drugs but can be autoimmune.

22 The classification, diagnosis and assessment of cancer

Introduction

Neoplasia is yet another example of derangement of normal biological mechanisms causing disease. Great progress has been made in our understanding of this group of diseases in recent years and in Chapters 22–29 it is hoped to demonstrate how the seemingly disparate strands of knowledge relating to neoplasia are now being unified as we learn more about the biology and chemistry of cellular behaviour. Neoplasia should be clearly contrasted with hypertrophy and hyperplasia, yet all these phenomena involve alterations in growth control mechanisms.

In this introductory chapter the basic terminology of neoplasia and the essential characteristics of tumours will be discussed. Subsequent chapters will consider:

- the biological features of neoplastic cells and how they differ from normal cells
- the relationship of genetic changes and tumours
- the role of carcinogens and other environmental factors
- the role of hormones and growth factors
- the role of viruses
- immune mechanisms
- the epidemiology of tumours.

Definition

Neoplasia means new growth and a *neoplasm* (also commonly known as a tumour) is an area of tissue whose growth has outstripped and become independent of the adjoining tissue. By far the most important group of neoplasms are those known generically as cancers.

Synonyms for cancer are 'malignant growth' or 'malignant neoplasm'. Willis provided a comprehensive definition of a tumour as 'a mass of tissue the growth of which exceeds and is uncoordinated with that of normal tissues and persists in the same excessive manner after cessation of the stimuli that evoked the change'.

Classification

Taxonomy tends to be regarded as the dullest part of any subject. In the study of neoplasia, however, taxonomy is crucial since the label given to a tumour by a pathologist based upon its histological appearances is a very important guide to the prospects of the patient being alive 1, 5 or 15 years later. Important decisions regarding the type of treatment that the patient will be given are also largely dictated by the histopathologist's report.

The most basic and important taxonomic decision about a neoplasm is whether it is *benign* or *malignant*. This is perhaps the pathologist's most important task in hospital practice. Whilst we speak of benign and malignant as distinct entities, it should be remembered that we are really talking of a spectrum of behaviour, the opposite ends of which are represented by these terms. This does not devalue their utility as concepts, but one should be aware that exceptions inevitably occur.

Cancers are classified according to the tissue and cell type from which they are originated. Examples of malignant tumours are:

- *carcinoma*— a cancer of epithelial cells
- *sarcoma*—a cancer of connective tissue or muscle cells
- *leukaemia, myeloma or lymphoma*—a cancer of the bone marrow and immune system.

Examples of benign tumours are:

- *chondroma*—a tumour of cartilage
- *lipoma*—a tumour of fat cells.

Cancers may be further classified by their degree of *cell differentiation*. This is important because the prognosis for poorly differentiated carcinomas is usually worse than that for well-differentiated cancers.

Immunocytochemical methods using monoclonal antibodies directed against cell surface determinants (e.g. B- and T-cell antigens) allow more precise classification of cancers (e.g. lymphoma) and improve patient management.

Table 22.1 shows that certain terms, e.g. carcinoma, sarcoma, lymphoma, invariably indicate a malignant tumour. It also shows that some tissues produce only tumours considered to behave in a malignant manner.

Table 22.1 Classification of tumours

Tissue of origin	Benign	Malignant
Epithelium	Adenoma	Carcinoma
	Papilloma	
	Pigmented naevus	Malignant melanoma
Mesenchyme		
Connective tissue	Fibroma	Fibrosarcoma
Smooth muscle	Leiomyoma	Leiomyosarcoma
Striated muscle	Rhabdomyoma	Rhabdomyosarcoma
Connective tissue	Myxoma	Myxosarcoma
Cartilage	Chondroma	Chondrosarcoma
Fat	Lipoma	Liposarcoma
Bone	Osteoma	Osteosarcoma
Vessels	Angioma	Angiosarcoma
Lymphoid tissue	—	Lymphoma
Haemopoietic tissue	—	Leukaemia
Mesothelium	—	Mesothelioma
Meninges	Meningioma	—
CNS glial cells	—	Glioma
Nerve sheath	Neurofibroma	Neurofibrosarcoma

A complex system of classification for the different types of epithelial neoplasm is employed. Here attention is given both to the cell type and to the organ from which the tumour originates, e.g. gastric adenocarcinoma. This means a malignant epithelial tumour (carcinoma), derived from glandular epithelium (adeno) of the stomach. In contrast, malignant tumours arising from the normal epithelium of the oesophagus are termed squamous carcinomas. Correct use of conventional taxonomy is essential not only to distinguish benign and malignant tumours but also to identify different sorts of malignancies, since these vary in their clinical behaviour and response to treatment.

Benign tumours

A benign tumour:

- is slow growing
- is well demarcated from the surrounding tissues
- is composed of cells indistinguishable from those from which it is derived
- does not infiltrate into adjacent tissues or spread to distant organs
- does not threaten life unless it happens to interfere with some function necessary for survival.

In practice a benign tumour is dangerous only if it encroaches on a vital structure like the brain or if it produces something harmful, such as an excess of a hormone.

Features

The cells of benign tumours behave abnormally in their growth pattern but normally in their failure to breach natural boundaries. Benign tumours resemble the parent tissue closely and may be surrounded by a zone of compressed parent tissue or a fibrous 'capsule' such that they may be easily removed by the surgeon (Fig. 22.1). Such *enucleation* is not without potential hazards since some benign tumours do push out irregular small protrusions into this 'capsule' such that enucleation does not remove all the tumour and there may be a recurrence. In particular this can occur in the benign salivary gland tumour called a pleomorphic adenoma.

Behaviour

The cells of benign tumours are usually normal in their capacity to form their natural products, whether it be collagen or hormones. This can be an embarrassment to homeostasis, for example if hormones are produced in excess of bodily requirements, e.g. hypercalcaemia as a consequence of hyperparathyroidism due to excess and inappropriate

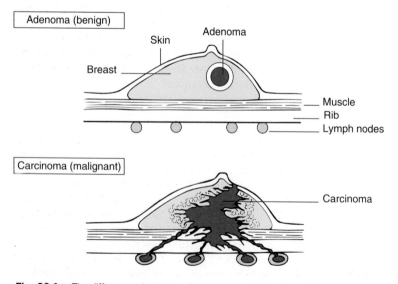

Fig. 22.1   The differences between a benign (adenoma) and a malignant (carcinoma) tumour of the breast.

production of parathormone by a parathyroid adenoma. In such cases surgical removal is usually necessary. The compression of some vital structure by a benign tumour may also necessitate removal, e.g. compression of the brain or spinal cord by a meningioma.

Complications

Perhaps the most important question from both the theoretical and the practical points of view about benign tumours is whether or not they become malignant, i.e. invade surrounding tissues, spread to distant organs and lose the features of the parent cell. The great majority of benign tumours never acquire any of these characteristics. There are, however, instances where a malignant tumour develops at the site of a tumour that was previously found to have the structural features of a benign tumour. This phenomenon is viewed as evidence that some neoplasms with the histological features of benign tumours are in fact in a 'preinvasive' phase and are destined to be malignant. This is supported by the fact that such transformations from benign to malignant almost always occur in specific, well-recognised situations. Perhaps the best example is adenomas in the large bowel; there is good evidence that, if not removed, these will progress to become overtly malignant.

Hamartomas

A hamartoma should be clearly distinguished from a benign tumour. A hamartoma may be defined as a developmental abnormality composed of chaotically arranged tissue but in an appropriate site. It may occur in any site but the best-known example is the pulmonary hamartoma which may cause concern as it usually presents as a solitary 'coin lesion' on chest X-ray.

Premalignant tumours

Multiple events are probably necessary for the formation of a malignant tumour. It is thus possible that a series of morphological changes will be discernible in tissues during this process. Some of these may allow the definition of *premalignant* states which could be of both theoretical and practical value. Their potential practical value lies in the possibility that exists for early detection and thus early cure, and their theoretical importance lies in the possible information that they provide about the early steps in oncogenesis.

The best examples of such states are to be found in epithelia but probably occur in many other tissues. In the squamous epithelium of the uterine cervix a series of histological changes may be seen, with increasing cytological and architectural *atypia* (or *dysplasia*) that progresses through to a state termed *carcinoma in situ* where the epithelial cells show all the cytological features of malignancy but there is no invasion through the basement membrane.

Cancer screening

The existence of the spectrum of changes mentioned above is put to clinical use in cervical screening where smears of cells from the uterine cervix are examined by pathologists in an attempt to detect preneoplastic changes and early cancers. Similar changes occur in the skin, the breast and in urothelium of the bladder and ureters. In addition some benign tumours may be considered preneoplastic as stated above.

Malignant tumours

A malignant tumour has, in general, characteristics which are the opposite of benign. Cancer typically (but not invariably):

- is fast growing
- is poorly demarcated from surrounding tissues
- is composed of cells which may differ markedly from the cells of origin
- infiltrates adjacent tissues and spreads to distant organs
- sooner or later invariably causes death if untreated, no matter where it arises.

Differentiation between malignancy and non-malignancy is obviously important and hence detailed classification of tumours is important. A broad classification of human tumours is given in Table 22.2.

What makes a tumour malignant?

Cancer results from a fundamental breakdown in the rules of cell regulation, which are necessary for the existence of a multicellular

Table 22.2   The characteristic features of benign and malignant tumours

Benign	Malignant
Slow growing	Fast growing
Non-infiltrating	Infiltrating
Resembles parent tissue	Differs from parent tissue
Cells normal	Cells abnormal
Does not spread to distant sites	Spreads to distant sites
Only kills if damaging vital function	Always kills if untreated

organism. Free living cells, such as bacteria, compete to exist, but cells in a multicellular organism must collaborate to ensure survival of the whole organism. Cancer occurs when cells mutate and compete with each other, ultimately destroying the multicellular organism.

Cancer represents a complex cellular phenotype resulting from multiple 'hits' or events. The view of a linear model of accumulated changes may be simplistic but facilitates an understanding of how they contribute to the malignant phenotype.

Each hit confers a selective advantage to the affected cell among a rapidly expanding and competitive Darwinian population. Cells thus progress to greater stages of malignancy characterised by:

- more rapid growth
- immortalisation
- invasiveness
- metastasis
- angiogenesis.

Uncontrolled cell multiplication in vivo, to which most of our understanding is confined, represents only one attribute of the malignant phenotype. That tumour cells inherit the malignant phenotype suggests a predominance of genetic hits. *Exogenous factors* or *carcinogens* can be regarded as acting on a *predisposed substrate*.

Cancer can be defined by the four following characteristics:

1. clonality (a cancer comprises a clone of malignant cells which have originated from a single cell)
2. autonomy (there is breakdown in normal feedback regulation of growth)
3. differentiation (cancer cells lack differentiation from each other)
4. metastasis (cancer cells can disseminate to other parts of the body).

These definitions may also apply at certain times to normal physiology (e.g. embryogenesis and wound repair). The difference between a benign and malignant tumour is that those that are benign remain differentiated and do not metastasise.

Clonality

By the time a tumour is causing symptoms, it usually contains a billion or more cells, but it is thought that primary tumours originate from a single abnormal cell (see also p. 281). The reasons for this are as follows:

- Virtually all solid tumours and the majority of haemopoietic malignancies have *chromosomal abnormalities*. These may be translocations of chromosomal fragments, additions or deletions of

Table 22.3   Examples of uniform chromosomal abnormalities in all cells within a tumour

Tumour	Chromosomal abnormality
Chronic myelogenous leukaemia	The Philadelphia chromosome. This is a translocation between chromosomes 9 and 22 with a break in chromosome 22 occurring at a gene site called the breakpoint cluster region
Nodular lymphoma	Translocations between chromosomes 14 and 18 are common and they involve the bcl 2 gene located on chromosome 18

parts of chromosomes, or even whole chromosomes. Translocations may produce characteristic proteins called fusion proteins. The presence of uniform chromosomal abnormalities in all cells within a tumour is strong evidence for the clonal origin of the tumour. Examples are shown in Tables 22.3 and 24.2.

- If tumours produce antibodies, they are always monoclonal (e.g. myelomas) and may be either lambda or kappa chains.
- Variations in the form of proteins (e.g. glucose-6-phosphate dehydrogenase) are rare in tumours and usually one form of protein is found. Two forms of the enzyme glucose-6-phosphate dehydrogenase are known; the gene for this enzyme is carried on the X chromosome and its expression is governed by the Lyonisation phenomenon, i.e. one allele is always expressed and the other repressed in any given cell. Glucose-6-phosphate dehydrogenase in leiomyomas from heterozygote women is either of the A or B subtype and never mixed, suggesting that the tumours are descended from a single parent cell.

Autonomy: how cancer avoids regulatory control

Cancer cells may avoid regulatory controls of cellular proliferation in a number of ways. These include:

- Growth factor production (p. 303): the cancer cells may secrete a polypeptide that can bind to a receptor on its surface and result in autostimulation. This is termed autocrine secretion. Transforming growth factor alpha is an example and is able to act as an analogue of epidermal growth factor (EGF).
- Increased expression of cell surface receptors: increased numbers of EGF receptors are commonly found in epithelial tumours, renal cell carcinomas and squamous lung carcinomas.
- Self-activation of internal biochemical pathways (e.g. tyrosine kinase): usually activation of these pathways is dependent upon

binding of a specific growth factor to a cell surface receptor. In this way cell surface receptor binding is bypassed.

- Cancer cells may also manipulate their environment by ensuring an adequate blood supply and this can be achieved by secreting angiogenesis factors.

Differentiation

A further feature that may be seen in transformed cells is loss of differentiation. Loss of differentiation and uncontrolled proliferation are phenomena which develop independently. Although interference with differentiation in some cultures often provokes cell proliferation, arrest of proliferation does not usually by itself induce the cultures to differentiate.

Cells which are already fully differentiated, e.g. keratinised squamous epithelium, cannot undergo neoplastic transformation. To be susceptible to transformation a cell must belong to the stem cell population of the organ from which it is derived.

Such cells have the capacity both to divide and to differentiate, as opposed to the fully differentiated forms which can no longer divide. In stratified epithelium there is an anatomical separation of the two populations, whilst in liver there is no obvious difference. In other organs which lack the power of cell replication, e.g. adult nervous tissue, stem cells are few or absent.

Transformation of a stem cell in vivo or in vitro means that it is diverted from the path of differentiation to that of continued cell proliferation. Uncoupling of differentiation and proliferation is an important component of tumorigenesis. The persistence of stem cells into adult life is of course essential for homeostasis in situations such as regeneration of epithelium. The ability of these stem cells to become autonomous and cause cancer is a further example of the way disease develops from perversion of a survival mechanism. In this instance, since most cancers develop after the reproductive stage of life, there is a clear survival advantage for the species in selecting regenerative powers at the expense of cancer developing in later life.

Cell surface changes may reflect loss of differentiation. There may be alteration of the receptors that transmit signals across the cell membrane and via cyclic nucleotides and other 'second messengers' to the nucleus. The process is known as signal transduction. Transport mechanisms at the surface are increased and there are decreased levels of glycoprotein, sialic acid and glycosyltransferase. These biochemical changes are those observed in normal cells exposed in vitro to growth factors such as insulin or certain serum fractions. The malignant cell could be said to behave as if it were permanently exposed to such factors even when they are not present.

The membrane changes in transformed cells are reflected in alterations of the surface antigens. Histocompatibility antigens are normally present on the cell surface and may be specific to the species, individual or tissue. Transformation may be accompanied by the appearance of new cancer-associated antigens both at the cell surface and within the cell. If the transformation is induced by a virus, then the antigens expressed tend to be the same for all tumour cells induced by the same virus, even in different species. If transformation is induced by chemicals, there is a great multiplicity of cancer-associated antigens at the cell surface that do not cross-react with other tumours induced by the same chemical, even in the same animal. In human cancer, malignant melanomas from different patients have been found to have tumour-specific antigens in common, and several types of soft tissue sarcoma have yielded cross-reacting tumour-associated surface antigens.

Another type of tumour-associated antigen found in transformed cells is that which also occurs in normal embryonic and fetal cells but not adult tissues. Examples of this phenomenon include *carcinoembryonic antigen* (CEA), associated particularly with carcinoma of the large bowel, and *α-fetoprotein*, associated with hepatocellular carcinoma and some testicular tumours. Such antigens may be released into the blood and their quantification can be used to assess the success of treatment and the presence of recurrent disease. These abnormal antigens, and the expression of normal antigens in the wrong place or at the wrong time, are a further reflection of the altered gene expression which is characteristic of the neoplastic phenotype.

Metastasis

Cancer cells become malignant when they are able to invade and colonise surrounding tissues. To do this solid cancers must change their cell adhesion properties, detach themselves from their neighbours, and enter the circulation, either through blood vessels or the lymphatics. The cell then needs to reverse the process and exit the circulation through a vessel wall in another part of the body in order to produce a metastatic colony.

The mechanisms involved in metastasis are thought to be very similar to those used by the lymphocyte in moving from one part of the immune system to the other. This process does not appear to be random and certain cancers have a predilection for metastasis to certain organs (e.g. gut cancer to the liver, breast cancer to bone, sarcoma to lungs). Tumours may spread to adjacent organs and tissues by direct extension and by *invasion*. Alternatively spread may occur to draining lymph nodes by embolisation or permeation of lymphatic channels; into body cavities by shedding of free cancer cells; or to distant organs by way of the blood stream following penetration of veins. All such extensions of the tumour beyond its primary site of origin are known as *metastasis* or secondary growth, and in general carry a poor prognosis. Indeed, the occurrence or non-occurrence of metastasis is a major factor in determining the curability of a given patient with malignant disease.

Three factors are important in determining the likelihood of secondary spread of a tumour. These are:

1. the nature of the tumour itself
2. the resistance of the host
3. the susceptibility of the organ to which the tumour cells spread.

Nature of the tumour

The propensity of different tumours to spread is very variable. The factors governing this are only poorly understood. Tumour cells must enter the lymphatic or vascular channels in some way, either in clumps or as single cells. Presumably the tendency to do this relates in some way to the invasive properties of the tumour cells. Having reached the circulation the tumour cells must survive and become impacted in some distant vascular bed. Here the tumour may start growing. In general, sarcomas, i.e. malignant tumours of connective tissues, tend to spread early via the blood stream because they usually are rapidly growing, they invade veins and the sarcoma cells have low adhesiveness to each other. In contrast, carcinomas generally metastasise via lymphatics, at least initially.

Host resistance

Host resistance is of possible importance in determining the potential for metastasis. Both adaptive and non-specific resistance mechanisms may be involved. It is known that mononuclear phagocytes may be involved in resistance to tumour spread, and a correlation between macrophage content of a series of tumours and their propensity to metastasise has been noted. Natural killer cells (NK cells) (p. 47) have been implicated as being of some importance in experimental systems. The role of lymphocytes and humoral mechanisms is less clear but protective effects and potentiating effects have been described.

Organ susceptibility

The organ in which the wandering cancer cell lodges also plays an important part in determining whether a secondary deposit develops. Every malignant tumour probably discharges showers of tumour cells into the lymph and blood but only a small proportion of these potential seedlings take hold and grow. It may be that some of this is due to immunological mechanisms. However, it is clear from post mortem studies and experimental work that this can be only part of the story. Some organs, for example skeletal muscle, kidney and spleen, only rarely allow secondary deposits to develop, whereas others, such as bone, liver and brain, are very common sites for metastatic deposits. Certainly relative blood flow differences cannot be the explanation since the kidney receives about 20% of the cardiac output. The most plausible explanation seems to be that some tissues provide a suitable micro-environment whilst others do not. The role of growth factors in such events may be important.

Diagnosis and assessment

The way in which cancer becomes apparent (i.e. how it presents clinically) depends on the nature of the tumour and on the site of growth. It may be found as a painless lump, e.g. in the breast, or it may produce loss of weight and general ill-health, or cause some specific and often alarming symptom such as haemoptysis (coughing up blood). There may also be inappropriate expression of the genomic repertoire, for example there may be hormone production (e.g. ACTH production by carcinoma of the lung) causing Cushing's syndrome. Such events may also be due to trivial diseases but, needless to say, they must always be managed with great seriousness by attending clinicians.

Features

In the diagnosis and assessment of a malignant tumour the pathologist attempts to identify the cells from which the tumour is derived, if possible by observing the junction of normal and neoplastic cells. He then records the extent to which the individual tumour cells resemble the cells and structures from which the tumour appears to be derived. This is called the 'degree of differentiation' of the tumour. If the cytological features and architectural features (i.e. the formation of glands, tubules, sheets, etc.) are indistinguishable from those of the parent tissue then the tumour is said to be *well differentiated*. If the cells bear no resemblance to their cells of origin and no normal structures can be discerned, the tumour is said to be *undifferentiated* or *anaplastic*. There are of course all degrees of intermediate differentiation. It should be noted that the degree of differentiation may vary within a tumour, and in general the grade of the tumour is determined by the area of least differentiation.

Behaviour

Two fundamental histological features of cancer cells are:

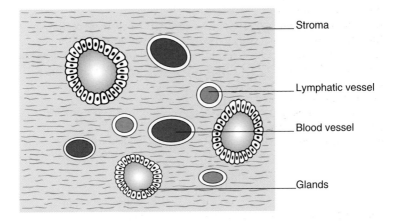

Fig. 22.2 Normal glandular tissue, e.g. in breast or large intestine, showing normal architecture of epithelial glands and related structures.

- their architectural and cytological abnormalities—this is demonstrated in their diminished ability to form appropriate structures such as glandular acini (Fig. 22.2)
- that the ratio of the nuclear size to the cytoplasmic size is usually raised and the nucleus may have increased amounts of deeply stained chromatin.

There may be great variation in size and shape between the cells of a malignant tumour and *bizarre forms* may be present, e.g. irregular multinucleate giant cells or very large single nuclei whose chromosomes are increased in number and show structural abnormalities.

The number of *mitoses* in tumours is very variable. It must be remembered that cell division is a normal process and occurs with great frequency in many normal tissues. Indeed mitotic figures are extremely numerous in the basal layers of the skin, in the glands of the gut and in the germinal centres of lymph nodes, for example. Numerous mitotic figures can often be present in malignant tumours but this is not an invariable finding. Bizarre mitotic figures with abnormal morphology may on occasion be seen in tumours and are very rare in normal tissues. In very poorly differentiated tumours bizarre forms may be numerous.

Complications

Further examination of malignant cells reveals that not only have they lost their proper orientation to each other but they have also lost their

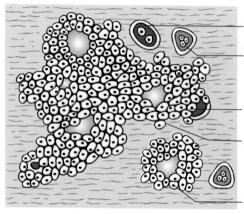

Blood vessel containing
cancer emboli

Lymphatic vessel containing
cancer cells

Blood vessel invaded
by cancer cells

Stroma invaded
by cancer

Cancer cells forming
abnormal glands

Fig. 22.3   Cancerous glandular tissue involving adjacent tissues, lymphatics and blood vessels. Note loss of normal glandular arrangement.

orientation with respect to other cells of surrounding normal tissues, i.e. they often *invade* adjacent tissues. An adenocarcinoma of the large bowel arising in the colonic epithelium will, for example, often invade the underlying submucosa and muscle coats and even penetrate the peritoneal surface. Invasion of veins and lymphatic vessels is common. Thus in addition to cytological and architectural abnormalities the third and diagnostically the most important characteristic of malignancy is *infiltration* or *invasion* (Fig. 22.3).

Malignant tumours induce the *formation of new blood vessels* which keep them supplied with nutriment and this may be a factor in limiting their growth. The underlying mechanism involves the elaboration of a factor or factors by the tumour cells that incites the production of new vessels. Such factors are, of course, of biological value in normal tissues in situations such as wound healing; again we see that pathology involves subversion of normal processes. If the tumour outstrips its blood supply, its centre may become ischaemic and necrotic.

Leukocytic exudation of lymphocytes, macrophages and granulocytes is also sometimes apparent and may be a response to the production of factors by the tumour, or alternatively to damaged adjacent tissues.

KEY POINTS

- Neoplasia is an example of derangement of normal biological mechanisms causing disease, involving alterations in growth control mechanisms.
- A tumour is an area of tissue whose growth has outstripped and become independent of the adjoining tissue.
- The terms benign and malignant represent opposite ends of a spectrum of behaviour.
- Benign tumours are slow growing, well demarcated, well differentiated and do not infiltrate into adjacent tissues or spread to distant organs. They do not threaten life unless interfering with some function necessary for survival, encroaching on a vital structure or producing something harmful, such as an excess of a hormone.
- Malignant tumours tend to arise from a single cell as a result of carcinogens acting on a predisposed substrate. They are characterised by rapid growth, immortalisation, invasiveness, metastasis and angiogenesis.
- The role of the pathologist is to identify the cells from which the tumour is derived, and to assess the degree of differentiation. Cancer cells may show bizarre forms and an increased number of mitoses.

23 Understanding cancer: from the laboratory to the clinic

Investigating cancer cells

The cultivation outside the body of transformed cells, whether created artificially or obtained from pre-existing tumours, has provided an excellent opportunity to identify the features which distinguish a malignant cell from its normal counterpart.

The first point to emerge is that the essential change seems to occur in the transformed cell itself: malignancy is not merely the removal of competing normal cells so that a few hardy survivors can overgrow the rest. This has been shown directly by transforming a single cultured cell with a cancer-inducing chemical (carcinogen), then allowing the transformed cell to divide. It is observed that all of the cell's progeny retain their malignant potential in spite of the fact that the transforming chemical is no longer present.

Allowing a single cell to divide and collecting its daughter cells is known as cell *cloning*. Study of transformed cells in culture has shown that the properties of malignancy are passed from one generation to the next, so that the tumour is perpetuating itself even when the stimulus has been removed. This suggests that transformation involves a change in the genetic information of the affected cell. Not only is the cell transformed, so are all its progeny, although there may be an accumulation of differences in karyotype, phenotype and antigenic expression with successive generations.

The essential consequence of these alterations appears to be a lack of responsiveness to control mechanisms which regulate the behaviour of the normal cell. This lack of control affects an enormous range of cellular processes such as cell movement, replication and differentiation.

Cancer under the microscope

Cancer cells have readily detectable abnormalities under the microscope. *Cellular features* are:

- enlarged nuclei with prominent nucleoli
- increased mitosis
- multiple nuclei.

Histologically there is disarray with partial or complete loss of normal tissue architecture. The degree of derangement usually correlates with the extent of disease spread or metastatic potential of the cancer.

There may be a heterogeneous mixture of biologically distinct clones of cancer cells, each of which is capable of replication. There is considerable evidence for this variation within a tumour. For example, it is known that the histological appearance often varies from place to place within any given tumour; there are often differences also in antigen expression in different parts of the tumour. Although, in general, all the tumour cells have the same karyotype, differences may be observed. Variation may occur in the level of hormone receptors in different parts of a tumour and in the sensitivity of cells within a tumour to different drugs, radiation or temperature.

Finally, there can be marked differences in the proliferative activity of cells within a tumour and in their propensity to metastasise. Hence 'dedifferentiation' may be considered as the outgrowth of a particular population of cells within a tumour that has some selective advantage and thus becomes the predominant cell type.

Biochemical differences

Metabolic differences may be observed: for example cancer cells tend to be much more dependent on glycolysis than their normal counterparts which utilise aerobic respiration to a large extent. It is, however, important to appreciate that differences of this sort are more likely to be a result of malignant change than its cause.

Occasionally, loss of differentiated phenotype can be shown to be accompanied by disappearance of a specialised biochemical function. In primary carcinoma of the liver the malignant cells appear to lose the ability to respond to the normal feedback mechanism that regulates blood cholesterol levels. Cells that do not have this regulatory mechanism presumably have a proliferative advantage over those that do and thus become the dominant population.

What happens if cancer cells are transplanted?

A test of whether a cell has suffered malignant transformation is its ability to survive and grow when transplanted to another living host;

non-transformed adult cells will usually not grow when transplanted into another animal. Indeed most normal adult cell lines grow with difficulty when transplanted to tissue culture even under ideal conditions. The direct result of their successful growth after transplantation to another animal is death of the host. This is ultimate proof that malignant transformation of the inoculated cells has taken place.

Cancer cells in culture

In cell culture, cells are kept in artificial media in incubators. In such conditions it is possible to keep some types of normal mammalian cells for limited periods of time. They proliferate, at least until they become confluent when their proliferation ceases (contact inhibition), and they can be induced to differentiate, at least to some degree. Neoplastic cells may also be grown in such conditions, and the behaviour of such cells is often rather different. Under these conditions the abnormal growth of tumour is matched by the proliferation of cancer cells compared to their normal counterparts. Cancer cells can be derived from:

- a spontaneously arising malignant tumour
- a similar tumour induced experimentally in an animal by exposing it to a virus or carcinogenic chemical or to ionising radiation
- normal cells in tissue culture made neoplastic by treating them in vitro with viruses or chemicals.

Cultures derived from any of these sources are described as *transformed*, although the term is most commonly used in relation to cells converted to malignant behaviour during in vitro culture.

Transformed cells may also show the abnormal karyotypes (chromosome patterns) observed in natural tumours. Cancer cells in culture will continue dividing until the mass reaches a critical size and ceases to grow. This brake is due to lack of nutrition of the innermost cells, for if a culture is transferred to a living animal host it acquires its own blood supply by stimulating growth of new vessels and will grow until the host is killed. Alternatively, if the in vitro culture is divided into portions and placed in other culture bottles with fresh medium and this process is repeated at intervals, then cell growth will continue indefinitely. This is in contrast to normal cells which will only proceed through a finite number of cell divisions before dying.

Changes at the cell surface are particularly noticeable in transformed cells. For example, one of the most obvious effects is loss of contact inhibition (sometimes known as density-dependent growth inhibition) of division. When normal cells are grown in tissue culture, they continue to divide and spread out until they are confluent, at which point movement and cell division cease. In contrast, when transformed cells under the same conditions become confluent they do not stop dividing or moving and thus form disordered multilayered heaps. This is perhaps analogous to the infiltrative behaviour of tumour cells in vivo. Transformed cells fail to recognise or to respond to the normal regulatory signals and continue to proliferate in spite of increased crowding.

Clinical presentation of cancer

It is possible to reconstruct some fairly typical natural histories of malignant disease. In carcinoma of the stomach a middle-aged or elderly man may present with loss of weight and appetite. He looks unwell and pale. Examination of the upper gastrointestinal tract by barium contrast X-ray or by fibreoptic endoscopy shows the presence of a tumour and a biopsy is taken. Histopathological examination reveals the presence of adenocarcinoma and the patient proceeds to gastrectomy. However, at operation numerous white nodules are found in the peritoneum and the mesenteric and aortic lymph nodes are enlarged and filled with tumour (metastasis). The liver is also enlarged and exhibits white nodules of tumour. The patient recovers from the operation but a few months later becomes ill and confused, is readmitted to hospital and dies of pneumonia. A post mortem examination reveals that the gastric cancer has spread to many organs including the brain.

A different type of case history is that of a woman who discovers a lump in a breast. It is removed and histological examination shows it to be adenocarcinoma. The woman is well for 14 years, then unaccountably develops illness and back pain. She is found to have numerous secondary deposits, one of which is biopsied. Histological examination reveals that it is very similar to the previous primary tumour. She dies soon afterwards of the consequences of extensive metastatic disease.

On a more cheerful note, a middle-aged man might present with rectal bleeding and investigation may show a mass in the rectum. The biopsy findings are of adenocarcinoma of the rectum and a proctocolectomy is performed. The patient remains symptom free and dies of old age many years later.

Case histories such as these illustrate some of the typical ways in which tumours present and behave. It is a useful exercise to try to consider the pathology of diseases in terms of the real cases that you see during your clinical training.

Non-metastatic manifestations of neoplasia

Hormone promotion

Patients may have systemic manifestations of tumours without there necessarily being disseminated disease. For example both benign and malignant tumours may generate hormones and hormone-like substances, as in the case of a *pituitary adenoma* which may produce ACTH and stimulate the adrenals to produce excessive quantities of steroid hormones, thus causing *Cushing's syndrome*. Alternatively small cell carcinoma of the bronchus may also produce ACTH and lead to a similar phenomenon, although the lung does not produce a significant amount of ACTH in normal circumstances. This is then referred to as the *ectopic production* of ACTH. Other hormonal effects are listed in Table 23.1, as are cutaneous, neurological and haematological manifestations of tumours.

Cachexia

Finally it should be noted that tumours may be associated with intense wasting of patients (cachexia); this may also be a result of the

Table 23.1 Non-metastatic manifestations of neoplasia

Manifestation	Tumour example
General	
Cachexia (wasting)	Many
Nausea	
Haematological	
Anaemia	Many
Thrombosis	Carcinoma of pancreas
Disseminated intravascular coagulation	Carcinoma of stomach
Microangiopathic haemolytic anaemia	Carcinoma of prostate
Polycythaemia	Renal carcinoma
Hormonal	
Hyponatraemia (ADH-like substance)	Small cell carcinoma of bronchus
Cushing's syndrome (ACTH)	
Hypoglycaemia (?Somatomedin)	Mesothelioma
Carcinoid syndrome	Carcinoid tumours
Hypercalcaemia (PTH-like substance)	Squamous carcinomas
Cutaneous	
Acanthosis nigricans	75% of patients have adenocarcinoma
Dermatomyositis	15% have malignancy
Herpes zoster (and other opportunistic infections)	Lymphomas
Exfoliative dermatitis	Lymphomas
Generalised pigmentation	Many tumours (?MSH-like activity)
Neuromuscular	
Myopathy	Many tumours
Neuropathy	
Dementia	

elaboration by the tumour of some factor or factors that severely disrupt normal physiology. It is possible that *tumour necrosis factor* (also known as cachectin) may be responsible for this and other systemic manifestations (p. 140). This substance may be of advantage to the host by mobilising energy stores and activating specific and non-specific immune mechanisms. Only when released in vast amounts (as in advanced cancer) does it threaten the individual. Again we come across the idea of pathology being understandable in terms of alterations in normal mechanisms.

What causes cancer?

Cancer is associated with genetic (sex, age and race) and environmental factors (geographical location, diet and exposure to chemicals and physical agents).

KEY POINTS

- Transformation to malignancy occurs within the cell itself and the properties of malignancy are passed from one generation of cells to the next.
- Malignant cells demonstrate a lack of responsiveness to control mechanisms which regulate the behaviour of the normal cell, including processes such as cell movement, replication and differentiation.
- Transformed cells have:
  — multiple nuclei
  — enlarged nuclei with prominent nucleoli
  — increased mitosis.
- Malignant cells grow chaotically, having lost contact inhibition of division. The only limiting factor on transformed cell growth in culture is lack of nutrition of the innermost cells.
- The natural history and clinical presentation of cancer is very varied.
- Non-metastatic manifestations of neoplasia include cachexia and hormonal effects.

24 Genetic and molecular mechanisms of cancer

Regulation of cell proliferation has some common mechanisms irrespective of cell type and in normal cells is achieved by *proto-oncogenes* and *suppressor genes*.

ONCOGENESIS

Introduction

The scientific study of neoplasia is an exciting and rapidly moving field. A central theme is that neoplasia is essentially a disorder of genetic information and its expression; it has been stated that 'Tumour cells are characterised by the presence of a *heritable lesion* that determines insensitivity to the normal restraints governing cell multiplication'. Disordered cellular differentiation and development are also important themes in neoplasia.

The role of genetics in cancer is perhaps best explained by the notion that in the normal genome there may be many genes which code for important regulatory proteins. If these genes are expressed in the wrong amount (too much or too little), or at the wrong time, or are expressed at the correct time and in the correct amount but in an abnormal form, or some combination of these, then abnormal control of cellular function may ensue. This may then be reflected in an abnormal phenotype and abnormal behaviour such as excessive proliferation and/or abnormal differentiation. This concept underlies the *oncogene hypothesis* of cancer.

Viral transformation and oncogenes

Many animals, and probably man as well, are susceptible to virally induced cancers. The *retroviruses* are an important group of cancer-

277

causing viruses. They have a simple structure, usually being made up of only three genes:

1. *Gag* (coding for a group antigen)
2. *Pol* (coding for a polymerase enzyme)
3. *Env* (coding for envelope proteins).

Two broad groups are known:

1. acute transforming viruses
2. slow transforming viruses.

The acute transforming viruses contain a fourth gene which can induce neoplastic transformation in a susceptible cell and may thus be called an *oncogene* (literally 'cancer-causing gene', see p. 309). The slow transforming viruses, so called because they only rarely and only after prolonged periods cause cancer, do not themselves contain an oncogene. In those cells that are transformed by slow transforming retroviruses, the virus is always integrated into the host genome, and always at the same site.

Proto-oncogenes and activation

The idea that single genes could cause cancer came from studies of virus-induced cellular transformation, but it had been suggested that similar genes might exist in all cellular genomes. Evidence in support of this view exists and indeed it is now believed that the oncogenes present in retroviruses (viral oncogenes or v-oncs) have been derived (transduced) from normal genes (proto-oncogenes) in the genomes of normal cells.

It has been found that in some tumours there are abnormalities of proto-oncogenes. There may be an alteration in the level or timing of gene expression, or structural abnormalities of the gene (mutations). When proto-oncogenes are aberrantly expressed or mutated they are termed cellular oncogenes (c-oncs). The function of these proto-oncogenes is not to cause cancer; rather they are involved in various different aspects of cellular function, many of which we do not yet understand. Again we come to the idea that pathology can be understood as disordered physiology: in this case the abnormal function of a gene can lead to neoplasia.

Insertional mutagenesis

That proto-oncogenes exist in the normal genome helps to explain the oncogenic action of slow transforming retroviruses. Insertion of such a virus at a particular site in the host genome may bring a cellular gene (proto-oncogene) under the influence of regulatory sequences in the viral genome (enhancers and promoters), such that there is an alteration in proto-oncogene expression. This is termed *insertional mutagenesis*.

Gene amplification

Karyotypic abnormalities may be associated with another method by which proto-oncogenes can be activated. Gene amplification is associated with the presence of karyotypic abnormalities called 'double minutes' or 'homogeneously staining regions'. Gene amplification involves excision of the segment of DNA carrying the proto-oncogene, end to end replication of that segment and reinsertion of the amplified segment. This is seen in neuroblastoma, for example, where the proto-oncogene N-*myc* is amplified.

Finally, mutations may be seen in the coding sequence of proto-oncogenes such that they produce an abnormal product. An example of this is mutation of the oncogene *ras*, which is typically at position 12, 13 or 61. It may be that some chemical carcinogens have a particular propensity to cause mutations at particular sites although this has not yet been confirmed.

Chromosome rearrangements

Another way in which proto-oncogenes can be activated involves chromosomal rearrangements. It is found that some karyotypic abnormalities are characteristic of particular types of tumour. Examples of malignancies in which these abnormalities are found include chronic myeloid leukaemia and Burkitt's lymphoma; the mechanisms involved are described below (see p. 282).

Presence or absence of oncogenes as a cause of cancer

More than 40 different mammalian genes are now thought to be oncogenes but only a few are well understood. Some are listed in Table 24.1. It is important to remember that whilst we talk of oncogenes, it is their products (*oncoproteins*) that are important. In general the products of oncogenes are involved in some way in regulatory cascades that control cellular differentiation and proliferation. Some code for receptor proteins, particularly growth factor receptors (e.g. *erb*B which codes for epidermal growth factor), whilst a few are known to code for growth factors themselves (e.g. *sis* which codes for platelet-derived growth factor). Others code for proteins with enzymic function, notably tyrosine kinase (e.g. *src*) or for proteins with GTP binding properties (e.g. *ras*). Some code for nuclear proteins whose function is unknown (e.g. *fos*).

The types of oncogene so far described all cause cancer as a consequence of altered or enhanced function, but there is evidence to

Table 24.1   Some oncogenes

Oncogene	Notes
Growth factor related	
sis (simian sarcoma virus)	Platelet derived growth factor
Growth factor receptor	
erbB (erythroblastosis virus)	Modified epidermal growth factor receptor
fms (feline McDonagh sarcoma virus)	Modified M-CSF receptor
Enzyme	
—Tyrosine kinase	
src (Rous sarcoma virus)	Protein kinase activity, membrane-
abl (Abelson sarcoma virus)	associated or cytoplasmic. Some ? growth
fes (feline sarcoma virus)	factors
—Serine/threonine kinase	
ros (Rochester sarcoma virus)	Cytosolic kinase
rel (reticuloendotheliosis virus)	
GTP binding	
ras: 3 types, Harvey, Kirsten and N (after strains of virus and Neuroblastoma)	GTP binding proteins ?? role in 2nd messenger signalling
Nuclear	
myc (myelocytomatosis virus)	Possibly DNA binding proteins
fos (FBJ osteosarcoma virus)	
myb (myeloblastosis virus)	
Other	
bcl-1, bcl-2 (B cell lymphoma)	Identified at sites of chromosal rearrangments
bcr (breakpoint cluster region)	Seen at breakpoint on Philadelphia chromosome

Note that the names of oncogenes are derived from the name of the retrovirus from which they are obtained, or from some characteristic that they possess.

support the idea that other genes may be involved in oncogenesis by their *absence*. For example, suppose that one gene is an important inhibitor of the function of other genes, i.e. it produces a repressor protein of some kind; its absence therefore may lead to altered activity of certain cellular functions, including differentiation and proliferation. Mutations due to chemicals or radiation, or some other event such as chromosomal deletion or rearrangement, or the insertion of a retrovirus might lead to the loss of such a gene in a somatic cell. Furthermore, such a loss of an allele may occur in the germ line such that all progeny cells are hemizygous (a state where only a single allele occurs at a locus, as opposed to the homozygous state where two identical alleles are present and the heterozygous state with two dissimilar alleles). In such a situation, where only a single allele exists, only one allele need be lost in order for tumours to develop. Such concepts can be used to explain some hereditary cancers such as retinoblastoma and familial adenomatous polyposis.

Suppressor genes

These genes can either inhibit cell growth or induce programmed cell death (*apoptosis*). Their involvement in oncogenesis occurs when they are either lost or inactivated. Suppressor genes may act normally by binding transcription factors required for cell cycle progression or may serve themselves as transcription factors that activate genes inhibiting cell cycle progression or proliferation.

p53

p53 is a 53 kD protein and is at present the most commonly found mutated gene in human tumours. It is one of the most important members of the tumour suppressor gene family. Of the 6.5 million people diagnosed with cancer each year worldwide, about half have p53 mutations in their tumours.

p53 acts as a molecular policeman helping to coordinate a complex system of responses to prevent DNA damage that might otherwise lead to cancer. It does this by preventing cell cycle progression if DNA needs repairing; once DNA is repaired, the cell cycle resumes. If repair is not carried out, then p53 triggers cell suicide by apoptosis. When mutated, however, p53 can be dangerous as DNA repair may not be carried out and oncogenesis may result.

Genetic factors

Genetic factors are important in some types of cancer. Alterations in genetic information appear to be the basis of neoplasia, and a number of mutations may be required to cause cancer.

During a human lifetime it is estimated that there are 10^{16} cell divisions. It is remarkable, therefore, that cancers are not more common. This is probably because a number of mutations are needed to turn a normal cell into a cancer cell and because cancer develops (oncogenesis) by progression from mild abnormality to malignancy. This is why there is a long delay between the causal event and the onset of the disease (e.g. leukaemia following radiation exposure).

The rate at which cancer develops therefore depends on the gene mutation rate and the selective advantage that this mutation confers on the cell.

Evidence for genetic alterations causing cancer

Evidence that genetic alterations play an essential role in oncogenesis includes the following:

- familial aggregations (e.g. retinoblastoma)
- chromosomal abnormalities carried in the germ line that confer increased risk of developing certain types of cancer (e.g. leukaemia and trisomy 21/Down's syndrome)
- the demonstration of specific somatic rearrangements of chromosomes or genes in certain cancers (e.g. the Philadelphia chromosome in chronic myeloid leukaemia and Burkitt's lymphoma)
- the increased risk of malignancy associated with an incapacity to repair DNA damaged by mutagens (such as occurs in xeroderma pigmentosum)
- associations between chemical mutagens and their carcinogenic affect (see Table 25.1)
- evidence that mutation or unregulated expression of particular genes (amplification) converts cells that behave normally into cells that behave in a malignant fashion.

It is commonly found that cancer cells contain chromosomal abnormalities which can be detected in metaphase spreads (p. 181). Furthermore, tumours of a given type often show the same abnormality. Characteristic chromosomal abnormalities are listed in Table 24.2. The genes involved are only partly understood, but they, or rather their products, seem to be important in neoplasia. For example:

Chronic myeloid leukaemia

In chronic myeloid leukaemia a consistent translocation between chromosomes 9 and 22 occurs; the resultant abnormal chromosome is called the Philadelphia chromosome. In this disease the molecular pathology is now becoming clear (Fig. 24.1). A gene on chromosome

Table 24.2   Some recognised chromosomal abnormalities in cancer

Tumour	Karyotypic abnormality
Chronic myeloid leukaemia	t(9,22)
Burkitt's lymphoma	t(8,14)
Acute promyelocytic leukaemia	t(15,17)
Follicular lymphoma	t(14,18)
Meningioma	monosomy 22
Retinoblastoma	deletion long arm 13
Neuroblastoma	deletion short arm 1
Nephroblastoma	deletion short arm 11
Small cell lung cancer	deletion short arm 3

t = translocation

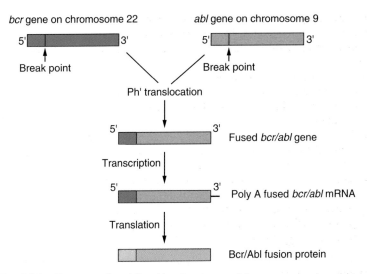

Fig. 24.1 The conversion of the *abl* proto-oncogene into an oncogene in patients with chronic myelogenous leukaemia. The chromosome translocation responsible joins the *bcr* gene on chromosome 22 to the *abl* gene form chromosome 9, thereby generating the Philadelphia chromosome. The resulting fusion protein has the amino terminus of the Bcr protein joined to the carboxyl terminus of the Abl tyrosine protein kinase. In consequence, the Abl kinase domain presumably becomes inappropriately active, driving excessive proliferation of a clone of haemopoietic cells in the bone marrow.

9 (called *abl*) is translocated to, or near to, a point on chromosome 22 called the breakpoint cluster region (*bcr*). *bcr* normally codes for a protein but when *abl* is translocated to this point a new, abnormal protein is produced with an abnormal function (it phosphorylates tyrosine). How this leads to neoplasia, or indeed whether it is an initiating or secondary event, is unclear. Since it occurs in 100% of cases it seems likely that it is important in the development of the tumour.

Burkitt's lymphoma

In Burkitt's lymphoma, a tumour of B lymphocytes, a translocation occurs between a gene on chromosome 8 (called *myc*) and the locus on chromosome 14 that codes for immunoglobulin heavy chain. There is great production of immunoglobulin in B lymphocytes so, when *myc* is placed near the immunoglobulin genes, it falls under the influence of the immunoglobulin gene's controlling elements. As a consequence there is an increased expression of *myc*, the function of which is unknown but may be involved in the development of the tumour.

Amplification of proto-oncogenes

Amplification of a gene or genes may occur in some tumours. The mechanism underlying this is not understood; although it may represent a non-specific phenomenon, it occurs quite frequently in some particular types of tumour. Moreover, the genes involved tend to be proto-oncogenes (see above). For example, amplification of N-*myc* occurs in neuroblastoma. Whilst the significance of this in terms of the development of the tumour is unclear, it has been shown that there is a good correlation between the number of amplified copies of N-*myc* and the stage of the disease (and hence prognosis). A similar relationship has been noted between amplification of the oncogene *erb*B and the prognosis in breast cancer. It may be that, in the future, such molecular pathology may provide a great deal of clinical information of diagnostic and prognostic value.

A further aspect of gene amplification is its relationship to drug resistance. Exposure of transformed cells to chemotherapeutic agents can lead, in time, to development of drug resistance. This process is of obvious clinical significance.

Genetic alteration and disease progression

The idea of tumour progression has been considered earlier but genetic alterations may be seen in this phenomenon. For example, in some types of lymphoma a series of karyotypic alterations are seen with progressive disease. The cause of the alterations in chromosomes is not known. It may be that the consistency of the sites involved in translocations, deletions and other changes in particular tumours reflects the sensitivity of the chromatin at those sites to some external factor; for example it may be that some mutagens (chemicals, radiation, etc.) preferentially attack 'fragile sites' in the genome.

Specific genes involved in cancer

It is important to note that not only are the chromosomes involved in these changes characteristic of given tumours, the points on the chromosome at which abnormalities occur are relatively fixed. Since the position of genes on chromosomes is fixed, this is an important piece of evidence supporting the notion of the involvement of particular genes in cancer. The identification of consistent karyotypic abnormalities in tumours is a useful clue to the identification of genes that may be involved in the development of these tumours. For example, the identification of an abnormality of chromosome 5 in a case of colorectal cancer arising in familial adenomatous polyposis was an important step to identifying the gene locus involved in this condition.

Single gene defects

The rare occurrence of genetic cancers buttresses the view that defective DNA is a central theme in neoplasia. There are several rare inherited diseases known as *chromosomal breakage syndromes* where autosomal chromosomes are aberrant and DNA repair is defective, including:

- xeroderma pigmentosum
- Fanconi's anaemia
- ataxia telangiectasia
- Bloom's syndrome.

The molecular defects in some of these diseases are now understood; for example in Bloom's syndrome there is a defect in the DNA repair enzyme DNA ligase I as a consequence of a mutation in the gene that codes for this enzyme. All of these conditions are associated with a high cancer risk in a variety of different organs.

Other, more common *chromosomal abnormalities* may also confer an increased risk of cancer. In Turner's syndrome there is an increased risk of ovarian tumours, in Klinefelter's syndrome of male breast carcinoma and in Down's syndrome of chronic myeloid leukaemia (CML).

There are few examples of tumours due to a simple *gene inheritance* and showing Mendelian transmission through the generations. The two most important are:

1. retinoblastoma, a tumour of the eye, which can be familial and is then transmitted as an autosomal dominant characteristic
2. familial adenomatous polyposis, starting as multiple benign tumours (adenomas) which become malignant with the passage of time; the inheritance is autosomal dominant.

Genetically determined malignancies might be expected to eliminate themselves by natural selection since most sufferers would die before producing children, and this probably explains their relative rarity. The conditions enumerated above may be attributable to a high mutation rate in the affected genes or, in the case of familial adenomatous polyposis, to its relatively late onset. Although rare, these conditions are of great interest since such 'experiments of nature' may provide important clues to the biology of the more common sporadic forms of the disease.

Retinoblastoma

Retinoblastoma occurs in two forms: one is sporadic and unilateral; in the other the predisposition to tumour development is inherited in an autosomal dominant fashion and/or the tumour is bilateral. It was postulated that the genetic loss in both forms of the disease was the same. In unilateral cases, loss of both copies of the inhibitory gene must occur by somatic mutation. In bilateral or hereditary cases, one event is already present in the germ line and only one further event is required. These predictions have been confirmed at the molecular level.

The Rb1 gene is located at chromosome 13q14, encoding a 928 amino acid protein. It is expressed in normal tissue but mutated in all retinoblastomas.

Breast cancer

Breast cancer is the most common cancer and the leading cause of death from malignant disease in women. The average prevalence worldwide is 1/1500 women. There are 21 000 new cases per year in England and Wales, and 143 000 cases in the USA. In the USA 40 000 women died of breast cancer in 1990 and the incidence appears to be rising. Breast cancer is 100 times less common in men than in women.

Five per cent of breast cancer is clearly inherited and linked to two candidate genes, BRCA1 and BRCA2. The BRCA1 and BRCA2 genes have been mapped to loci 17q12–21 and 13q12–13, respectively. BRCA1 is found in 40% of familial breast cancers and 80% of families with an increased risk of both breast and ovarian cancer. The contribution of BRCA2 is roughly equivalent, but does not influence the rate of ovarian cancer.

The BRCA1 gene is comprised of 21 exons and encodes a protein which contains 1863 amino acids and a zinc finger domain. The gene appears to encode a tumour suppressor protein that is a negative regulator of tumour cell growth.

Other genes, including p53, probably account for the remaining familial susceptibility to breast cancer. Almost all breast cancers are typical adenocarcinomas and arise from the glandular epithelium lining the lactiferous ducts and ductules. By the time of diagnosis most primary cancers have invaded the stroma and present as breast lumps.

Polygenic defects

Whereas single gene defects are rare, *polygenic inheritance* is probably a more important factor in the development of cancer. Polygenic inheritance in this instance means that the total parcel of inherited genetic information favours the operation of environmental carcinogens on a particular organ.

An important example is cancer of the large bowel, where 'cancer families' can be identified, many members of which develop carcinoma (this is distinct from familial adenomatous polyposis). By contrast, lung and bladder cancer, for example, do not show any obvious familial tendencies.

Furthermore, it is important not to confuse environmental factors with inherited ones. Many cancers, e.g. gastric cancer, are more common in social class V and so may appear to cluster in families who remain impoverished for many generations. Others may be related to family tendency to take up the same occupation.

Another way in which genetics may influence cancer causation is the possible variation in the levels of enzymes and the activities of metabolic pathways that detoxify and/or remove possible carcinogens. For example, in mice genetically determined variations in the level of aryl hydroxylase alter the amount of hydrocarbon available to act as a carcinogen. It is possible that similar variations may influence the relative susceptibility of man to carcinogens.

KEY POINTS

- Proto-oncogenes and suppressor genes regulate cell proliferation in normal cells.
- When proto-oncogenes are aberrantly expressed or mutated by various mechanisms they are termed cellular oncogenes. Proto-oncogenes are involved in various cellular functions, coding for:
  — receptor proteins, particularly growth factor receptors
  — growth factors themselves
  — proteins with enzymic function, notably tyrosine kinase
  — proteins with GTP binding properties
  — nuclear proteins.
- Oncogenes cause cancer as a consequence of altered or enhanced function; other genes may be involved in oncogenesis by their absence.
- Genetic factors are important in some types of cancer. They throw light on the role of mutation in carcinogenesis and provide support for the 'multiple hit' or 'multistage' theory of neoplasia. Furthermore, they emphasise the role of DNA in neoplasia.
- Alterations in genes and their products (i.e. proteins) and their functions in normal and abnormal cells are the key to understanding neoplasia.

25 Cancer: chemicals, radiation and other environmental factors

CHEMICALS

Chemical carcinogens may take a long time to produce their effects and it required Percival Pott, an observer of genius, to discover the connection between chemicals and cancer 200 years ago. His observation, that soot lodged in the scrotal skin during boyhood caused squamous carcinoma of the scrotal skin in adult chimney sweeps, initiated not only systematic cancer research but also industrial and environmental medicine and led to the discovery of the major group of cancer-causing chemicals.

After Pott's discovery, other occupations and other soots, tars and oils were found to be linked to cancers, as were aromatic amines used in dyes, chromium ores and asbestos. The close correlation between cigarette smoking and lung cancer is evidence that this tumour is due to a chemical carcinogen or carcinogens in the inhaled smoke.

Carcinogens in man

As regards the number of chemicals which induce tumours in man, it could be said that very many are suspected but relatively few are unequivocally proven! The most important proven examples are:

1. aromatic amines, e.g. β-naphthylamine
2. pitches, tars and oils containing polycyclic hydrocarbons
3. asbestos
4. ores such as chromium and nickel
5. Thorotrast, an agent formerly employed as a radiological contrast medium
6. diethylstilboestrol.

Carcinogens in animals

On the other hand, the number of chemicals known to be carcinogenic in animals and therefore theoretically carcinogenic in man is very great and increasing almost daily. Some of these chemicals occur naturally, such as aflatoxins from the mould *Aspergillus flavum* which grows on rotten peanuts, but most are synthetic. It is, of course, dangerous to extrapolate from one species to another with regard to carcinogenic potential or any other biological activity.

Initiation and promotion of chemical carcinogenesis

Two processes are involved in chemical carcinogenesis: *initiation* and *promotion*. It is difficult to define these concepts in other than operational terms. If we consider chemically induced tumours of the skin of mice, a substance such as methylchloranthrene will not usually induce tumours on its own, irrespective of the number of applications or quantity used. However, if a single application of methyl-chloranthrene is followed by applications of phorbol ester to the same site, then tumours will ensue. Conversely, if the methylchloranthrene is applied *after* the phorbol ester no tumours develop. How can this be interpreted?

An initiating agent causes a change in the genome of the cells to which it was applied, which is necessary but not sufficient to lead to a tumour. Further events are required, in particular further cellular proliferation which may be produced by application of a promoting agent.

Some chemical carcinogens are both initiating and promoting agents, i.e. complete carcinogens, whilst others are incomplete in that they require the assistance of a promoting agent. An important consequence of these observations (which have been repeated in other animal systems and in man) and this interpretation, is that carcinogenesis is, in general, a *multistep process*.

All chemical carcinogens require a latent period to elapse between administration and the development of the tumour, although this varies with the chemical and the doses. As regards natural cancers, there is often a long latent period of 10–40 years before the tumour becomes clinically apparent. This is well seen both in cigarette smokers who develop lung cancer, and in those occupationally exposed to aniline dyes who develop bladder cancer.

Detecting carcinogens

The testing of foodstuffs, food additives, environmental pollutants, etc., for cancer-inducing effects is a difficult and expensive process. As will be explained later, the induction of mutation in bacteria is a useful screening test for carcinogenicity. Certainty only prevails, however, when ignorance allows the experiment to be unwittingly performed on man, as in the induction of lung carcinoma by cigarettes.

Working from animal experiments, one has to consider the potency of the carcinogenic substance, the type of tumour it produces, how it has to be given to do so, the type and number of species in which the tumour can be provoked and the importance of the substance to man. When the risk of a particular substance causing cancer is small, the benefit to society gained by using that substance might be considered to be worth the disadvantage. The sweetening agents saccharine and cyclamates may or may not be carcinogenic in man but their use certainly helps to reduce obesity which has an unquestioned mortality and morbidity.

Why do chemicals cause cancer?

A glance at any list of chemical carcinogens reveals a great diversity of chemical structure. This suggests either that many types of molecules may transform cells or that carcinogens are converted in the body to a final common active product. In fact most carcinogens need to be acted upon by bodily enzymes before they are effective cancer-producing agents. The final active product is known as the *ultimate carcinogen*, and its intermediary precursor as the *proximate carcinogen*. All the available evidence suggests that there are many different ultimate carcinogens.

At first sight it seems strange that chemicals which are ingested as active carcinogens are much less important than those taken in as inactive precursors. However, because they are all very reactive molecules, the former interact with the lining epithelium of the respiratory and alimentary tracts which are constantly shed and discarded, taking the carcinogen with them (at least in the majority of cases). The inactive precursors do not react with the lining cells and are innocently absorbed. This is a simplification, since we know that some of the most important neoplasms are those of the lining epithelium of the gut and respiratory tract. Here the importance of the cells that are not shed, in particular stem cell populations, must be emphasised.

Formation of cancer provoking agents

Bodily enzymes

We are faced therefore with a situation in which chemicals are converted by the body's own enzymes to cancer-provoking agents. The enzymes in question are the *microsomal hydroxylases*, the same catalysts that have a role in some liver diseases. These drug metabolising enzymes undoubtedly evolved as a method of detoxifying harmful substances ingested or manufactured by the body. They are unusual in that their level can be increased by feeding them with certain substrates, i.e. they are inducible enzymes.

The *process of detoxification* involves:

1. oxidation
2. hydrolysis
3. conjugation.

Unfortunately the oxidation and hydrolysis which neutralise many poisons cause some otherwise harmless substances to form highly reactive intermediates which are cancer-producing. It might be argued that activity in these enzymes should be selected against in evolution since they cause cancer. However, undetoxified poisons would be likely to kill children or young adults of reproductive age, whereas cancer is largely a disease of middle and old age, affecting those who have already reproduced the species. Survival advantage therefore lies with retention of the enzymes.

The *polycyclic hydrocarbons* are found in soot and cigarette smoke and are the most important potential carcinogens in man. They are converted to metabolic derivatives called epoxides by the microsomal hydroxylases, the epoxide being the ultimate carcinogen (Figs 25.1, 25.2).

Aromatic amines, e.g. 2-naphthylamine, and *azo compounds*, e.g. dimethyl aminobenzene, are also converted to the active carcinogenic forms by the action of microsomal hydroxylases. In the case of 2-

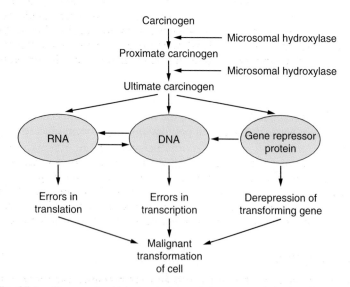

Fig. 25.1   The ways in which chemicals may induce cancer in body cells.

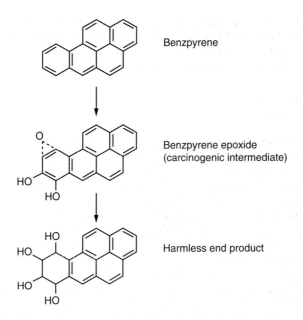

Fig. 25.2 The conversion of polycyclic hydrocarbon, benzpyrene, to the carcinogenic intermediate, benzpyrene epoxide, and eventually to a harmless metabolite, by the enzymic action of host tissue microsomal hydroxylases.

naphthylamine the active product is the N-hydroxy derivative which is then esterified by sulphate to form the ultimate carcinogen. This active form is then detoxified by the addition of glucuronide and excreted in the urine. Unfortunately the transitional epithelium of the bladder in man (but not in dogs) contains the enzyme glucuronidase; thus the active ultimate carcinogen is re-formed and has its action on the transitional epithelium.

Nitrates and nitrites

Some foodstuffs contain nitrates and nitrites. Nitrates can be converted to nitrites by the action of bacteria, and nitrites may react with amines to form nitrosamines, which may be carcinogenic. It is possible that such factors are of relevance to the development of carcinoma of the stomach, and the geographical distribution of this neoplasm may in part reflect dietary intake of nitrites/nitrates and agents that influence the formation of nitrosamines in gastric juice.

Bacterial enzymes

Bacteria in the intestine may also convert potential carcinogens to active cancer-inducing agents. Cycasin (methyl-azoxy-methanol glucoside) is a compound obtained from plants. In the presence of bacteria which contain a glucosidase it liberates methyl-azoxy-methanol, the carbonium ion of which acts as an ultimate carcinogen, just as it does in nitrosamines. The formation of a highly reactive electrophilic product (note: epoxides are very electrophilic) may possibly be of importance in the formation of large bowel cancer.

Endogenous compounds may possibly be metabolised by bacteria to ultimate carcinogens. There is some evidence that bile salts may be metabolised by bacteria in the large bowel and this may also be of some significance in the genesis of carcinoma of the large bowel.

Cancer related to occupation

Mention has already been made of occupations with increased risks of neoplasia of various sorts. Other examples include angiosarcoma in workers exposed to vinyl chloride monomer, and adenocarcinoma of the nasal and paranasal sinuses in furniture makers. Occupational exposure to asbestos causes malignant mesothelioma as well as fibrosing lung disease. Dramatic evidence for this came from Nottingham where many women exposed to asbestos in the manufacture of gas masks during World War II developed mesothelioma many years later.

With the increasing use of many new materials in modern industry, it is important to keep an open mind to the possibility of new dangers, particularly given the latent period often associated with chemical carcinogenesis.

Proof of mutagenicity

The proof of the mutagenicity of known human carcinogens such as -naphthylamine was established by what is commonly called the 'Ames test', after its discoverer. A mutant strain of bacteria, usually *Salmonella typhimurium*, is used which is abnormal in that it cannot grow in the absence of histidine. Chemical mutagens reverse this bacterial mutation so that when they are added to the cultures some of the bacteria begin to grow. Many carcinogens failed to show any mutagenic activity until it was realised that they first had to be converted to the active ultimate carcinogen by microsomal enzymes. When this is done, by incubating the suspected substance with liver extract before adding it to the bacterial culture, 90% of chemical carcinogens are found to be mutagenic and 90% of non-carcinogens are found to be non-mutagenic.

Why is cancer not more prevalent?

Considering the prevalence in the environment of compounds that can be shown to be mutagenic in the Ames system, it has to be asked why even more people do not succumb to cancer. It is possible that part of the explanation lies in the microsomal enzyme system itself. There is considerable variation between individuals in the degree to which particular substances induce this system to become active. There is similar variation between different components of the system. In some individuals, the enzyme reactions leading to the formation of mutagenic intermediates are stronger than those causing final detoxification (Fig. 25.2) and in others the situation is reversed.

The molecular basis of carcinogenesis

The molecular basis of the ability of carcinogens to cause somatic mutation is in most cases an intimate reaction with DNA. Some carcinogens link themselves directly to guanine as do polycyclic hydrocarbon epoxides. Some add methyl groups to guanine, some remove amino groups from cytosine, and others cross-link between the two chains of a DNA molecule. The chemical alterations in DNA cause faulty pairing of bases to occur whenever DNA is replicated. For example, guanine which has been methylated is 'mistaken' for adenine so that when the affected DNA is replicated an A–T base pair is formed instead of the GC base pair that was needed. When an epoxide is added directly to a guanine base, a massive distortion of the DNA molecule results, with inevitable faulty replication.

Failure of DNA repair mechanisms

In spite of these severe effects, chemical interference with DNA molecules by carcinogens is by no means always followed by cellular mutation. This is because cells have a battery of enzymes devoted to the excision and repair of damaged DNA.

It seems quite likely that somatic mutation and hence cancer occurs only:

- when the repair mechanism fails
- when the cell is forced into errors of DNA repair
- when the mechanism is simply swamped by the frequency of mutational events.

It may be that it is faulty repair, rather than the chemical reaction of mutagen and DNA, which is the direct cause of carcinogenic mutation. Errors in DNA repair are more likely to occur when the affected cells are dividing quickly rather than more slowly and this may be why cancer develops preferentially in organs where cell turnover is high, such as the intestine, rather than where it is low, such as skeletal muscle. This cannot be the entire story, however, since some tissues with high turnover rates, e.g. the small bowel, have far fewer tumours than other tissues with relatively high turnover rates, e.g. the large bowel. Most important mutational events occur when cells are dividing.

Excessive replication promotes cancer

Mutation (alias initiation) is obviously crucial in understanding cancer but promotion also is important. The essence of promotion is accelerated cell division. It can be demonstrated experimentally that after administration of a mutagenic carcinogen, cancer follows more quickly if the skin is irritated or wounded, if the liver is forced to regenerate, or if cell division in thyroid or ovary is accelerated by hormonal treatment. In humans, an increased risk of cancer is associated with ulcerative colitis, where the bowel epithelium regenerates excessively for many years; with exaggerated proliferation of the epithelium of the tongue; and with Paget's disease of bone where the bone turnover is much increased.

Why should excessive replication promote cancer in cell populations which are dividing rapidly? Mutation (initiation) must precede promotion, so the effect has to be to augment the effects of mutation. The answer is not known. Hurried cell division could increase the chances of faulty DNA base repair. It could also increase the possibility of mistakes in cell division, so that a cell is left with two copies of a mutant gene instead of only one, by a kind of non-dysjunction (p. 182) or as a result of exaggerated somatic recombination. Promotion could also be due to activation of latent genes which happen to have undergone carcinogenic mutation.

Cancer latency

In contemplating the role of initiation and promotion in cancer in man one returns again and again to the phenomenon of latency. The daughters of mothers who received diethylstilboestrol during pregnancy did not develop adenocarcinoma of the vagina until they were 15–20 years of age. The reasons for this very long latency in this example of 'transplacental carcinogenesis' are unknown. The long latent periods associated with industrial cancer and cigarette smoking have been already mentioned. A long latent period is the norm with pleural mesothelioma associated with asbestos exposure. It should be noted that asbestos is not known to be a mutagen and the mechanism by which it causes tissue damage and incites neoplasia is unknown.

Synergy of carcinogens

The interplay between carcinogens should be noted. For example those exposed to asbestos have about a 5-fold increased risk of lung cancer (in addition to the risk of mesothelioma). Smokers have a 10-

fold increased risk of lung cancer. Those who are both exposed to asbestos and who smoke have a 50-fold increased risk of lung cancer. Fortunately such examples of true synergy are rare.

Genetic and non-genetic mechanisms of cancer

Although mutation figures prominently in current thinking about chemical carcinogenesis, we must not forget non-genetic or epigenetic mechanisms. Chemical carcinogens react with RNA and proteins as well as DNA and this may possibly have some relevance to the processes underlying neoplasia.

IONISING RADIATION

There is unequivocal evidence that both electromagnetic radiation, e.g. ultraviolet and X-rays, and particulate radiation, e.g. electrons, neutrons and α-particles, cause cancer in man (Table 25.1).

Table 25.1 Agents known to produce cancer in man

Agent	Site of cancer
Various polycyclic hydrocarbons	Scrotum
Ionising radiation	Skin, bronchus, marrow and most if not all organs
Ultraviolet light	Skin
β-naphthylamine	Bladder
Benzidine	
Asbestos	Bronchus, pleura and peritoneum
'Chrome ore'	Bronchus
'Nickel ore'	Bronchus, nasal sinuses
Bischloromethyl ether	Bronchus
Hardwood dust (?)	Nasal sinuses
'Isopropyl oil'	Nasal sinuses
Benzene	Marrow
'Betel mixture'	Mouth
Chlornaphazine (treatment of myeloma)	Bladder
Arsenic (when used as a medicine)	Skin, bronchus
Phenacetin (in study of analgesic nephropathy)	Renal pelvis
Tobacco	Bronchus; also mouth, pharynx, larynx, oesophagus, bladder
Mustard gas	Bronchus, larynx, nasal sinuses
Vinyl chloride	Angiosarcoma of the liver
Stilboestrol	Male breast, vagina in child exposed in utero
Aflatoxin	Liver

The most important is *ultraviolet light* because it is probably the most common cause of skin cancer. The evidence here, as in the case of the relationship between cigarettes and lung cancer, is epidemiological. It comes from a statistical association between UV irradiation on the one hand and cancer of exposed lightly pigmented parts of the skin on the other. Thus skin cancer is much more common in the sunny states of the USA than in the north but is rare in the black population.

UV light induces tumours in animals and provokes mutations in many forms of life in direct proportion to its ability to cause tumours. This suggests that it launches a direct attack on the genetic apparatus and it has indeed been confirmed that UV irradiation forms bonds between adjacent bases in cellular DNA with the formation of abnormal thymine dimers. It is reasonable to assume that this deformation of DNA leads to malignant transformation.

The best evidence for this cause and effect relationship comes from genetically determined diseases such as *xeroderma pigmentosum* (p. 285). The genetic abnormality is a lack of an enzyme which normally repairs defects in DNA. Patients with the disease have an extremely high incidence of skin cancer in those parts of the body exposed to sunlight. The inference is that UV irradiation regularly causes defects in cell DNA in the skin, but that these abnormalities are normally repaired by a specific enzyme that is missing or defective such that mutations can occur and tumours arise.

Radioactive emissions

Radioactive emissions such as X-ray irradiation are well known as potent carcinogens. Many of the early pioneers in this field, including Roentgen, developed skin cancer. Miners engaged in the excavation and extraction (and hence possible inhalation) of radioactive ores, such as uranium, had a high rate of lung cancer, even in the pre-cigarette era when the disease was rare. Workers licking brushes dipped in radium-containing paint used for luminous watch dials had a high incidence of osteosarcoma of the jaw. Bone marrow tumours (leukaemia) were common amongst the early radiologists, and the therapeutic use of even small doses of X-rays for a variety of diseases was frequently followed years later by cancer of the treated part. All these examples date from the days before the hazards were recognised.

Mechanisms of radiation damage

Forms of radiation other than UV light cause mutations by breaking chemical bonds in DNA rather than forming new bonds. It is possible that these breaks are due to the formation within the cell of very active free radicals, derived for example from intracellular water (p. 32). X-rays are relatively weak and cause single chain breaks which are relatively easily repaired. As with UV light, mutation probably occurs only when two such breaks occur simultaneously and the repair mechanism fails. Because this demands two independent events, cancer-inducing mutation increases with the square of the dose of X-rays. In the case of high energy particles, such as neutrons, a single interaction with the particle will cause two breaks which cannot therefore be repaired. As a result the mutation rate increases in direct proportion to the dose.

Survivors of the atomic bombs probably received more radiation than anyone in history. The Nagasaki bomb produced mostly X-rays and the subsequent incidence of leukaemia was proportional to the square of the calculated dose received by the patient. The Hiroshima bomb produced a heavy output of neutrons and the subsequent leukaemia incidence was directly proportional to the dose received. However, the amount of genetic mutation occurring in children was much less than expected with only a handful of detected cases.

Radiation in the natural environment

Exposure to radiation from the natural environment should not be ignored. For example the granite of Cornwall or Aberdeen leads to the local populace being exposed to high radiation levels in the form of radon gas and many people in these areas are exposed to more radiation than nuclear power workers. Radon has been estimated to cause up to 1500 deaths from lung cancer in the UK annually. 'Man made' radiation, for example emissions from Sellafield and other nuclear installations, may add to this.

Whilst there is no doubt that medium and high level radiation exposure, such as was encountered after the Japanese atomic bombs or the Chernobyl accident, may cause an increased incidence of cancer, the significance of low level radiation is still a matter of controversy. Although radioactivity induced cancer is evidently dose-dependent, it cannot truly be said that there is a safe lower limit of response. A study of workers at the nuclear submarine base at Rosyth showed chromosome defects in direct proportion to exposure to γ-rays. In particular, aberrations were found at levels of exposure well below internationally agreed environmental and occupational maximal permissible limits. However, chemical exposure may be more important as chromosomal abnormalities have been found to be even higher in coal-fired power stations.

CHRONIC IRRITATION

This is often put forward as a predisposing cause of cancer but the concept does not sustain close scrutiny. The smoking of clay pipes with hot stems or the practice of some tribes of holding hot dishes to the bare abdomen over long periods of time results in carcinoma of the lip and abdominal skin respectively and has been attributed to chronic irritation. Oesophageal cancer has also been tentatively linked to the regular drinking of very hot drinks. The most likely explanation for most of these instances is that they act as promoters, increasing the chance that some somatic mutation in the affected cells will lead to malignant transformation.

Oncogenesis may also be environmental. Different surroundings or habits could vary the chance of developing a cancer (Table 25.2) and account for the variable incidences of certain cancers in different countries (see Ch. 29).

Table 25.2   The variation in incidence of certain cancers in different countries

Cancer	Country	Incidence*
Skin	Australia	20
	India	< 0.1
Lung	England	< 11
	Nigeria	0.3
Liver	Mozambique	8
	England	0.08
Rectum	Denmark	2
	Nigeria	0.1

*Number of new cases/1000 population/year, adjusted for age distribution.

KEY POINTS

- Chemical carcinogens may take a long time to produce their effects (latency).
- A large number of chemicals are known to be carcinogenic in animals though relatively few have been definitely proved to be carcinogens in man.
- Most carcinogens require the action of body enzymes to transform them into effective cancer-producing agents (ultimate carcinogens).
- Susceptibility to the effect of a carcinogen varies between individuals because of variation in activity of the microsomal enzyme system or its components.
- Carcinogens cause somatic mutation in most cases by reacting with DNA, resulting in faulty replication. UV irradiation forms bonds between adjacent bases in cellular DNA. X-rays cause single chain breaks. High energy particles such as neutrons cause irreparable damage to DNA.
- Many occupational and environmental carcinogens have now been recognised. The risk posed by low level radiation or chemicals from various sources has not yet been fully quantified.

26 Cancer: hormones and growth factors

It is likely that complex regulatory systems involving the coordinated action of a range of growth factors control cellular proliferation and differentiation in normal tissues. Such factors act in a variety of ways (Fig. 26.1):

- endocrine signal transmission, that is the secretion into the blood stream of some agent that acts on distant cells
- paracrine responses, involving the secretion by a cell of some agent which acts locally on nearby cells
- autocrine responses, involving the release by a cell of factors which act on itself.

These ideas are of importance in the modern understanding of the function of cells, their interactions with each other and the development of neoplasia and other disorders of growth control. In some ways the distinction between hormones and growth factors is rather artificial and it is logical to consider them together.

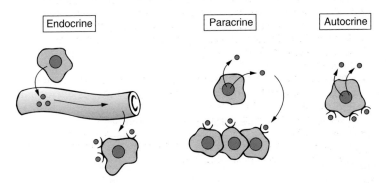

Fig. 26.1   Methods of inter-cell communication.

The action of hormones

The majority of hormones act by binding to an extracellular receptor which transmits a signal through the cell membrane which is in turn sent via a chemical signalling system (such as cAMP) to the nucleus where a change in mRNA (increase or decrease in production or production of different species) occurs. The exceptions are steroid and thyroid hormones which, on binding to an extracellular receptor, are internalised and moved to the nucleus where they act directly. Now growth factors act in a similar way to most hormones, behaving as ligands for specific receptors. Whilst there is clear evidence of the role of hormones in cancer, at least in a permissive manner, this is not the only way in which extracellular messengers can influence the behaviour of transformed cells.

Breast and prostatic cancer

Certain organs in the body respond to hormones such as oestrogens, testosterone or prolactin by *hyperplasia* and *hypertrophy*. Two of these organs, the breast and the prostate, are commonly the site of cancer. Both breast and prostatic cancers are well known to undergo regression if action is taken to withdraw the hormones that stimulate these organs, and this property of hormone responsiveness is employed therapeutically. Thus many cases of breast cancer show some response if the ovaries are removed or a drug such as tamoxifen is given that has anti-oestrogen effects. Many cases of prostatic cancer can be shown to regress under the action of female sex hormones. Thus there is good evidence that tumours of these organs are in some way influenced by the action of hormones or are dependent on hormones for their continued growth.

The role of prolactin, oestrogen and progesterone in mammary tumours

The role of hormones has also been demonstrated in the case of some tumours in animals. Mice of a susceptible genetic strain who receive the mouse mammary tumour virus (or so-called Bittner agent) in their mothers' milk will not develop breast tumours if prolactin, oestrogen and progesterone are denied them by removing their pituitary, adrenals and ovaries. In the presence of the hormones all the mice develop tumours.

A similar situation holds for chemical carcinogens. Thus in some strains of rats, a single injection of a polycyclic hydrocarbon (dimethylbenzanthracene, DMBA) will induce breast tumours in almost 100% of cases. If, however, the ovaries, adrenals and pituitary are removed, then the tumours do not occur and will disappear if already induced. Injection of oestrogens causes the tumours to recommence their growth, unless the pituitary has been removed. This indicates that some pituitary factor is involved: it now seems certain that it is the peptide hormone prolactin. There is evidence also that oestrogens induce the release of prolactin from the pituitary and enhance its effect on breast tissue. There is also evidence that high levels of prolactin in the blood enhance the growth of mammary cancer only when oestrogens are present.

The general conclusion is that prolactin, oestrogen and possibly progesterone are all necessary for the induction of mammary tumours by viral or chemical carcinogenesis. Furthermore, there is evidence that the response of human breast cancer to therapeutic hormonal manipulation is determined to some extent by the presence of hormone receptors in the tumour cells.

Hormones as cancer promoters

In all these cases the role of hormones appears to be permissive, i.e. they permit carcinogenesis to occur rather than themselves causing it. This suggests that, in terms of the previous chapter, they are promoters rather than initiators of malignancy. In certain organs hormones are essential for DNA synthesis, even under carcinogenic stimulation. The effect of ovarian hormones on breast tissue is to increase the number of cells in mitosis rather than accelerate the rate of individual mitosis, i.e. shorten the cell cycle. The permissive role of these hormones is supported by work in which breast tissue in organ culture has been transformed by the action of DMBA but only in the presence of suitable amounts of oestrogen, prolactin and progesterone, the hormones alone having no transforming properties.

Inappropriate secretion of hormones by tumours

Another aspect of hormones and cancer is the production by some tumours of biologically active hormones in inappropriate amounts and without the normal controlling mechanisms of homeostasis. This has already been mentioned in Chapter 23, page 274. This is not likely to have any beneficial effect from the tumour's point of view but in some cases may be of diagnostic value.

Growth factors

A list of physiologically important growth factors is shown in Table 26.1. Only some of the better characterised factors are listed and many more are likely to be described. In any given tissue there may be multiple growth factors operating. For example in the bone marrow several different factors act—erythropoietin, macrophage colony stimulating factor (M-CSF), granulocyte CSF, granulocyte and

Table 26.1   Growth factors

Growth factor	Notes
Epidermal growth factor (EGF)	Affects wide variety of cell types (53 amino acids)
Transforming growth factor α (TGFα)	Affects wide variety of cell types (48 amino acids)
Transforming growth factor β (TGFβ)	Action modulated by TGFα— sometimes acts as an inhibitory factor (homodimer)
Platelet derived growth factor (PDGF)	Glial and some mesenchymal cells and platelets
Fibroblast growth factors (FGF I, II, III)	Derived from endothelial cells and some mesenchymal cells
Erythropoietin	Regulates erythropoiesis (166 amino acids)
Interleukin-2	T-cell growth factor
M-CSF	Macrophage colony stimulating factor
G-CSF	Granulocyte colony stimulating factor
GM-CSF	Granulocyte and macrophage colony stimulating factor
Interleukin-3 (multi-CSF)	All haemopoietic progenitor cells
Nerve growth factor (NGF)	Nerves, especially sensory and sympathetic
Glial growth factor (GGF)	Astrocytes and Schwann cells

macrophage CSF, etc. Furthermore, growth factors may modulate the action of each other, i.e. the action of one may alter the way in which a cell responds to another. These responses involve proliferation and differentiation and are as yet only poorly understood. However it is clear that the correct, ordered functioning of these factors is important for the normal control of proliferation and differentiation. Some growth factors influence the transition of a cell from G_0 to G_1 and on into the cell cycle (p. 162).

The significance of growth factor function in neoplasia

In view of the role of growth factors and in the light of our thesis that pathology involves the subversion of normal mechanisms, what evidence is there that disordered growth factor function is of significance in neoplasia? An important clue came from the realisation that an oncogenic retrovirus called simian sarcoma virus contained a gene with sequence homology with the mammalian gene that codes for a growth factor called PDGF (platelet derived growth factor, p. 223). It has been known for some time that neoplastic cells have, in general, reduced requirements for serum which untransformed cells need for survival in vitro. It was thus suggested that neoplastic cells may produce an abnormal form of PDGF as a result of a mutation in the gene (called *sis*), and that this abnormal form may act in an autocrine manner on the cell which produced it, leading to abnormal growth control. Since PDGF action is but the first step in signal transduction, it may be that the subversion of other genes may lead to disordered growth control.

Oncogenes and growth factor receptors

Further studies have shown that a number of oncogenes code for abnormal growth factor receptors. For example *erb*B oncogene codes for an abnormal form of the receptor for epidermal growth factor (EGF). In some tumours, notably squamous carcinoma, this aberrant molecule has been truncated and acts abnormally. Rather than responding normally to EGF, it is constitutively activated, i.e. turned on all the time, and thus sends an abnormal signal. Other oncogenes also code for abnormal proteins which have roles in signal transduction. As emphasised in Chapter 24, the normal products of the proto-oncogenes are vital to normal cellular function if expressed in the correct quantities at the correct times. It is only when these normal genes are dysregulated (by mutation in controlling sites, amplification), or undergo structural mutation such that an abnormal product is formed, that they have oncogenic potential.

Growth factors and cancer promotion

An important consequence of our increased knowledge about growth factors and cancer is the explanation of some previous observations. In particular the effect of some promoters in chemical carcinogenesis is understandable. Phorbol esters (Ch. 25) are now known to activate an enzyme called *protein kinase C* which is involved in signal transduction.

A further and very important consequence is the possibility of new therapeutic modalities. For example it is now well established that small cell lung cancer produces and responds to the hormone (growth factor) bombesin in an autocrine manner. Thus there is potential for the use of bombesin antagonists in the therapy of this tumour. It may be that the application of other growth factor antagonists has a place in curing other tumours.

KEY POINTS

- Hormones are promoters rather than initiators of malignancy.
- Organs in the body respond to hormones such as oestrogens, testosterone or prolactin by hyperplasia and hypertrophy. Regression of tumours occurs on withdrawal of the hormones that stimulate these organs, depending on the level of hormone receptors in the tumour.
- A number of oncogenes code for abnormal growth factor receptors and may result in the receptor being permanently 'switched on'.
- Some chemical carcinogens may act as promoters by activating growth factors.
- Hormone/growth factor antagonists may have a place in the therapy of tumours that are hormone responsive.

27 Cancer: viruses

In recent years this particular area of cancer research has been very fruitful and the contribution of virologists has been crucial to our modern understanding of the biology of neoplasia. Indeed the concept of oncogenes arose from studies of virally induced cell transformation.

Viruses causing cancer

There are three important groups of virus which have been associated with cellular transformation in vitro and with neoplasia in vivo. These are listed in Table 27.1. Some appear to cause tumours in their natural hosts, others are oncogenic only when infecting other species, whilst a number have only been observed to cause cellular transformation in vitro.

It is important to consider the criteria which need to be fulfilled in order to show that a given virus is the cause of a given tumour. Koch postulated that to prove causality a microorganism must be isolated from the lesion that it is thought to cause, it should be grown in vitro, and on introduction into a suitable host it should produce the same lesion. One might suggest also that specific immunisation of the animal should prevent that lesion. It can be very difficult to fulfil these criteria in the case of viruses and cancer, particularly in man.

In addition, it is important to remember that the virus alone may not be sufficient to cause the tumour. A range of other factors may also be needed.

In animals, viruses that cause cancer can be transmitted 'horizontally' from animal to animal, like other infections. They can also be transmitted 'vertically' from parent to child, either as part of the germ cell genome or as an infectious agent, e.g. in mother's milk as in the case of the mouse mammary tumour virus.

Table 27.1   Oncogenic viruses

Family	Virus	Species affected
Large DNA viruses		
Adeno		
Herpes	Saimari, ateles	Simian
	Marek's	Chicken
	Lucke	Frog
	Herpes simplex ??	Man
	Epstein–Barr ??	Man
	HBLV-1 ??	Man
	CMV ??	Man
Small DNA viruses		
Papova	Polyoma	Mouse
	Papilloma	Man, others
	SV40	Rodents
Hepadna	Hepatitis B	Man
RNA viruses		
Retroviruses		
Type B	Mouse mammary tumour virus	
Type C	Avian sarcoma virus (Rous)	
	HTLV-1	
	Feline leukaemia virus, etc.	

DNA and RNA viruses

There are two broad categories of virus: those with genomes composed of DNA and those with genomes composed of RNA. Both types cause tumours in animals. However, whilst several types of DNA virus can cause cancer and transform cells in vitro, only one type of RNA virus, the *retrovirus*, has the ability to cause tumours and transform cells in vitro. This is because, of the RNA viruses, only the retroviruses have the enzyme reverse transcriptase (RNA-dependent DNA polymerase), which allows the cell to make a DNA copy of the RNA viral genome which can then be incorporated into the host cell genome. That this is a crucial step will be illustrated shortly.

It is known that the viruses of the Hepadna group also have a reverse transcriptase activity and convert their double-stranded DNA genome into an RNA template from which more DNA is produced.

Oncogenic retroviruses

Oncogenic retroviruses (oncoviruses) are divided into two groups on the basis of their morphology: Type B and Type C. They may also be classified, according to the speed and efficiency with which they transform cultured cells, into acute and slow transforming viruses.

Acute transforming viruses

Acute transforming viruses rapidly cause cell transformation in permissive cells. It has been found that this is due to a single gene (an oncogene) in the viral genome whose expression in the cell leads to transformation. In the case of the Rous sarcoma virus this gene (called *src* for sarcoma) is present in addition to the three normal genes of the retrovirus (*Gag*, *Pol*, and *Env*, see Ch. 24). Since the full genetic machinery of the virus is present, the complete replicative cycle occurs. In all other acutely transforming retroviruses the oncogene exists together with only part of the normal viral genome and the virus cannot, by itself, go through the full replicative cycle. However, because of the oncogene, it can transform a permissive cell. In order for this 'defective' virus to replicate, a second virus (a helper virus) is needed to supplement the defective or missing genes. As a consequence, isolation of the virus from transformed cells can be difficult.

Oncogenes and tumour suppressor genes

The life cycle of retroviruses provided the first clues for identifying cellular genes that might participate in tumorigenesis. Integration of viral DNA is in itself potentially mutagenic, a phenomenon described as *insertional mutagenesis*. Secondly, recombination between cellular and retroviral genomes can implant cellular genes into the viral genome, and in this new setting the cellular genes may become oncogenic (see Ch. 24).

Progressive multiplication in vivo

Progressive cell multiplication may result from mutations of cell cycle regulators in two ways:

- gain-of-function mutations of positive regulators
- loss-of-function mutations of negative regulators.

Gain-of-function mutations represent the majority of the originally described oncogenes, mutations of proto-oncogenes implicated in the transduction of growth regulatory messages. Such mutations would generate a continuous unregulated stimulus for cell division; *ras* gene products were among the first oncogene products to be implicated in human cancers.

Loss-of-function mutations behaving in a recessive fashion might result in uncontrolled cell proliferation. Tumour suppressor genes (otherwise termed anti-oncogenes), in their unmutated form, arrest cell division.

Evidence that malignancy might be a consequence of recessive mutations came from cell fusion experiments where the malignant phenotype was suppressed following fusion with non-malignant cells.

Study of hereditary tumours gave additional support for this view. Analysis of familial retinoblastoma led to the formulation of Knudson's two-hit hypothesis, now a paradigm for inherited tumour development. Observation of the incidence and age at presentation of tumours suggested a model in which two events must occur in a single retinal cell for a tumour to develop.

Slow transforming viruses and insertional mutagenesis

Retroviruses of the other group are called slow transforming viruses since they only rarely, and only after some delay, lead to cellular transformation in permissive cells in vitro. These viruses do not contain a transforming oncogene. How then do they lead to transformation? To understand this, one needs to consider the viral genome in a little more detail. The genome is linear with the structural genes (*Gag*, *Pol* and *Env*) in the centre. At the ends of the genome are a series of controlling elements which influence the transcription of the viral genes. These elements are called long terminal repeats (LTRs). As mentioned before, retroviral replication involves integration of the viral genome into the host cellular genome. It has been found that the integration site is randomly spread through the host cell genome, but that in those cells which are transformed the integration site is always the same. This suggests that an important cellular gene is present at this site which, if incorrectly expressed (due to the influence of the viral LTRs), results in cellular transformation.

Although more difficult to demonstrate experimentally, it is also possible that viral integration at a specific site may lead to the destruction of the cellular gene at this site. This may be a way of removing the effect of a tumour suppressor gene and thus allowing transformation to occur. Identification of the sites of integration of slow transforming retroviruses has allowed the identification of a number of cellular genes whose abnormal expression can lead to transformation, and thus they may be termed oncogenes. Examples include the *Wnt*-1 gene that is present at the insertion site of the mouse mammary tumour virus (Fig. 27.1). The process of retroviral genome insertion into the host cell genome leading to some mutational event is known as insertional mutagenesis (see p. 278).

The X gene and cell transformation

A further method by which retroviruses can cause cell transformation has recently been described in human T-cell lymphotropic viruses (HTLV). In addition to *Gag*, *Pol* and *Env* a fourth gene, called *X*, may exist in some viruses. The protein for which this codes may function on the viral LTRs, altering the way in which these control viral gene

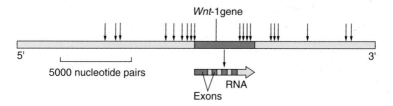

Fig. 27.1   Insertional mutagenesis. In this example the process activates a gene called Wnt-1 (formerly called int-1) and produces breast cancer in mice infected with the mouse mammary tumour virus (MMTV). The sites of MMTV integration observed in 19 different tumour isolates are indicated by *arrows*. Note that the insertions can activate transcription of the Wnt-1 gene from distances of more than 10 000 nucleotide pairs away and from either side of the gene. This effect is attributed to a powerful enhancer DNA sequence present in the terminal repeats of the MMTV genome.

expression. Thus X gene product is acting as another level of gene control.

The product of X may also act elsewhere on the host cell genome, perhaps even on another chromosome rather than nearby: that is, in a *trans* (at a distance) manner rather than *cis* (locally, as in the example of insertional mutagenesis). Thus host cell gene regulation may be altered by the viral products at a distance, and this can lead to neoplasia. In particular, expression of growth factors and growth factor receptors may be increased and the cell may then enter an autocrine loop where it is producing both growth factor and growth factor receptor and thus stimulating itself. This is seen in T cells infected by HTLV-1, where increased production of interleukin-2 and interleukin-2 receptor (p. 67) occurs as a consequence of transacting viral products modulating the cellular genome.

It is possible that the immunosuppression associated with infection by viruses such as the human immunodeficiency virus (HIV, p. 57) may lead to neoplasia as a consequence of infection with other viruses.

Cellular consequences of DNA virus infection

In general, infection of a cell by a DNA virus results in viral replication and the death of the cell. In some cases, however, a persistent infection occurs with the virus residing in the cell, without productive infection. In some cases integration of the DNA viral genome into the host cell DNA genome occurs. Viral integration appears to be essential for DNA viruses to cause cellular transformation, in the same way that it is needed for retroviruses to cause transformation.

Some viruses and the diseases they cause (Table 27.2)

Human papilloma viruses (HPV)

These viruses are known to cause a self-limiting proliferation of epithelial cells called warts. Such lesions remain benign and usually regress spontaneously. In rare cases, usually in association with defective cell-mediated immunity and with ultraviolet radiation possibly acting as a cofactor, widespread warts occur. This is called *epidermodysplasia verruciformis*, and *squamous carcinoma* occurs in many cases. A similar phenomenon occurs in cattle where bovine papilloma viruses, together with bracken acting as a cofactor, can lead to alimentary tract tumours.

The role of papilloma viruses in other human tumours is not proven, but there is considerable epidemiological evidence and some experimental evidence to support a role for HPV 8, 11 and 16 in *carcinoma of the cervix*. This is, however, as yet unproven.

Herpes simplex viruses (HSV)

HSV Type II has also been implicated in the pathogenesis of *carcinoma of the cervix*. Again, epidemiological data has been the major pointer to such an association. HPV is widely viewed as likely to be the more important but a role for HSV cannot be absolutely discounted.

Epstein–Barr virus (EBV)

The role of other herpes viruses in neoplasia is more clearly established. The Epstein–Barr virus (EBV) was isolated from cell lines of *Burkitt's lymphoma*. It has also been associated with *nasopharyngeal carcinoma* occurring in some parts of southern China.

Table 27.2   Human cancer and viruses

Virus	Cancer
DNA viruses	
Papilloma virus	Benign warts
	Cancer of uterine cervix
Hepatitis B virus	Hepatocellular carcinoma
Epstein–Barr virus	Burkitt's lymphoma
RNA viruses	
Human T-cell leukaemia virus Type I (HTLV-1)	Adult T-cell leukaemia/lymphoma
Human immunodeficiency virus (HIV)	Kaposi's sarcoma

EBV infects human B lymphocytes and causes *infectious mononucleosis* in some individuals. This involves a polyclonal proliferation of B lymphocytes which is self-limiting due to the effect of cell-mediated immunity. In some families where there is a major defect in T cells and, as a consequence, in cell-mediated immunity, the proliferation of B cells goes unchecked. After some time a monoclonal population develops from this polyclonal proliferation and an overt *B-cell lymphoma* develops to which the patient succumbs.

In Burkitt's lymphoma (a tumour of B lymphocytes), EBV infection can be demonstrated in the majority of cases. There is an epidemiological association with malaria, and this may possibly have a role in causing chronic low grade immunosuppression. This is not sufficient to lead to the tumour; cytogenetic alterations are known to occur, notably a translocation between chromosome 8 and 14. Again we have evidence that viral infection may not be sufficient, by itself, to cause neoplasia. A final example of EBV-induced lymphoma is the development of lymphomas containing EBV genomes in transplant patients. Immunosuppression may have an important role here.

Cytomegalovirus

Other herpes viruses have been implicated in the development of human tumours, most notably cytomegalovirus, which has been linked to the development of *Kaposi's sarcoma*.

Hepatitis B virus

Hepatocellular carcinoma caused by hepatitis B virus is, in some parts of the world, an enormous social and economic problem. It causes more than 50% of cancer deaths in some parts of Africa and Asia, particularly in young adults. There is considerable epidemiological and experimental evidence that the hepatitis B virus is an important factor in the pathogenesis of this tumour. Similar viruses have been shown to be the major factor in causing hepatocellular carcinoma in animal models (notably the woodchuck).

Again there appears to be a need for persistent infection with integration of the viral DNA genome into the host liver cell genome, however the mechanism whereby this leads to cellular transformation is unclear. In addition there seems to be a need for other factors. For example, dietary factors such as aflatoxins, derived from the mould *Aspergillus flavus*, have been implicated in some cases; alcohol may also be important.

Absolute proof of the role of hepatitis B virus in the causation of hepatocellular carcinoma, in terms of fulfilling Koch's postulates, is still lacking. The availability of an effective immunisation against this virus may however lead to a substantial reduction in acute and chronic hepatitis due to the virus and also to a reduction in deaths from cancer.

Environmental cofactors in neoplasia

It is important to note that cases of hepatocellular carcinoma without evidence of hepatitis B virus infection do occur, in the same way as cases of Burkitt's lymphoma occur without evidence of EBV infection. It seems, therefore, that whilst some human tumours may be caused by viruses (with the help of cofactors), other pathways to the neoplastic phenotype may exist for any given tumour type.

The problem is to identify specific environmental risk factors and their mode of action. Some may work as tumour initiators, others as tumour promoters. Tobacco smoke is probably an initiator, whereas phorbol esters (e.g. tetradecylphorbol acetate) are thought to act as promoters: they are not mutagenic, but can cause skin cancer in areas previously exposed to a tumour initiator.

KEY POINTS

- There are three important groups of virus which have been associated with neoplasia:
  — large DNA viruses
  — small DNA viruses
  — RNA viruses (retroviruses)
- Infection with the virus alone may not be sufficient to cause a tumour. A range of other cofactors may also be needed.
- The oncogenic retroviruses are divided into two groups: Type B and Type C. They may also be classified as acute and slow transforming viruses.
- Acute transforming viruses rapidly cause cell transformation due to a single gene (oncogene) in the viral genome whose expression in the cell leads to transformation.
- Viruses implicated in the pathogenesis of cancers include:
  — Human papilloma viruses (HPV) and HSV Type II: carcinoma of the cervix.
  — Epstein–Barr virus: Burkitt's lymphoma
  — hepatitis B virus: hepatocellular carcinoma.

28 Cancer: immune mechanisms

Immune surveillance

The possibility that the immune system may have a role in the destruction of tumour cells has been suggested for some time. In its most general form this concept is termed *immune surveillance*. It is based upon a series of propositions. For example, many tumours, induced by chemicals or viruses or occurring spontaneously from unknown causes, acquire on the surface of their constituent cells new, tumour-specific antigens (TSA) not present in normal tissues. These antigens are exposed on the cell surface, are alien to the immune system and the body's defences have not previously been exposed to them, therefore they should elicit an immune response. This prediction is largely based on experience with the rejection of tissue grafts such as skin or kidney. In this case the graft has surface histocompatibility antigens which differ from those of the recipient (p. 81).

Immunogenicity of tumours

The concept that tumours are immunogenic is supported by the demonstration in many patients of circulating antibodies and sensitised lymphocytes directed against their own tumours. *Malignant melanoma* seems to be particularly effective in inducing this immune response but many other types of cancer have been shown to produce similar effects.

The efficiency with which foreign tissue grafts are destroyed has led to suggestions that the speedy reaction to alien histocompatibility antigens has evolved as a survival mechanism directed against the emergence of cancer cells. It has also been suggested that a continuous process of immune surveillance exists in which circulating lymphocytes monitor the tissues for such antigens and destroy the intruding cells; although an attractive idea, this view has little support today. None the less, immunological factors do seem to have a role in the development and progression of some tumours.

Immunosuppression and cancer

The theory of immune surveillance would predict that experimentally induced tumours should be initiated more readily in animals without an intact immune apparatus. In practice the incidence of tumours induced in experimental animals by viruses is indeed greatly enhanced if immunosuppression is induced. The incidence of tumours reverts to normal if immune lymphocytes are transfused into the immunosuppressed animals. The effect appears to be mainly due to *cell-mediated immunity* (p. 44). A similar fall in tumour incidence has been observed after lymphocyte transfusion to animals in which neoplasms are induced by X-rays.

On the whole, immunosuppression produces much less dramatic effects on the incidence of tumours induced by chemical carcinogens. This observation is supported by clinical experience in immunosuppressed patients (for example after renal transplantation). There is no excess incidence of the majority of neoplasms, including the common cancers such as breast, stomach or colon. There is however an increased incidence of rarer neoplasms such as lymphomas and some epithelial tumours, notably skin cancer. Both these groups of tumours may have viruses involved in their pathogenesis, as illustrated in Chapter 27.

It has been suggested that the age distribution of most tumours (old age and infancy) reflects the periods when the immune system is at its least effective, and furthermore that immunosuppression (whether spontaneous or caused by drugs or radiation) should increase the observed incidence of neoplasia.

Examples of spontaneous regression of tumours of various sorts are also well recognised. This may be associated with the presence of immunologically competent cells (lymphocytes) at the site of the tumour. A good example of this is malignant melanoma. These ideas were taken as further support for the hypothesis of immune surveillance.

Blocking antibody and tumour enhancement

The main flaw in the theory of the immune control of cancer is the failure of the immune system to destroy clinical cancer more effectively than it appears to do. Tumours may be less immunogenic than we have postulated or may be successful in provoking some diversion of the immune response which prevents their destruction. There is ample evidence for the latter suggestion. It has been shown that whereas it is cellular immunity, i.e. sensitised lymphocytes and macrophages, which kills tumour cells, tumours also induce the production of circulating antibodies. This antibody forms complexes with the tumour antigens and the resulting immune complexes prevent the immunological destruction of the tumours by lymphocytes and macrophages. The antibody is called *blocking antibody*. This mechanism could actually increase the growth of the tumour (a phenomenon called tumour enhancement). Tumour enhancement may also be produced by antigen, lost from tumour cells, blocking antigen receptors on immunocompetent cells.

Stimulation of tumour growth by lymphocytes

Another possible explanation for the lack of success of the immune response against cancer is provided by in vitro experiments in which small numbers of sensitised lymphocytes were found to stimulate tumour growth, whereas large numbers inhibited the tumour cells. The mechanism is unknown but the phenomenon can be reproduced in vivo. It would seem that a combination of a large tumour with a weak or slow immune response leads to enhancement of tumour growth instead of suppression.

The problem remains of why early tumours should arouse only weak responses. One explanation is that they tend to arise in *privileged sites*, i.e. areas of the body where even foreign antigens fail to evoke an immune response. Thus, in the mouse, the mammary gland is a privileged site and a tumour growing there becomes immunogenic only when it extends beyond the confines of the mammary fat pad. By this time, of course, it is too large to be susceptible to immunological attack. The same may be true of human breast cancer and also of many epithelial tumours.

Preferential growth of tumour cells of low antigenicity

Finally, since tumours or individual tumour cells vary in their antigenicity, it seems inevitable that if destruction by the immune system is only partially effective, a process of natural selection will lead to preferential growth of tumour cells of low antigenicity. Similarly, if enhancement by the immune system were predominant, natural selection would favour those tumour cells responding best to immunostimulation at the expense of those susceptible to immunodestruction. In either case the tumour could be predicted to adjust its antigenicity to the level best suited for its continued growth.

Failure of the immune system to eliminate malignant tumours

It can be seen that there is no shortage of explanations for the failure of the immune system to eliminate malignant tumours in spite of their new antigenic expression. The concept of immune surveillance, i.e. that tumours are prevented from developing by an intact immune system, is thus no longer generally accepted.

It would be wrong, however, to exclude the possibility that the immune system may have some role in the biology of cancer:

- It is known that tumours may be associated with macrophages and lymphocytes which may elaborate substances such as tumour necrosis factor (TNF, p. 140) which influence the behaviour of the tumour cells and the response of the body to cancer.
- There is good evidence that cases of colorectal lymphoma associated with a lymphocytic response nearby have a better prognosis than those that do not.
- Mention has already been made of spontaneous regression in some tumours. This may have an immunological basis.

Taking these clinical observations together with the experimental findings discussed above, it would seem that immunity is effective mainly against virus-induced tumours and against tumours of the immune system. Defects in immune regulation may be important in the development of lymphoid tumours. Immune mechanisms are relatively ineffective against most cancers of man but there is still much to be learnt about possible interactions between the specific and non-specific arms of the immune system and neoplasia.

Immunology and diagnosis of cancer

Immunology does have an important role in the diagnosis of cancer. The antigens that are expressed by neoplastic cells may be abnormal or may be normal but expressed at an inappropriate time. For example, *carcinoembryonic antigen* (p. 264) is expressed by carcinoma of the colon but not by normal colonic epithelium. It is however expressed during development of the gut.

The demonstration of antigens such as carcinoembryonic antigen or similar substances may provide the pathologist with a means of investigating and diagnosing tumours. This has been put to great advantage in the technique of *immunohistochemistry*, where an antibody that recognises the antigen of interest is itself demonstrated by a labelled antibody that recognises an epitope on the first antibody. This approach of using immunological reagents for the study of cancer is fundamental to modern cancer research.

Antibodies can also be used in the *radiological localisation of tumours*. Antibody can be tagged with a radiolabel, injected into a patient where it binds to cells that express the antigen in question, and then localised by a suitable radiological detection system.

Immunotherapy and cancer

Antibodies may also be used as therapy. For example, bone marrow affected by lymphoma can be extracted from the patient and mixed with an antibody and complement which then lyse the tumour cells expressing the antigen to which the antibody has bound. The 'cleaned' bone marrow is then reimplanted into the patient.

KEY POINTS

- Many tumours acquire on the surface of their constituent cells tumour-specific antigens (TSA) which are alien to the immune system and should therefore elicit an immune response. However, the immunogenicity of tumours varies and the action of the immune system may on occasion even enhance tumour growth.
- The concept of immune surveillance, i.e. that tumours are prevented from developing by an intact immune system, is no longer generally accepted, but studies in immunosuppressed subjects indicate that immunity is effective against virus-induced tumours and against tumours of the immune system.
- Immunology has an important role in the diagnosis and therapy of cancer.

29 Epidemiology of cancer

Epidemiology is the study of disease in populations and dates back to 1660 when John Graunt studied causes of death in the city of London. Many of the major advances in cancer studies have had their basis in observations concerning the incidence of a particular tumour in a particular population, such as:

- scrotal cancer in chimney sweeps of the 18th and 19th centuries
- bladder cancers in the aniline dye industry
- bronchial cancer in cigarette smokers
- skin cancer in X-ray pioneers
- mesothelioma in asbestos workers
- Burkitt's lymphoma in inhabitants of East Africa.

All the above are instances of how an alert observer can open a door to fresh understanding of the cancer problem.

It is useful to consider the incidence of malignant tumours as a whole and the incidence of the more common varieties in men and women. About 600 000 people die in the UK every year, and about 140 000 of them die of cancer-related causes. In men the most important tumours numerically are:

- lung cancer (26 000 deaths)
- colorectal cancer (8000)
- carcinoma of the stomach (6000)
- carcinoma of the prostate and of the pancreas (5000).

The data for women are:

- breast cancer (12 500 deaths)
- lung cancer (9000)
- colorectal cancer (8000)
- ovarian cancer (4000)

- carcinoma of the endometrium (2000)
- carcinoma of the cervix (2000).

It is worth putting these figures in the context of, say, deaths from *myocardial infarction* (90 000 in men and 67 000 in women), or from *cerebrovascular disease* (44 000 in men and 27 000 in women).

Interpretation of epidemiological data

There is more to the epidemiology of cancer than simple description but the interpretation of epidemiological data can be very difficult.

Cancer of the uterine cervix is much less common in Jewish women than in other members of the population and this led to the speculation that circumcision of the sexual partner was a protective factor. This would seem to be borne out by the lower incidence of the disease in the circumcised Moslems of Yugoslavia than in the non-Moslem population of the same country. However, cloistered nuns have a very low incidence, as do Seventh Day Adventists. There is also in many countries a strong inverse correlation with socio-economic group, the lowest income groups in general having the highest incidence of the tumour.

Analysis of all these and other sets of data revealed two factors which seemed to spell a high risk of cervical cancer and which seemed to cut across all other group affinities. The two factors are:

1. an early age at first intercourse
2. a high number of sexual partners.

These factors operate largely regardless of race, religion, circumcision or economic status.

The association of cervical cancer with frequent intercourse with many sexual partners from an early age suggests the operation of a sexually transmitted infective agent, most effective if introduced when the patient is young. *Herpes simplex virus (HSV) Type II* has been considered for some time to be a sexually transmitted agent that may possibly be involved in the pathogenesis of cervical cancer.

An even more likely candidate is the *human papilloma virus (HPV)*; in this case epidemiological evidence is now supported by some experimental data. However the direct role of this agent has still to be finally proven. If this does indeed turn out to be an important factor in the development of this common form of cancer, then it will be the epidemiologist who led the virologists and molecular biologists to their goal!

Geographical variation

One of the most fascinating and important aspects of the cancer problem is the enormous differences that exist between the frequency

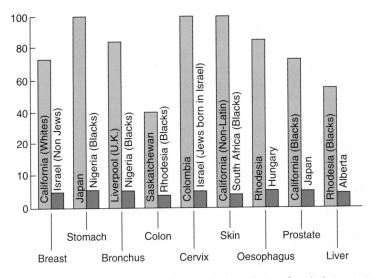

Fig. 29.1 Some striking differences between incidence rates of particular cancers in different parts of the world (modified from R. Doll).

of occurrence of particular tumours in different parts of the world (Fig. 29.1).

Liver cancer is common in the Bantu of Southern Africa, but rare in the black population of the USA of Bantu origin and it was concluded many years ago that this must mean that an environmental factor was responsible, not a racial one. However the situation is complex and involves a variety of factors, including endemic *hepatitis B virus* infection and the possible role of a variety of dietary (chemical) factors such as *aflatoxins*.

Indeed the vast majority of geographical differences in cancer rates are due to environmental features which in theory could be identified and neutralised. This is another way of saying that most cancer is potentially preventable if the clues presented by epidemiology are followed. Where clear-cut racial factors operate they seem to be protective, as in the rarity of cancer of the testis in the Congo-Kordofaminian group, whether resident in Africa, the USA or the West Indies.

Risk differentials can be used to find out whether patients with a particular cancer have things in common, whether they live in areas of high or low frequency of the cancer. Thus cases of bronchial carcinoma occurring in either a high risk or low risk area anywhere in the world show a close correlation with cigarette smoking. The conclusion is that in the low risk area, either few people smoke, or they smoke less dangerous cigarettes, or that other things make smoking less carcinogenic than it is elsewhere.

Geographical variation of breast cancer

There are great differences in the geographical incidence of breast cancer: studies in the UK, USA, Brazil, Japan, Greece, Yugoslavia and Taiwan have shown that this appears to be due to variation in factors such as age of first pregnancy, age of menarche and age at menopause. In other words, pregnancy at an early age and relatively few reproductive cycles confer a high degree of protection against some other causative factors, for example an oncogenic RNA virus. Lactation practices such as the duration of breast feeding, once thought to be important, now seem to be of little significance. Another fascinating aspect of breast cancer is the age variation (see below).

Epidemiological study of particular populations

Japan is a magnet for cancer epidemiologists. Apart from the low incidence of breast cancer there is also the striking rarity of cancer of the prostate and the equally marked frequency of carcinoma of the stomach. Both these differentials are as yet unexplained. Of particular use in establishing the importance of environmental factors has been the study of migrant populations. When the Japanese with a very high rate of gastric cancer migrate to the USA, they at first retain their high incidence. With the next generation of US-born Japanese, however, the incidence falls dramatically, even when all marriages are within the original Japanese ethnic group. Conversely, Japanese with a low rate of large bowel cancer acquire the high incidence of the US population after migration.

These observations and others make it quite plain that some environmental factors, probably dietary habits, and not a genetic determinant are responsible for the differential incidence of these forms of cancer, since the risk correlates with the environment and customs rather than with race. Breast cancer in Japanese migrants to the USA also shows an increased incidence compared with the low levels in Japan, but the increase is slower and less dramatic than is the case in cancer of the large bowel.

Geographical risk differentials

Some other geographical differences, especially the incidence of skin cancer in Australia, are easily explained by exposure to sunlight. Other geographical risk differentials are quite bizarre. In the Caspian littoral of Iran there is a dramatic gradient in the incidence of oesophageal cancer with differences up to 20-fold between the eastern and western ends of the coastline. The risk of oesophageal cancer seems to correlate with rainfall, the lowest rainfall being associated with the highest incidence of cancer. It may be that the rainfall determines the nature of the vegetation and hence the diet. It must be remembered however that the presence of an association does not necessarily imply a causal relationship.

Geographical similarities of cancer

The geographical diversity in tumour incidence worldwide led Doll and Peto to estimate that at least 65% of cancer deaths could be attributed to the environment (30% being due to tobacco alone). These figures would imply that a large proportion of cancers are, in theory, potentially preventable.

Whilst many tumours show great geographic variation in incidence, of equal interest are those tumours that have the same incidence throughout the world, for example *primary brain tumours*.

It is important to consider the effect of variations in diagnostic accuracy which may profoundly influence epidemiological data. For example, in underdeveloped countries *acute lymphoblastic leukaemia* may not be readily diagnosed, thus suggesting that it is less common than in the developed world. Furthermore, if children die of intercurrent infection or endemic infectious diseases, true incidences will be obscured. This tumour is of particular interest since it would appear to have the same incidence in all populations that have been rigorously investigated, suggesting that environmental and genetic factors are of little importance. It may be that the occasional occurrence of this tumour is the price we pay for the massive lymphoid proliferation that occurs in childhood during the development of the immune system. This process involves new mutations occurring in order to develop the full range of immunological responses: rare mistakes occur and possibly lead to neoplasia.

Relationship of cancer to age

The relationship of cancer to age also provides important information. In general, cancers increase in incidence with age such that if age and incidence are plotted as a log–log plot the resultant age incidence curve is a straight line. Exceptions, however, occur and the most obvious is the case of tumours of childhood, some of which are due to genetic determinants, such as *retinoblastoma*, etc., or to events that occur in childhood as in the case of *acute lymphoblastic leukaemia*.

Another example is *breast cancer*. If a log–log age incidence curve is plotted for breast cancer, then a kink in the line occurs at the menopause. Indeed it would appear that events at the menopause (presumably hormonal) are protective and that postmenopausal women have a lower incidence of breast cancer. The biological explanation for this epidemiological observation is still unclear but may reflect alterations in the hormonal milieu or the responsiveness of the breast epithelium to its environment.

Another type of age incidence curve is that of *lung cancer* with a peak in late middle age and then a decline in incidence. The interpretation of age incidence curves can be difficult and the possibility of *cohort effects* must be considered. This means that if one looks at the incidence of lung cancer in a given age group in different decades, one sees a change in incidence that is reflected in mortality. This variation reflects alterations in the smoking habits of the individuals in these cohorts of patients.

Some tumours have a *bimodal age distribution*; for example *Hodgkin's lymphoma* is common in young people then declines in incidence until a second, smaller peak in old age. A similar age distribution is seen with *osteosarcoma*. Osteosarcoma is, in general, a tumour of childhood and young adults; however it can be seen in old age when it is associated with Paget's disease of bone, a disorder of the elderly.

Why is cancer related to age?

In the examples of breast, lung and gastric cancer, statistical analysis shows that the relationship of incidence with age is due not to ill-defined ageing processes or to increased somatic mutation, or to loss of potency of the immune system, but to a greater or lesser exposure to environmental carcinogens:

- In gastric cancer we can conclude that the longer we live the greater the exposure.
- The break in the curve of lung cancer is due to the relatively sudden increase in the popularity of cigarettes affecting cohorts of the populace. In other words, the old acquired the habit of smoking too late in life to influence their cause of death.
- The change in rate of increase in incidence of breast cancer in middle age may well reflect a change in the hormonal status of women at the menopause, and the role of hormones as promoters in this tumour.

Some epidemiological associations are difficult to identify and to understand. For example the variation in incidence of *testicular germ cell tumours* appears to have a relationship with the prevalence of *cryptorchidism* (undescended testis). In addition there is an association with in utero exposure to exogenous steroid hormones, and a relationship to maternal weight (increased incidence in children of fat mothers) and low birth weight (increased incidence in small children). The identification of these associations has required careful study of affected patients and the previous generation! However such investigations have led to a plausible hypothesis that exposure to excess steroids during the period of testicular organogenesis may result in future testicular neoplasms.

Ageing, latency and genetic mutation

The death rate from *carcinoma of the large bowel* rises 1000-fold between the ages of 30 and 80 years; this is typical of many tumours. The combined effects of latency and the passing of years can produce complex age distribution curves for tumours. These various graphs and curves have been studied intensively by statisticians and they are in virtual agreement that the observed facts can be explained only by accepting that malignant transformation occurs as the end result of a series of steps, taking place at different times during the life span of an individual.

One generally held view is that each cell contains genes (or switches), the expression of each of which needs to be altered (turned on or off) in order for the neoplastic phenotypes to be expressed. The chance of any single mutation is 'spontaneous' or related to exposure to some carcinogen or other mutational insult (e.g. radiation). Thus the likelihood of cancer will rise in direct proportion to age to the power of 'n'. If the number of genes that must be altered in expression (switched on or off) is 4, then the risk of cancer would increase with age to the power 4. This means that the logarithm of cancer incidence should be linearly related to age, which in many cases it is. The slope of the curve will be proportional to the number of genes, i.e. for large bowel cancer it is 6 and thus at least 6 genes must be involved.

The protective effect of smoking

A further epidemiological association that is difficult to understand is that of smoking and a protective effect on endometrial cancer observed in a number of studies. It is known that an important factor in the causation of *endometrial cancer* is the action of inappropriate levels of steroid hormones. The association of obesity and endometrial cancer may be due to the metabolism of steroids to active oestrogens in fatty tissue (perhaps of relevance in germ cell tumours, see above). It seems that at least in vitro the products of cigarette smoke can inhibit this peripheral metabolism and thus reduce the levels of available oestrogen. Although not yet proven, this idea is the result of careful epidemiological work.

Socio-economic factors

The relationship of cancer to socio-economic status is complex. Within a fairly homogeneous population such as the UK or USA, most cancers (with the exception of breast and ovary) are more common in the less affluent and less well educated (p. 349). There are many reasons for this, such as smoking habits, dietary and drinking patterns and exposure to industrial carcinogens.

Taking the world as a whole, the inverse relationship between affluence and cancer incidence is not always present. *Carcinoma of the large bowel* shows a linear correlation between its age-corrected incidence and indices of prosperity, notably the proportion of the diet taken as beef. An important positive relationship is between the per capita consumption of animal fat and the incidence of *breast cancer*.

The striking differences in the relationship of cancer to occupation, habits, geography and age all emphasise that the majority of tumours are due entirely or at least predominantly to environmental factors which are theoretically identifiable and preventable. For the most part, these environmental factors consist of:

- dietary practices
- social customs
- habits such as smoking
- exposure to industrial processes.

We are therefore talking mainly of a micro-environment which, except for the constraints of poverty, men may abandon or retain as they wish.

KEY POINTS

- The aetiology of a particular tumour is often revealed by its increased incidence within a particular population.
- Interpretation of epidemiological data can be very difficult. The aetiology of a tumour may involve interplay of a variety of factors, environmental, racial, dietary, etc.
- Geographical risk differentials may result in dramatic gradients in the incidence of certain cancers. On the other hand, some cancers show little or no variation in incidence worldwide, suggesting that environmental and genetic factors are of little importance in their aetiology.
- Increasing incidence of many cancers with age is related to latency and exposure to environmental carcinogens.

30 Nutritional pathology

Fetal and infant growth and adult disease

A number of recent studies have shown that an infant's height and weight at 1 year of age are related to the subsequent risk of a number of chronic diseases including hypertension, heart disease and diabetes. The hypothesis is that failure to 'adapt' efficiently to nutrition in the first months of life is a marker of later failure to adapt efficiently to a Western diet. People who were small infants are more likely to manifest heart disease at age 60. The basis for these findings is still unclear but they underline the importance of being able to balance our nutritional environment.

MALNUTRITION

Malnutrition is defined as *insufficient intake of protein or energy to meet metabolic demands*. This will result in impairment of normal physiological processes.

Causes include:

- inadequate dietary intake
- increased metabolic demand, e.g. because of disease
- increased nutrient loss.

It should be noted that efficient use of dietary protein requires energy from non-protein calories. Adaptive responses will function over a short time but they are finite as specialist protein has no storage form.

Protein-energy malnutrition (PEM): a worldwide perspective

Children between 1 and 2 years of age are most susceptible as they are dependent upon others for food. *Gastrointestinal infection* is a significant precipitant of PEM in children. The World Health Organization (WHO) estimates that at least 300 million children have growth retardation secondary to malnutrition.

In developed nations those most at risk are the institutionalised elderly and children of the poor. PEM can be found in patients admitted to hospital and, for example, may result in an increased incidence of post-operative infections.

Circumstances in which protein-energy malnutrition can occur

Stress   The inflammatory response to infection and trauma results in increased energy metabolism and protein turnover and predisposes to PEM. For example, the resting metabolic rate may be about twice normal in patients with burns, 1.5 times normal in patients with infection and 1.3 times normal in patients with bone fractures.

Considerable amounts of nitrogen are lost during an acute illness. In the healthy adult about 12 g of nitrogen is lost in the urine each day in a fasting state; this can be doubled in sepsis and trauma. One gram of urinary nitrogen corresponds to approximately 30 g of lean body mass so it may be appreciated that a daily loss of 0.6 kg of lean body mass can occur during acute illness. This loss is caused by the mobilisation of amino acids from skeletal muscle and their redirection to organs critical for immediate survival. Hormones such as cortisol, adrenaline and growth hormone, and cytokines such as interleukin 1 and tumour necrosis factor alpha are involved in this physiological process.

Starvation   This occurs when circulating glucose, fatty acids and triglycerides, together with liver and muscle glycogen, provide less fuel than is needed for basal metabolism. Triglycerides may then be mobilised from adipose tissue and catabolised to fatty acids and ketone bodies. In the brain glycolytic pathways need to be used: the substrates required are either glucose or amino acids derived from skeletal muscle. As there is no storage form of protein in the body a significant loss of functional protein can occur each day. The body adapts to maintain the supply of adequate fuel substrates to vital tissues such as the brain whilst minimising the amount of protein broken down. Tissues such as the heart, kidney and skeletal muscle change their primary fuel substrate from glucose to fatty acids and ketone bodies. Other tissues—such as bone marrow, renal medulla and peripheral nerves—switch from the full oxidation of glucose to anaerobic glycolysis which results in the production of lactate and pyruvate. These compounds are converted to glucose in the liver with energy derived from fat oxidation. In this way, energy stored as fat can be utilised for glucose synthesis whilst conserving protein energy.

As starvation continues, physical exertion decreases to conserve energy and the resting metabolic rate drops by about 10%. The brain develops the ability to utilise keto acids. Protein turnover is reduced and amino acids are reused more efficiently. Eventually, however, these homeostatic compensatory mechanisms cannot cope with the negative caloric and/or protein balance.

The consequences of protein-energy malnutrition

The function of all organs is impaired:

- Gastrointestinal tract: structural and functional atrophy of the intestine can occur resulting in malabsorption.
- Immune system: both the cell-mediated and humoral immune systems are impaired, increasing susceptibility to infection which in its turn worsens the malnourished state.
- Endocrine system: primary gonadal dysfunction occurs in moderate to severe PEM; this may be in association with amenorrhoea.
- Cardiovascular system: the myocardial mass is decreased and this may result in conduction abnormalities.
- Respiratory system: muscle atrophy will result in a decrease in inspiratory and expiratory pressure and in the vital capacity.
- Wound healing: collagen deposition at the site of the wound is decreased.

OBESITY

Definition

There are a number of ways of defining obesity. Tables of ideal and desirable weight are available and are based upon actual area estimates as well as associations with longest life expectancy. Alternatively the body mass index—body weight (kg) divided by height (m²)—may be used. Body builders, who have excess weight due to lean tissue, would however be considered obese using this measurement. A better method is measurement of the percentage of body fat, which can now be calculated by a number of techniques including water baths, impedance and body composition scans. Fat distribution is also important. Central fat is an independent factor in a number of diseases.

Fat is a very efficient method of energy storage. One gram of adipose tissue is equivalent to approximately 38 kJ and an individual of normal weight can survive 2 months of total starvation. When food is scarce this is of value for survival; however, in developed society food is generally not scarce and the ability to store fat, with consequent obesity, is of negative survival value.

Any degree of excess adiposity imparts a health risk. The National Institutes of Health (USA) have concluded that a 20% increase in relative weight or body mass index (BMI—kg/m²) above the 85th percentile for young adults constitutes a health risk. This means that approximately 20–30% of adult men and 30–40% of adult women are obese. The highest rates of obesity occur among poorer minority groups. Rates of obesity are continuing to rise in men and women in most developed countries.

Obesity increases the risk of premature death, diabetes mellitus, hypertension, atherosclerosis, osteoarthritis, gall bladder disease and certain cancers.

Aetiology

Obesity results when there is an abnormality of either intake of energy or expenditure. If excess calories are stored in adipose tissue then obesity will eventually result.

The regulation of eating behaviour is not completely understood. Appetite control centres are found in the hypothalamus. There is a feeding centre in the ventrolateral nucleus of the hypothalamus which sends positive signals to the cerebral cortex to stimulate eating. There is also a satiety centre in the ventromedial hypothalamus which modulates eating by sending inhibitory impulses to the feeding centre. The hypothalamic centres may be influenced by a number of other regulatory processes. For example, increase in plasma glucose and/or insulin following a meal may activate the satiety centre. Also total adipose tissue mass has an influence on the activity of the hypothalamic centres. There seems to be a set point corresponding to body adiposity which may be one explanation as to why it is difficult to diet. A newly discovered protein, *leptin*, which is under genetic control is believed to activate the satiety centre.

The cerebral cortex, psychological, social and genetic factors all appear to interact to influence food intake and eating behaviour.

Daily caloric requirement ranges from 1/10 to 1/30 kJ (27–32 kcal) per kilogram of body weight. Physical activity modulates caloric balance, and obesity leads to inactivity. Reduced physical activity in mid life or due to illness or injury may also predispose to weight gain.

Is there a metabolic abnormality associated with obesity?

Major metabolic abnormalities have not been detected in obese individuals. There are three metabolic components comprising overall energy expenditure:

1. *Resting metabolic rate.* This accounts for between 60 and 75% of daily energy expenditure. The average resting metabolic rate in a 70 kg man is 6300 kilojoules (1500 kcal) per day. The resting metabolic rate is normal in most obese subjects.

2. *Exercise-induced thermogenesis.* The energy expenditure for a standard physical workload is normal or increased in obesity. It may be

increased due to the extra effort required because of the increased body mass. However daily energy expenditure due to exercise may be less in sedentary obese subjects because they take part in less physical activity.

3. *Thermic response to food.* This may also be called dietary thermogenesis; it refers to the energy utilised after a meal for digestion, absorption, metabolism and storage of foodstuffs. Energy utilisation may also be increased due to sympathetic nervous system activity. The thermic response to food is greater for protein and less for carbohydrates and may equal between 10 and 15% of the calories ingested. In human obesity it has been reported that there may be a decreased thermic response. This could be due for example to insulin resistance resulting in decreased glucose disposal in obese subjects. It is difficult to determine whether this contributes to obesity or whether it is simply associated with obesity.

Can the body adapt to excess calorie intake?

Normal individuals gain less weight than would be predicted on the basis of the excess calories ingested. This is significant when carbohydrate is consumed but less so when the excess calories consist of fat. This response is partially caused by an increase in the resting metabolic rate and is known as *adaptive thermogenesis*. Excess ingestion of carbohydrate leads to increased plasma levels of tri-iodothyronine (T_3) and decreased levels of reverse tri-iodothyronine (rT_3). The reverse happens in starvation. Adaptive thermogenesis is thought to be associated with an increased concentration of T_3 relative to that of T_4 and rT_3.

Over-nutrition may also cause increased central and peripheral sympathetic outflow: this leads to increased catecholamine-induced caloric utilisation resulting in increased heat production, and this may result in adaptive thermogenesis.

Adaptive thermogenesis can result in a 10–15% increase in resting metabolic rate. All influences of adaptive thermogenesis are the same in normal and obese subjects during periods of over-nutrition.

Adipose tissue lipoprotein lipase (ATLPL)

This enzyme is involved in the control of adipose tissue mass. Attached to the luminal surface of endothelial cells, ATLPL hydrolyses fatty acids from triglycerides of circulating triglyceride-rich lipoproteins. The released fatty acids are taken up by adipose sites, converted to triglycerides and stored. It is thought that in obesity there are excessive levels of ATLPL which result in preferential deposition of fat calories in adipose tissue. This enzyme does not appear to reduce following weight reduction which may explain why obese patients have difficulty maintaining reduced weight.

Environmental, cultural and genetic influences also contribute to obesity. In adults up to 50% of the variation in weight is believed to be associated with genetic factors. The level at which genes work is unclear: they could affect any of the pathways already discussed.

Secondary obesity may occur in the following conditions:

- hypothyroidism
- Cushing's syndrome
- insulinoma
- hypothalamic disorders, e.g. Fröhlich's syndrome characterised by obesity, hypogonadotrophic hypogonadism, diabetes insipidus, visual impairment and mental retardation.

Pathology

Adipose tissue stores are found subcutaneously around internal organs, within the omentum and in intramuscular spaces. There is also expansion of lean body mass with increased size of kidneys, heart, liver and skeletal muscle. Fatty liver is common in severe obesity.

Sites of adiposity, size and number

During childhood and puberty, both the size and number of adipose sites may increase. During adulthood mild to moderate obesity is usually due to adipose site hypertrophy, however severe obesity may cause an increase in number of adipose sites. Interestingly, when weight reduction occurs, a decrease in the size of existing adipose sites occurs but there is not a decrease in adipose site number; thus, when a given complement of adipose sites is attained, this number is fixed and cannot be reduced.

Effects of obesity on metabolism

Hyperinsulinaemia and insulin resistance

Hyper- or euglycaemia and hyperinsulinaemia indicate insulin resistance, a common feature in obesity. There is a correlation between the degree of obesity and the magnitude of hyperinsulinaemia. Insulin resistance may be due to:

- an abnormal beta cell product
- circulating insulin antagonists
- tissue insulin insensitivity.

Tissue insensitivity is thought to be the primary abnormality. It may occur in two ways: firstly there seems to be a decreased number of insulin receptors in mild hyperinsulinaemia and insulin resistance;

secondly, as the insulin resistance state worsens, a post-receptor defect emerges and may predominate.

Diabetes mellitus

About 80–90% of non insulin-dependent diabetics are obese. Obesity-induced insulin resistance is an important contributory factor to the diabetes in these patients and exacerbates the diabetic state. Fat deposits in the central abdomen appear to be the most important.

Cholesterol

Total body cholesterol is increased in obesity and is mostly found in adipose tissue cholesterol stores. Low density lipoprotein contains most of the plasma cholesterol and this may be mildly elevated in obesity. Cholesterol turnover may also be increased, leading to increased biliary excretion of cholesterol and possibly resulting in gallstone formation.

Triglycerides

Hyperglyceridaemia is common and is correlated with a degree of obesity. Very low density lipoprotein contains most of the circulating triglyceride in the fasting state and is elevated. This is due to increased hepatic VLDL production, promoted by hyperinsulinaemia.

Plasma free fatty acid (FFA)

Increased FFA turnover exists in obesity, acting as an important precursor for hepatic triglyceride synthesis.

Manifestations and complications of obesity

Hypertension

There is a strong association between hypertension and obesity, with as many as 60% of cases of hypertension being attributable to excess weight. Hypertension probably arises from increased blood volume as peripheral vascular resistance is normal. Weight loss usually leads to reduction of systemic blood pressure.

Hypoventilation syndrome

In some obese individuals there is upper airways obstruction during sleep which leads to hypoxaemia and hypercapnia. This causes the individual to wake and normal respiration to resume. The condition thus results in chronic sleep deprivation and daytime somnolence. In severe cases, polycythaemia, pulmonary hypertension and cor pulmonale may ensue.

Adrenal function

Differential diagnosis of Cushing's disease may be difficult; 24-hour urinary 17-hydroxycorticosteroid excretion may be elevated, as may plasma cortisol levels.

Growth hormone

There is reduced secretory response of growth hormone to stimuli such as hypoglycaemia and starvation.

Atherosclerosis

Obesity is a significant risk factor for the development of coronary artery disease and stroke. This may be due to obesity itself but the main association is with hypertension, hyperlipoproteinaemia and diabetes.

Osteoarthritis of the knees

There is a 5-fold increased risk in the obese, the risk increasing by 10–30% for each 5 kg gained.

Treatment for complications of obesity

Treatment is with weight reduction. This causes significant amelioration of hyperinsulinaemia, insulin resistance, diabetes, hypertension and hyperlipidaemia.

ANOREXIA NERVOSA AND BULIMIA

These are eating disorders occurring in young healthy women who develop a fear of becoming fat. Patients are most commonly white women from middle-class backgrounds. In anorexia nervosa there is restriction in caloric intake whilst in bulimia there is binge eating followed by vomiting and use of laxatives. The cause is unknown. Hypothalamic abnormalities are present but revert to normal with weight gain. Psychological factors probably play a predominant role in the aetiology of these disorders.

VITAMIN DEFICIENCY AND EXCESS

Vitamin deficiency usually occurs as part of a generally malnourished state. This may result from:

- food faddism
- another disease, e.g. malabsorption
- treatment, e.g. haemodialysis
- total parental nutrition
- an inborn error of metabolism

Vitamin excess is becoming more common.

General points to be made before a discussion of specific vitamin deficiencies are that:

1. The requirement for a vitamin to be obtained from the diet is a result of an evolutionary inborn error of metabolism. This may be found in a wide range of animals, e.g. the limited ability to synthesise thiamine, whereas the single gene defect that prevents ascorbic acid synthesis is present in only a few species, e.g. humans and the guinea pig.

2. In contrast to essential amino acids and essential fatty acids only small amounts of vitamins are required. This is because vitamins are not tissue building blocks or substrates for energy production; instead they act as prosthetic groups for quantitatively minor tissue constituents or as catalytic co-factors for biological reactions.

3. Some vitamins never seem to be deficient in humans, e.g. pantothenic acid. This may be because they are ubiquitous in foods or are stored efficiently by the body.

4. Alcoholism is a major cause of vitamin deficiencies. This may be due to diminished intake or impairment of absorption and storage. There may also be associated genetic factors.

5. It may not be possible to ascertain biochemically that there is a deficiency, therefore it is important to recognise manifestations of vitamin deficiency and monitor response to replacement therapy in order to confirm the diagnosis.

6. Excess vitamin consumption may be indirect as a result of diet or as a result of deliberate ingestion. Some toxicity syndromes are well documented, e.g. fat soluble vitamins A and D, but symptoms of excess of other vitamins, e.g. water soluble vitamins, are inconsistent unless well understood.

Deficiency states (Table 30.1)

Niacin: deficiency state—pellagra

Niacin is the generic term for nicotinic acid and its derivatives. It is formed from tryptophan. 1 mg of niacin is formed from 60 mg of dietary tryptophan.

Table 30.1   Vitamin deficiency states

Vitamin	Source	Clinical effect
A (retinol)	Carrots, fish, eggs, liver	Night blindness, dry eyes, mucosal infection
B_1 (thiamine)	Cereals, fruit, dairy produce	Beriberi, neuropathy, heart failure, psychosis and encephalopathy
B_2 (riboflavine)	Cereals, fruit, dairy produce, liver	Mucosal damage
B_6 (pyridoxine)	Cereals, meat, fish	Confusion, glossitis, anaemia and neuropathy
B_{12} (cobalamin)	Meat, fish, dairy produce	Megaloblastic anaemia, spinal cord damage
C (ascorbic acid)	Fruits, green vegetables	Scurvy, tiredness, bleeding gums and bruising
D (cholecalciferol)	Dairy produce, fish, sunlight	Rickets, osteomalacia
E (tocopherol)	Cereals, eggs, oils	Anaemia, neuropathy
K	Vegetables, liver	Blood clotting defects
Niacin	Dairy produce, beans, peas	Pellagra, dermatitis, diarrhoea, dementia
Folate	Green vegetables, fruit	Megaloblastic anaemia, small bowel atrophy, ulcers

Action   Niacin is an essential component of nicotinamide adenine dinucleotide (NAD) and nicotinamide adenine dinucleotide phosphate (NADP), co-enzymes for oxidation reduction reactions.

Clinical manifestations   Pellagra was previously an endemic disease associated with high intake of maize or millet. The aetiology is not straightforward as some populations existing on a maize diet do not develop pellagra. It may be that the disease is due to a complex deficiency state.

Pellagra is a chronic wasting disease associated with dermatitis, dementia and diarrhoea. Dermatitis is due to photosensitivity. Initial mental changes may include fatigue, insomnia and apathy. An encephalopathy then develops characterised by confusion, disorientation, hallucination, loss of memory and organic psychosis. Diarrhoea is caused by inflammation of mucosal surfaces and may also cause achlorhydria, glossitis, stomatitis and vaginitis. Skin lesions are characterised by hyperkeratosis, hyperpigmentation and desquamation. Death is usually due to a secondary complication.

There is no diagnostic test for niacin deficiency. Plasma tryptophan and erythrocyte NAD and NADP levels are low but no lower than in patients with generalised malnutrition.

Treatment   Nutrition education and niacin supplementation are successful in treatment. If there are adequate amounts of dietary tryptophan a small amount of niacin—10 mg per day—is sufficient to cure endemic pellagra.

Thiamine: deficiency state—beriberi

Thiamine consists of pyrimidine and thiazole moieties. The body absorbs about 5 mg per day and can store between 25 and 30 mg, principally in skeletal muscle, heart, liver, kidneys and brain.

Action Thiamine is a co-enzyme for a number of reactions that cleave carbon–carbon bonds, e.g. oxidative decarboxylation of α-keto acids (pyruvate and α-ketoglutarate) and keto analogues of leucine, isoleucine and valine and the transketolase reaction in the pentose phosphate pathway. Thiamine may also have a role in neuronal function. Thiamine deficiency results in inhibition of enzymic reactions and accumulation of proximal metabolites.

Source Thiamine has a widespread distribution in food, especially in vegetable products.

Clinical manifestations In developed nations thiamine deficiency occurs in alcoholics and food faddists and in patients receiving clinical treatment, e.g. chronic peritoneal dialysis, haemodialysis. In developing countries it is commonly due to consumption of milled rice or foods containing thiaminases.

Clinical deficiency affects the cardiovascular and nervous systems and is known as wet beriberi and dry beriberi/Wernicke–Korsakoff syndrome respectively). The typical patient has mixed symptoms.

Beriberi heart disease is marked by:

- peripheral vasodilation leading to a high output state
- retention of sodium and water leading to oedema
- biventricular myocardial failure.

An acute fulminant cardiovascular syndrome may occur leading to cardiovascular collapse and death within hours or days.

Nervous system beriberi consists of:

- peripheral neuropathy: symmetrical sensory motor neuropathy affecting peripheral limbs
- Wernicke's encephalopathy: vomiting, nystagmus, rectus muscle palsy leading to ophthalmoplegia, fever, ataxia and progressive mental disorientation, eventually progressing to coma and death
- Korsakoff's syndrome: retrograde amnesia, impaired ability to learn and confabulation.

Biochemical diagnosis Whole blood or erythrocyte transketolase activity is measured. This will be enhanced in deficiency when thiamine diphosphate is added.

Treatment   Intramuscular thiamine followed by oral treatment together with other water soluble vitamins.

Pyridoxine (vitamin B_6)

The reactive moiety is pyridoxal 5-phosphate which is found in all foods, e.g. meat, liver, vegetables and wholegrain cereals.

Action   Pyridoxine is a co-factor for enzymes involved in amino acid metabolism, e.g. transaminases, synthetases and hydroxylases. It is of particular importance in metabolism of trytophan, glycine, serine, glutamate and sulphur containing amino acids and is also required for synthesis of the haem precursor δ-aminolevulinic acid. The body store is principally in muscle. Pyridoxine is also associated with neuronal excitability.

Clinical manifestations   Pure deficiency is rare unless the vitamin is destroyed during food processing. A number of drugs, e.g. isoniazid and penicillamine, act as pyridoxine antagonists. Deficiency may result in encephalopathy together with seborrhoeic dermatitis, cheilosis, glossitis, nausea, vomiting, weakness and dizziness.

Biochemical diagnosis   There are a number of tests for deficiency, e.g. red blood cell glutamic pyruvic transaminase in the presence or absence of pyridoxal phosphate.

Treatment   Management is with dietary prevention. Supplements may be required in pregnancy unless the patient is taking isoniazid (30 mg per day).

Riboflavin

Function   The co-enzymes flavin mononucleotide (FMN) and flavin adenine dinucleotide (FAD) are involved in oxidative reduction reactions. They are covalently attached to enzymes such as succinate dehydrogenase and monoamine oxidase which are essential for their action.

Source   Riboflavin is absorbed from the gastrointestinal tract.

Clinical manifestations   Deficiency of riboflavin usually occurs in combination with deficiencies of other water soluble vitamins. A diet deficient in riboflavin will cause sore throat, hyperaemia and oedema of oral mucous membranes with cheilosis, angular stomatitis, glossitis, seborrhoeic dermatitis and normochromic, normocytic anaemia.

Drug interactions   Thyroid hormones and adrenal steroids enhance FMN and FAD synthesis. Phenothiazines and tricyclic antidepressants competitively inhibit flavin co-enzyme biosynthesis but on their own do not cause deficiency.

Vitamin C

Source   Most animals have the enzyme L-gluconolactone

oxidase which enables them to synthesise vitamin C from glucose. Humans, other primates and guinea pigs are unable to synthesise ascorbic acid and require vitamin C from the diet.

Action Ascorbic acid is involved in oxidation reduction reactions; it reduces metal ions associated with enzymes and acts as an anti-oxidant by removing free radicals. It is also involved in synthesis of collagen. Absence of vitamin C leads to impairment of peptidyl hydroxylation of pro-collagen and reduction in collagen formation and secretion by connective tissue. Non-hydroxylated collagen cannot form a triple helix. This defect results in many of the clinical features found in scurvy.

Source Vitamin C is present in milk, meat (kidney, liver, fish), fruit and vegetables. Deficiency is usually associated with poverty in urban areas. Those at increased risk are infants between 6 and 12 months of age being fed processed milk formulas unsupplemented with citrus fruits or vegetables and the elderly who are unable to adequately care for themselves.

Clinical features:

- Perifollicular hyperkeratotic papules—hair becomes fragmented and buried.
- Perifollicular haemorrhages—purpura at the back of the legs which may become confluent.
- Haemorrhage into muscles of arms and legs and joints. Splinter haemorrhages in nailbeds. Swelling of gums, friability, bleeding, secondary infection, loosening of teeth, poor wound healing, petechial haemorrhages in the viscera.
- Emotional changes.
- In children there may be painful bony swelling and the sternum may sink inwards.
- Normochromic/normocytic anaemia will result due to bleeding.

Diagnosis Plasma levels of vitamin C do not correlate well with clinical state. Platelet ascorbic acid levels are useful.

Vitamin A (retinol)

Source Vitamin A is found in liver, milk and kidneys. It may be synthesised from carotenes derived from plants.

Actions The vitamin is associated with carotenoid proteins that provide the molecular basis for visual excitation and is also associated with growth and reproduction. Its mode of action is thought to occur by binding to a transcription regulation protein that controls gene expression.

Clinical deficiency This is usually related to diet and occurs in conjunction with deficiency of other nutrients. It may also be associated with intestinal malabsorption, abnormal liver storage or enhanced destruction or excretion of vitamins (e.g. proteinuria). Night blindness is the earliest symptom; visual loss then develops in association with ulceration and necrosis of the cornea. Dryness and hyperkeratosis of the skin may also be present.

Vitamin D

Source   Vitamin D is derived either from the diet (milk, fish, margarine) as vitamin D_2 (ergocalciferol) or from sunlight which converts 7-dehydrocholesterol to cholecalciferol (D_3) in the skin. The precursors are hydroxylated in the liver and kidneys to the active form—1,25-dihydroxycholecalciferol.

Deficiency   This may be due to:

- inadequate sunlight
- inadequate diet
- intestinal malabsorption
- eating chapatis (which bind vitamin D)
- impaired hydroxylation due to kidney or liver disease.

Clinical deficiency:

- in children causes rickets—simpaired growth and mineralisation of the skeleton
- in adults causes osteomalacia—weakness and pain in muscles, spontaneous fractures of spine and pelvis
- in the elderly mild deficiency increases the risk of osteoporotic fractures.

Diagnosis   There are low blood vitamin D levels, high parathyroid hormone levels and high alkaline phosphatase levels with a low normal calcium.

Treatment   Vitamin D supplements orally or by injection.

Vitamin E (tocopherol)

Vitamin E is absorbed from the gastrointestinal tract in a similar way to other fat soluble vitamins.

Action   It is an anti-oxidant inhibiting oxidation of essential cellular constituents and prevention formation of toxic oxidation products.

Source   Vitamin E is widely distributed in foodstuffs.

Clinical deficiency   This usually occurs because of malabsorption and hence in association with deficiency of other fat soluble vitamins.

Manifestations include:

- areflexia

- gait disturbance
- decreased proprioceptive and vibratory sensation
- paresis of gaze.

Vitamin K

The basic structure is a quinone ring with side chain variation depending upon the source of the vitamin. Vitamin K is present in green leaves and may be produced by intestinal bacteria.

Function The vitamin is a component of the microsomal enzyme system that affects the post-translational γ carboxylation of glutamic acid in proteins of plasma, bone, kidney and urine. This includes the precursor proteins for the clotting factors 7, 9, 10 and possibly 5. Warfarin anti-coagulant drugs induce hypoprothrombinaemia by inhibiting the γ carboxylation of the precursor protein.

Deficiency may result from fat malabsorption and long-term treatment with oral antibiotics which may eliminate intestinal bacteria. Newborn infants tend to be deficient in vitamin K and hence have low plasma levels of several coagulation factors in the prothrombin complex.

Vitamin excess

Dietary supplementation with vitamins and minerals is common. Fat soluble vitamins are stored and hence may cause adverse effects. Water soluble vitamins are readily excreted in the urine and have limited storage.

Vitamin A and carotenes

Symptoms are caused by excess intake of vitamin A precursors in foods, principally carrots, resulting in carotenaemia, or occasionally in eskimos by eating polar bears.

Manifestations of hypervitaminosis include yellowing of the skin.

Manifestations of acute toxicity include:

- abdominal pain
- nausea
- vomiting
- headache
- dizziness
- sluggishness
- papilloedema.

There may be generalised desquamation of the skin.

Vitamin E

The manifestations of excessive intake are generally harmless but may include malaise, gastrointestinal upset, headaches and perhaps hypertension. In those taking oral anticoagulation, large amounts of vitamin E may antagonise vitamin K causing prolongation of the prothrombin time which will potentiate oral anticoagulants.

Vitamin K

Vitamin K may block the effects of oral anticoagulants and can cause jaundice in the newborn when given to pregnant women.

Pyridoxine

In large doses pyridoxine may cause severe peripheral neuropathy, ataxia, perioral numbness and clumsiness of hands and feet, with loss of position and vibration sense but normal reflexes and sensory function. It may also antagonise the effects of levodopa in Parkinson's disease and decrease the anticonvulsant effect of phenytoin and barbiturates.

Vitamin C

Vitamin C has been believed to minimise symptoms of the common cold but controlled trials have not demonstrated this. Long-term use may interfere with the absorption of vitamin B_{12}, enhance blood levels of oestrogen in women on exogenous oestrogens, cause uricosuria and predispose to the formation of oxalate kidney stones.

Niacin

Large doses of niacin used for the treatment of hypercholesterolaemia cause release of histamine which may cause flushing, pruritis and gastrointestinal upset and aggravate asthma. Excess intake is associated with acanthosis nigricans.

Vitamin D

Overdose, usually by medication, causes hypercalcaemia, nausea and kidney stones.

KEY POINTS

- Protein-energy malnutrition may result from inadequate dietary intake (starvation), increased metabolic demand, e.g. due to disease, or increased nutrient loss. Certain tissues compensate to an extent by changing their fuel substrate but eventually all body systems are compromised.
- Obesity for most patients is an eating disorder with a major genetic component and is a life-long illness requiring continuous treatment.
- Obesity is associated with diabetes, hypertension, heart disease and osteoarthritis.
- Behavioural modification and an appropriate exercise regimen are theoretically useful but of limited use for the majority. For the moment the epidemic of obesity is likely to continue.
- Insulin resistance is common in obesity, together with other metabolic and hormonal abnormalities.
- Vitamin deficiency is a common cause of disease around the world. In developed countries alcohol is a major cause.

31 Psychosocial factors in pathology

Everybody knows that disease is caused by ignorance, overcrowding, poverty, malnutrition and filth and that much of the world's population is still in the grip of these agents. They also know that high living standards and efficient public health eradicate rickets, plague, typhus, cholera, typhoid, puerperal fever and tuberculosis. The same high standards of living have, however, caused a crop of different diseases such as obesity, diabetes and coronary thrombosis.

Almost all the extraordinary increase in life expectancy that occurred in most Northern European countries between the seventeenth and early twentieth centuries was due to social change rather than advances in medical science or pathology. The contribution of these latter factors has been much more recent. Even the introduction of antibiotics and chemotherapy has had a minor effect on diseases such as tuberculosis or pneumonia compared with changes in nutritional and housing standards which were brought about as much by industrialisation and relative personal prosperity as by governmental action. In contemplating these events however we must not confuse population statistics with the enormous impact of medical advances on the survival prospects of individual patients, who must always be the doctor's first concern. This is classic social pathology.

Less well documented are the psychological effects of industrialisation, urbanisation and the nuclear family on men and women. It seems that once man is sure of food and shelter his expectations usually rise continuously with each improvement in his lot.

The role of psychological factors

The original concept of 'psychosomatic' medicine as proposed by Freud and Pavlov was that specific associations existed between unconscious conflicts or personalities and certain illnesses. These ideas have now largely been replaced by multifactorial concepts of disease, and the belief that psychosocial factors play a role in the onset and subsequent course of many medical conditions. It is also clear that the psyche and the body can no longer be regarded as distinct entities and that complicated interrelationships undoubtedly exist between the two at all levels.

The role of psychosocial factors in disease is attracting increasing interest. Many diseases have been proposed as having underlying psychological or social factors which trigger them although most of the evidence is inconclusive because of the difficulties in quantifying stress, life events and personality. Nevertheless, certain findings have emerged with some consistency.

Emotional factors and neoplastic disease

Many clinical observations have suggested that emotional factors play a role in neoplastic disease. Several studies have found an increased level of prior stressful life events in women with breast cancer. Personality studies have also shown women with breast cancer to be more likely to be 'passive', lacking an ability to express hostile or aggressive emotions. An increased frequency of prior life stress events has also been found in other neoplasms and in chronic diseases such as rheumatoid arthritis and schizophrenia. There is growing evidence, however, that supportive social environments, including family and friends, can buffer the impact of stress on the individual.

Psychological factors and immunity

The finding that certain cancers or autoimmune diseases may be modified by the psychological state of the individual has prompted research into links between the immune system and the human psyche. Human immune responses have been experimentally suppressed in vivo by psychological techniques such as hypnosis or meditation. Several recent studies have suggested that lymphocyte response may be reduced in depressive illness and that natural killer cell activity (which may be important in tumour suppression, p. 316) was low in individuals who coped poorly with stress. These studies, although far from conclusive, have demonstrated important links between emotion and disease and suggest that a positive approach to life may also be protective against certain diseases.

Myocardial infarction and personality

The most convincing evidence of psychosocial factors acting as a primary cause of illness occurs with myocardial infarction.

Associations have been found between certain psychological variables and blood lipid levels, coronary artery spasm and autonomic nervous control of the cardiovascular system. Certain personality types have been shown to be at greater risk of infarction, especially those classified as Type A. Type A personality is a rather ill-defined group of traits characterised by ambition, 'time urgency' (e.g. driving through amber lights) and hostility. The implications of this are unclear, although interestingly a study has successfully modified Type A behaviour in survivors of myocardial infarction, with resultant reduction in cardiovascular morbidity and mortality.

Sociological factors

The usual meaning of social pathology relates to diseases of individuals in which the main cause lies in the shortcomings or demands of society. These sociological factors are not necessarily as obvious as those which disgraced the Industrial Revolution. Stressful life events of all sorts—bereavement, retirement, moving home or changing or losing a job—can precipitate or exacerbate illness, not just depression but also streptococcal pharyngitis, rheumatoid arthritis and accidental trauma.

In the classic type of social pathology, i.e. disease due to socio-economic conditions, the worst examples have been solved in advanced societies, firstly by social change and secondly by scientific discoveries. There were for example only 500 deaths annually from tuberculosis in the UK in the 1990s compared with almost a quarter of a million deaths from heart disease.

This comparison is particularly interesting because a very large part of the death toll from diseases such as coronary thrombosis and carcinoma of the colon is associated with what we now regard as Western standards of nutrition and hygiene, whereas death from infectious diseases used to be inversely related to the same factors. The rising mortality from 'Western' conditions such as ischaemic heart disease and bronchial carcinoma correlates so closely with the coincident decline in deaths from diseases of poverty that it is almost as if an ecological balance were being struck.

Health and social class

Affluence, however, is a relative term. Great Britain at the end of the 20th century bears little resemblance to the grim Dickensian world of the mid-nineteenth century, nevertheless age-corrected death rates from all causes, for virtually all individual diseases and also infant mortality, still show a strong inverse correlation with socio-economic class. For 1991–93, in social class I (i.e. the higher professionals) the standardised mortality ratio from all causes for the ages 20–64 years was 66. For class V (unskilled workers) it was more than double—189. Even wider differences were seen for stroke, suicide and lung cancer, and the gap between the classes has widened since the 1970s. As can be seen from Table 31.1 there is a continuous gradation through the social classes. The same is true of infant mortality (Table 31.2).

The subdivision of the population into social classes is one of the most crucial aspects of social pathology. The system in use in the UK and many other countries is crude but valid. Various modifications have been proposed and the original social class III is often subdivided into 'junior' non-manual workers and skilled manual workers. In the USA, social class for research is based on income or years of education. Whatever its shortcomings, the system provides a very effective measure of the influence of socio-economic status on disease. The question of what causes the striking differences seen in Table 31.1 is one of the most interesting problems in social pathology. Social class correlates inversely with *cigarette smoking*, i.e. social class I has 17% male smokers, class V 49%. It correlates inversely with consumption of white bread, sugar and potatoes and positively with consumption of wholemeal bread and fruit. Social class I in 1977

Table 31.1   Mortality ratios of men in England and Wales between the ages of 20 and 64 years, in 1991–93, expressed by socio-economic group. Standardised mortality ratio for total male population = 100

Social class		All causes of death
I	(professional)	66
II	(employers, lesser professions)	75
III N	(non-manual workers)	92
III M	(skilled manual workers)	117
IV	(semi-skilled workers)	116
V	(unskilled workers)	189

Table 31.2   Infant mortality in England and Wales by social class. Expressed as deaths per 1000 live births

Social class		Perinatal (1st week of life)	Post-neonatal (1 month to 1 yr)
I		7.7	2.4
II		7.5	2.8
III N	(non-manual workers)	8.8	2.6
III M	(skilled manual workers)	9.2	3.2
IV		11.1	4.0
V		12.4	5.2

consumed 33 oz of fresh fruit per person per week, social class V only 17 oz. There is a dramatic inverse correlation between social class and participation in indoor and outdoor sports and games. In 1983 social class I had a participation index of 35 for outdoor sports and 34 for indoor games; social class V had corresponding figures of 9 and 15.

Not all health differences between classes can be explained by such easily measurable indices as smoking and diet. The incidence of *depression* in middle-aged woman in inner cities was found by Brown to be 8% in the middle class (I and II) and 25% in classes IV and V. Brown attributes these differences to poorer marital communication, fewer opportunities for escape from young children and lower self esteem.

There are many other expressions of increased morbidity (non-fatal illness) than depression. In men in the 45–64 year age group there is a dramatic rise in rates of acute and chronic sickness as the social class declines. This is reflected in a roughly corresponding rise in the consultation rate with general practitioners, as can be seen in Table 31.3.

In interpreting all these tables it would be wrong to assume that we are merely witnessing the effects of poverty. Only social class V can be said to be poor in the sense of nutritional and social deprivation and would be seen as 'well off' compared to their peers in the 1950s. Most of the differences can be attributed to different occupations and styles of living. Some of these factors are unavoidable by those concerned, others might be altered by education. The dramatic inequalities between social class V and the rest of the populace are undoubtedly related to deprivation. In the UK the differences in mortality and morbidity between the social classes appear to have widened over the last two decades, although the numbers of individuals in social class V have diminished. Unemployed males of all social classes also have

Table 31.3 Rates of acute and chronic sickness and consultations with general practitioners by social class, in men aged between 45 and 64 years, from 1974–76 in Great Britain. Acute illness is expressed as days per person per year, chronic illness rates per 1000. GP consultations as consultations per person per year.

Socio-economic class	Acute illness	Chronic illness	General practitioner consultations
I	13	168	2.6
II	13	161	2.6
III N	21	261	4.0
III M	23	248	3.7
IV	21	275	4.0
V	29	380	5.4

markedly higher rates of mortality and morbidity than their employed counterparts.

Other factors

It thus appears that economic and environmental factors have a far greater role in determining the wellbeing of a country than anything the health services alone can achieve. Nevertheless even in a socialist Utopia we could expect to find a proportion of the population whose health and life expectancy would be well below average because of their personal inadequacies. Public health messages and health scares appear to be mainly effective in the 'worried well', who are usually at low risk. Influencing individuals at high risk is much more difficult and constitutes a major challenge.

There are other examples of the way medical advances seem to unmask new types of social pathology. For many doctors a common clinical problem in their practice is the depressed, middle-aged married woman. Such a patient probably married young, is sufficiently well off to have no material worries but now finds that her children no longer need her and that she has made no intellectual or professional provision for such a day. It is not surprising that, feeling baffled and useless, she should accept the label of depressive illness. She may in fact be helped to deal with her situation by drugs which counteract her disabling depression but no one would pretend that they offer more than symptomatic relief. The point here is that until quite recent times only a minority of women survived the hazards of childbirth, infection and poverty to reach middle age. Those that did would be unlikely to have avoided widowhood and re-marriage, or might merely be grateful and surprised to have outlived their contemporaries. In any event it is unlikely that psychological depression would have been a problem for this small band of survivors.

As we have said, the second type of social pathology involves the application to socio-economic problems of the methods of analysis that have proved successful in understanding disease. One of the cornerstones of pathology, the detection of a progressive failure of adaptation, fits very obviously to the wage–price spiral of inflation. Pathology and natural selection are very closely linked, as this book should have made plain. Darwinian forces are at work in social pathology too but it would be unwise to draw premature conclusions as to where they are leading. The survival of society does not depend only upon economic success. As an example we can quote a country which becomes so successful that it finds its neighbours are too poor to buy its goods. For a time it will discover new customers but eventually adaptation will fail, unemployment will increase to unacceptable levels and security, prosperity and freedom may